VETERINARY
TECHNICIAN
EXAM

VETERINARY TECHNICIAN EXAM

2nd Edition

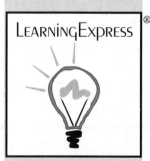

LEARNING EXPRESS®

NEW YORK

ISBN-13: 978-1-57685-961-2

For more information or to place an order, contact LearningExpress at:
    80 Broad Street
    4th Floor
    New York, NY 10004

CONTENTS

CONTENTS

CONTENTS

CONTENTS

CONTRIBUTORS ▶

Allen R. Balay, BS and DVM from Michigan State University; he is the past president of Association of Veterinary Technician Educators. A veterinary technology educator for 30 years, he is Director of Veterinary Technology, Ridgewater College in Willmar, MN.

Laura Earle, DVM from the University of Florida; she is the Program Manager of Brevard Community College's Veterinary Technology Program in Cocoa, FL. She was a small animal/exotic practitioner for 16 years with certification in animal chiropractic through the AVCA with special interest in dentistry, canine sports medicine, physical rehabilitation, homeopathy, and clinical nutrition.

R. Scott Keller, DVM from the University of Illinois College of Veterinary Medicine. He practiced in a small animal hospital until 1999, and since then he has been the coordinator of the Veterinary Medical Technology Program at Joliet Junior College in Joliet, IL, where he teaches surgery, anesthesia, and small animal nursing.

Jane Lewis, BA Williams College, DVM Cornell University College of Veterinary Medicine. She was a large and small animal practitioner for 15 years, and since 2007 has been a veterinary technology educator. She is the Program Coordinator for Veterinary Technology at Northwestern Connecticut Community College where she teaches small animal nursing, animal pathology, pharmacology, laboratory procedures, and dentistry.

Cindy Somerville, RVT from St. Clair College of Applied Arts and Technology in Windsor, Ontario, Canada. She has worked in small animal practice for 20 years as well as in emergency clinics for the last decade. Her special interest is in anesthesia and pain management. She is presently veterinary technician at the Bronte Road Animal Hospital in Oakville, Ontario, Canada.

HOW TO USE THIS BOOK ▶

Working as a veterinary technician is an exciting and promising career. Yet, preparing to become a veterinary technician can seem like a daunting process. This book will help in many ways. Ch. 1 covers all of the facets of becoming and working as a veterinary technician. Passing the Veterinary Technician National Exam (VTNE) is an essential part of becoming a veterinary technician. Some states require their own exam in addition to the VTNE to become a veterinary technician. Check your state's Department of Professional Regulations for their specific requirements. Ch. 2 will walk you through a system to help you hone your study skills, combat test anxiety, and improve test taking techniques. The rest of the book provides some of the most pertinent veterinary medical information needed to take the VTNE, and to practice taking a veterinary technician exam.

This book is not a substitute for your textbooks and vet tech program education, or a source for actual VTNE exam questions. However, this book will be a great review of material, plus the questions and answers are similar in rigor, content, and format of the actual VTNE. Also, see page 415 for your special access code that offers more practice online. The general pass rate for the VTNE is often close to 75%. Utilizing all that this book offers can significantly improve your own success.

Before taking the VTNE you should know as much as you can about the test, and the application process. All candidates should go to www.AAVSB.org/VTNE/. This web site has the VTNE application, candidate handbook, and additional preparation materials for the VTNE. Don't miss two very helpful PDF documents that can be found on their website. One PDF is "VTNE References," a list of current textbooks and journals that are used to validate every question on the test. The second PDF is "List of Abbreviations Used in VTNE." Successful completion of these exams leads to the credentialing process within an individual state and their rules, regulations and guidelines. Depending on which state you are pursuing credentials in, you could be given the designation of Certified Veterinary Technician (CVT), Licensed Veterinary Technician (LVT), Registered Veterinary Technician (RVT), or Licensed Veterinary Medical Technician (LVMT).

Chapter 2 explains the secrets of test-taking and how to improve your scores on multiple-choice exams through strategic planning. LearningExpress has developed a system to help you prepare for your exam by

- becoming familiar with the format of the exam(s),
- planning to have sufficient time to practice taking the exam(s),
- learning how to overcome test anxiety and exam fear,
- learning critical test-taking skills, such as pacing yourself through the exam, using the process of elimination, and knowing when to guess,
- planning to get enough rest and exercise before the test (and while preparing as well), and
- preparing your test supplies and having last-minute details ready.

Chapters 4 to 11 comprise the core of the book, reviewing the important topics of Pharmacology (4), Surgical Preparation and Assisting (5), Dentistry (6), Laboratory Procedures (7 and 8), Animal Care and Nursing (9), Diagnostic Imaging (10), and Anesthesia and Analgesia (11).

At the heart of the book are the three practice exams, in Chapters 3 and 12 and online. Prepare yourself as if for the actual exam with all the pencils, erasers, and other supplies you will need. Wear an accurate wristwatch or carry a stopwatch to allow yourself time to answer questions and skip those that hold you up. Chapter 3 is the place to start. Take the first 100-question exam, allowing yourself enough time to complete it. Since the VTNE allows three hours for 170 multiple-choice questions, you should aim to complete this practice test in about 90 minutes.

Once you are finished in the allotted time, turn to the section called Answers and Explanations. Score your exam carefully. Now, take note of the sections in which you did particularly poorly. You will want to review these with extreme care. We suggest that your exam preparation include all eight core chapters (4 through 11), but you may want to concentrate on those where you are weakest. Review each topic chapter here and in your textbooks as well. At the end of each topic chapter in this book, you will find a set of 50 questions. Remember to time yourself. Score these questions as you did the practice test in Chapter 3 to see how solid your knowledge of this topic is.

At the end of the eight reviews, take the second practice test, in Chapter 12. Remember to time yourself. Score the test and identify which topics still need improvement.

You have taken the first step toward veterinary tech success by buying this book—congratulations! Good luck with your studies and with your exam.

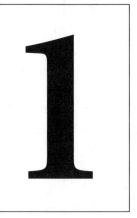

CHAPTER 1

VETERINARY TECHNOLOGY AS A PROFESSION

CHAPTER OVERVIEW

Veterinary technicians can perform many roles in many fields, from assisting the veterinarian in a private practice to working with pharmaceutical and pet food companies, zoos, and wildlife centers, to teaching. In the past, many veterinary technicians, learned the job simply by doing it, now called veterinary assistants but now it is required in nearly every state and province to get proper training and certification. That is the reason you are reading this book. The VTNE is the national certification exam, and some states require additional testing. Veterinary specializations and other degrees are available as well. There are a number of veterinary technology associations that keep members informed about things veterinary such as educational opportunities. Technicians must always maintain a professional and safe appearance. Finally, this chapter discusses veterinary technician salaries and benefits.

Veterinary technology is a very exciting career with endless opportunities for advancement and lifelong learning. The functions of a technician in the veterinary hospital include animal care and nursing, radiography, laboratory tasks, surgical assisting, dentistry, anesthesia, pharmacologic calculations and administration, clinic maintenance, business managing, grief counseling, and public health duties. The technician is the clinic employee who spends the most time with patients and clients—it is often the technician's job to translate doctor-speak to plain language that the client can understand. Often, the technician is the liaison with pharmaceutical sales representatives as well as being responsible for managing inventory and maintaining equipment in the practice. In short, veterinary technicians can do everything but diagnose, make a prognosis of the expected outcome of a disease, prescribe drugs, and perform surgery. They are an integral part of the veterinary healthcare team.

Education and Certification

A veterinary technician is a graduate of an AVMA (American Veterinary Medical Association) or CVMA (Canadian Veterinary Medical Association) accredited program in veterinary technology who successfully passed the VTNE. In most cases, the graduate is granted an associate's degree or certificate. Typically, a student can complete a program in 2 years. However, there are exceptions, and each school's admissions office can clarify the time it takes for completion. The AVMA Committee for Veterinary Technician Education and Activities (CVTEA) is the accrediting body of the AVMA and performs inspections of facilities and programs at least every six years at every accredited institution in the United States and Canada. Annual or biennial self-study reports are also submitted by each institution to address any deficiencies noted by the site team. Accreditation by this body indicates that quality education, facilities, and institutional support are present and that students receive the education expected by the AVMA.

Passing the VTNE and graduating allows the students to call themselves CVTs (Certified Veterinary Technicians). Some states require their own exam in addition to the VTNE to become a veterinary technician. Check your state's Department of Professional Regulations for their specific requirements. Depending on a particular state's veterinary practice act, a CVT may also be called an RVT (Registered Veterinary Technician) or an LVT (Licensed Veterinary Technician). For maintenance of licensure, CVTs in some states may be required to take continuing education credits every two years. The number of credits varies by state. These credits may be obtained at local, state, or national veterinary meetings or veterinary technician schools or associations.

Opportunities for further education and advancement are widely available. A number of schools offer a bachelor of science (BS) degree in veterinary technology. The bachelors degrees are usually more specialized than two-year programs and may focus on office management, laboratory animal medicine, or animal care. Most degreed programs articulate into the BS programs. That degree generally requires additional courses in communications/English, the social sciences, and the humanities.

Specialization certifications are also available for technicians in practice or with special interests through the National Association of Veterinary Technicians in America (NAVTA). Veterinary Technician Specialist (VTS) is the certification offered; it usually requires intensive training, including case studies and certification testing in the specialty field. VTSs are offered in eleven fields: anesthesia, emergency medicine and critical care, equine medicine, zoo medicine, dentistry, veterinary behavior, internal medicine, surgery, clinical pathology, clinical practice, and nutrition. The list is always growing. These specializations generally lead to higher salaries.

Specialization in laboratory animal medicine is offered through the American Association for Laboratory Animal Science (AALAS) based on continuing education in laboratory animal medicine, certification testing, and experience (number of years in lab animal practice).

Functions of a Veterinary Technician

Veterinary technicians with or without a specialization are extremely valuable in many fields. CVTs/LVTs/RVTs are employed at veterinary hospitals, specialty practices, government, pharmaceutical and medical equipment companies, pet food companies, sales departments, research facilities, teaching programs, zoos, wildlife management centers, animal behavior centers, and many other institutions. The opportunities are endless.

Government jobs for CVTs include research, food and site inspection, animal cruelty investigations, shelter medicine, service-dog training, evaluation of zoo facilities, and public health. Government jobs tend to come with higher salaries and include excellent benefits such as health, dental, vacation, paid continuing education, and regular hours.

Pharmaceutical companies usually employ CVTs in sales or research. Again, the benefits are high wage-earning potential with good benefits. Experience with laboratory animal medicine is important in research jobs. Pharmaceutical sales teams often use CVTs because they are well trained in client education and have good communication skills as well as expertise in pharmacology. High wages are possible, but are often based on sales commissions, and travel may be required.

Most of the larger pet food companies operate research facilities that are staffed by CVTs who are in charge of animal care and research. These companies also use CVTs for education and to answer the food hotlines, which give information about the foods (whether prescription or maintenance).

Zoos, wildlife centers, and animal behavior centers are usually looking for CVTs with experience in the field or with specialty certification. Many also request a few years of clinical experience, which gives the CVT more real-world application of skills.

Teaching positions may also be available to CVTs. To teach at the community college level, most schools require a minimum of a CVT and at least two years of experience in the field. University or state colleges usually require a CVT with a BS or a BA (bachelor of arts) plus two years of experience. Clinical teaching positions are also available at veterinary schools. Technicians employed at vet schools are often involved in teaching the veterinary students clinical skills and laboratory medicine. Because clinical teaching technicians are usually employed as staff, the educational requirements are not as stringent.

Veterinary Technician Associations

Veterinary technician associations are excellent means of networking with other technicians and opening up job opportunities. NAVTA has branches in most states—for example, the Florida Veterinary Technician Association (FVTA)—and most veterinary technology programs have student affiliations with the national association.

Many veterinary associations also have technician chapters, and every veterinary technician specialty has a college or academy associated with it that will accept associate (nonspecialty) members. These associations all have scientific meetings, and some have workshops and clinical laboratories that can help the CVT to become certified in the specialty. Although continuing education seems expensive, many employers are willing to help the CVT with part or all of the educational expenses if it will benefit the practice or company.

Technician Professionalism and Safety

Whatever roles veterinary technicians choose to pursue, they must always remember that they are representing their profession. Maintaining a professional appearance is always important. Many practices have dress codes that may include uniforms and rules regarding jewelry and tattoos. Adherence to these rules not only helps to maintain a professional appearance but shows respect for the practice and the profession.

Safety is also a major concern in veterinary medicine. Long, loose hair can be a hazard when dealing with animals. It can also irritate already stressed animals. Hair should be pulled back away from the face. Piercings may also be a hazard. Technicians with piercings and other jewelry should ensure that rings have flat settings and that earrings be the stud type to prevent animals from getting caught in the jewelry. Bracelets and necklaces can also get caught and cause injury to the technician or to the animal. Shoes should be nonslip and should not have open toes. Artificial nails can trap bacteria, making it impossible to maintain sterile conditions. Finally, animals have a better sense of smell than humans do. Perfume can be irritating to them and should be avoided.

Salaries and Benefits

Veterinary technology is among the top 20 fastest-growing occupations in the country according to the Bureau of Labor Statistics Occupational Outlook Handbook. The career is projected to grow by 52% by 2020. Full-time entry level CVT salaries range from $26,000 to $30,500 per year. This will vary by state. VTSs and CPMs (Certified Practice Managers) may command higher salaries depending on location and choice of specialty. The U.S. Government Bureau of Labor Statistics reported that there were 80,200 veterinary technicians employed in the United States in 2010. Assuming an average work week of 40 hours (2,080 hours per year), the median salary for a veterinary technician was $13.90 per hour. This ranged from $9.06 per hour (the lowest 10%) to $19.50 per hour (the top 10%). Annually, that translates into $28,920, ranging from $18,840 to $40,550 per year.

Generally, lower pay levels were in rural areas and higher levels in metropolitan areas, where the average wage is over $18 per hour. The top five metropolitan areas are Lansing–East Lansing, MI ($40,860), Fresno, CA ($40,690), San Diego–Carlsbad–San Marcos, CA ($39,790), Oakland–Fremont–Hayward, CA, Metropolitan Division ($39,690), and Kalamazoo–Portage, MI ($39,250). The best states for a veterinary technician are Connecticut ($34,810), Nevada ($34,700), the District of Columbia ($33,840), Michigan ($33,440), and California ($33,300).

In addition, veterinary technicians often receive benefits such as vacation, health insurance, and retirement plans, but these vary depending on the size of the employer and other factors. A typical employment benefits package can be worth over $20,000 per year in addition to salary.

2 ▶ THE LEARNINGEXPRESS TEST PREPARATION SYSTEM

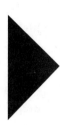

CHAPTER OVERVIEW

Taking any written exam can be tough. It demands a lot of preparation if you want to achieve a top score. The LearningExpress Test Preparation System, developed exclusively for LearningExpress by leading test experts, gives you the discipline and attitude you need to be a winner.

Taking this written exam is no picnic, and neither is getting ready for it. Your future career in veterinary technology depends on you passing the various parts of the test, but there are all sorts of pitfalls that can keep you from doing your best on this all-important exam. Here are some of the obstacles that can stand in the way of your success:

- being unfamiliar with the format of the exam,
- being paralyzed by test anxiety,
- leaving your preparation to the last minute or not preparing at all,
- not knowing vital test-taking skills: how to pace yourself through the exam, how to use the process of elimination, and when to guess,
- not being in tip-top mental and physical shape,
- doing poorly on test day by having to work on an empty stomach or shivering through the exam because the room is cold.

What is the common denominator in all these test-taking pitfalls? One word: control. Who is in control, you or the exam?

Now the good news: The LearningExpress Test Preparation System puts you in control. In just nine easy-to-follow steps, you will learn everything you need to know to make sure that you are in charge of your preparation and your performance on the exam. Other test-takers may let the test get the better of them; other test-takers may be unprepared or out of shape, but not you. You will have taken all the steps you need to take to get a high score on the veterinary technology exam.

Here is how the LearningExpress Test Preparation System works: Nine easy steps lead you through everything you need to know and do to get ready to master your exam. Each of the following steps includes both reading about the step and one or more activities. It is important that you do the activities along with the reading, or you will not be getting the full benefit of the system. Each step tells you approximately how much time that step will take you to complete.

Step 1. Get Information (30 minutes)

Step 2. Conquer Test Anxiety (20 minutes)

Step 3. Make a Plan (50 minutes)

Step 4. Learn to Manage Your Time (10 minutes)

Step 5. Learn to Use the Process of Elimination (20 minutes)

Step 6. Know When to Guess (20 minutes)

Step 7. Reach Your Peak Performance Zone (10 minutes)

Step 8. Get Your Act Together (10 minutes)

Step 9. Do It! (10 minutes)

Total time for the complete system is 180 minutes (3 hours).

Although we estimate that working through the entire system will take you approximately three hours, it is perfectly all right to work faster or slower. If you can take a whole afternoon or evening, you can work through the whole LearningExpress Test Preparation

System in one sitting. Otherwise, you can break it up, and do just one or two steps a day for the next several days. It is up to you—remember, you are in control.

Step 1: Get Information

Time to complete: 30 minutes
Activity: Read How to Use this Book (page xi)

Knowledge is power. The first step in the Learning-Express Test Preparation System is finding out everything you can about the veterinary technician exams offered. For example, the AAVSB website outlines all the details about taking the VTNE. Your local state veterinary technician boards will have information for you on local exam requirements, which vary from state to state.

What You Should Find Out

The more details you can find out about the exam, either from the national or from the state boards' publications, the more efficiently you will be able to study. Here is a list of some things you might want to find out about your exam.

- What skills are tested?
- How many sections are on the exam?
- How many questions are in each section?
- Are the questions ordered from easy to hard, or is the sequence random?
- How much time is allotted for each section?
- Are there breaks between sections?
- What is the passing score and how many questions do you have to answer right in order to get that score?
- Does a higher score give you any advantages, such as a better rank on the eligibility list?
- How is the test scored? Is there a penalty for wrong answers?
- Are you permitted to go back to a prior section or move on to the next section if you finish early?

- Can you write in the test booklet or will you be given scratch paper?
- What should you bring with you on exam day?

What is on the VTNE?

While the tests performed by individual states may vary, the Veterinary Technician National Exam (VTNE) is a standardized 170 multiple choice test that is taken on a computer. Of the 170 questions, only 150 will be used for your score. The other 20 are questions being tested for by AAVSB. You will not know which questions are which.

The VTNE questions can be categorized into 9 domains. These are listed below with a number that represent the percentage of those items on the test:

1. Pharmacy and Pharmacology-12%
2. Surgical Nursing-11%
3. Dentistry-7%
4. Laboratory Procedures-12%
5. Animal Care and Nursing-22%
6. Diagnostic Imaging-7%
7. Anesthesia-16%
8. Emergency Medicine/Critical Care-6%
9. Pain Management/Analgesia-7%

Important Facts about the VTNE:

- All multiple choice questions have 4 choices, with only one correct or best answer.
- Questions can include images. Be prepared for a few images that can include pictures, radiographs, charts, and images from a microscope. Quite often the source of these images will be the reference texts that the AAVSB has listed.
- Candidates are given 3 hours for the exam. The time remaining is displayed on the computer screen.
- Breaks are allowed, but the clock will continue to count down.
- Candidates can skip questions and come back to them. They can also change answers, use the strike-through feature to eliminate a choice, and mark questions for review.

- A calculator is available on the computer. It is like a standard Windows calculator. Practice using one before the day of the test.
- No scratch paper is allowed, but an erasable board is provided in place of scratch paper.
- A function key can be used to provide comment on a question. Take care to watch your time if commenting.

Other Things to Know about the VTNE:

- Arrive 30 minutes before the test time.
- Have Photo ID with the exact name that is on the application
- Read all of the *Candidate Information Handbook* supplied at the AAVSB website before applying.

If you have not already done so, stop here and read Chapter 1 of this book, which gives you an overview of the entire process of becoming a veterinary technician. Then move on to the next step and get rid of that test anxiety.

Step 2: Conquer Test Anxiety

Time to complete: 20 minutes
Activity: Take the Test Stress Quiz (page 9)

Having complete information about the test is the first step in getting control of the exam. Next, you have to overcome one of the biggest obstacles to test success: test anxiety. Test anxiety can not only impair your performance on the exam itself; it can even keep you from preparing properly. In Step 2, you will learn stress management techniques that will help you succeed on your exam. Learn these strategies now, and practice them as you work through the questions in this book, so they will be second nature to you by exam day.

Combating Test Anxiety

The first thing you need to know is that a little test anxiety is a good thing. Everyone gets nervous before a big exam—and if that nervousness motivates you to prepare thoroughly, so much the better. It is said that Sir Laurence Olivier, one of the foremost British actors of the twentieth century, threw up before every performance. His stage fright did not impair his performance; in fact, it probably gave him a little extra edge—just the kind of edge you need to do well, whether on a stage or in an examination room.

The Test Stress Quiz is on page 9. Stop here and answer the questions on that page, to find out whether your level of test anxiety is something you should worry about.

Stress Management Before the Test

If you feel your level of anxiety getting the best of you in the weeks before the test, here is what you need to do to bring the level down again.

- **Get prepared.** There is nothing like knowing what to expect and being prepared for it to put you in control of test anxiety. That is why you are reading this book. Use it faithfully, and remind yourself that you are better prepared than most of the people taking the test.
- **Practice self-confidence.** A positive attitude is a great way to combat test anxiety. This is no time to be humble or shy. Stand in front of the mirror and say to your reflection, "I am prepared. I am full of self-confidence. I am going to ace this test. I know I can do it." Say it into a tape recorder and play it back once a day. If you hear it often enough, you will believe it.
- **Fight negative messages.** Every time someone starts telling you how hard the exam is or how it is almost impossible to get a high score, start telling them your previous self-confidence messages. If the someone with the negative messages is you—telling yourself you do not do well on exams, that you just cannot do this—do not listen. Turn on your tape recorder and listen to your self-confidence messages.
- **Visualize.** Imagine yourself reporting for duty on your first day of veterinary technology training.

Think of yourself wearing your uniform with pride and learning skills you will use for the rest of your life. Visualizing success can help make it happen—and it reminds you of why you are doing all this work in preparing for the exam.
- **Exercise.** Physical activity helps calm your body down and focus your mind. Besides, being in good physical shape can actually help you do well on the exam. Go for a run, lift weights, go swimming—and do it regularly.

Stress Management on Test Day

There are several ways you can bring down your level of test stress and anxiety on test day. These techniques will work best if you practice them in the weeks before the test, so you know which ones work best for you.

- **Deep breathing.** Take a deep breath while you count to five. Hold it for a count of one, and then let it out on a count of five. Repeat several times.
- **Move your body.** Try rolling your head in a circle. Rotate your shoulders. Shake your hands from the wrist. Many people find these movements very relaxing.
- **Visualize again.** Think of the place where you are most relaxed: lying on the beach in the sun, walking through the park, or whatever. Now, close your eyes and imagine you are actually there. If you practice in advance, you will find that you only need a few seconds of this exercise to experience a significant increase in your sense of well-being.

When anxiety threatens to overwhelm you during the exam, there are still things you can do to manage the stress level.

- **Repeat your self-confidence messages.** You should have them memorized by now. Say them quietly to yourself, and believe them!
- **Visualize one more time.** This time, visualize yourself moving smoothly and quickly through the test, answering every question right, and fin-

TEST STRESS QUIZ

You need to worry about test anxiety only if it is extreme enough to impair your performance. The following questionnaire will provide a diagnosis of your level of test anxiety. In the blank before each statement, write the number that most accurately describes your experience.

0 = Never
1 = Once or twice
2 = Sometimes
3 = Often

_____ I have gotten so nervous before an exam that I simply put down the books and did not study for it.
_____ I have experienced disabling physical symptoms such as vomiting and severe headaches because I was nervous about an exam.
_____ I have simply not shown up for an exam because I was afraid to take it.
_____ I have experienced dizziness and disorientation while taking an exam.
_____ I have had trouble filling in the little circles because my hands were shaking too hard.
_____ I have failed an exam because I was too nervous to complete it.
_____ **Total: Add up the numbers in the blanks above.**

Your Test Stress Score

Here are the steps you should take, depending on your score. If you scored:

- **Below 3:** Your level of test anxiety is nothing to worry about; it is probably just enough to give you that little extra edge.
- **Between 3 and 6:** Your test anxiety may be enough to impair your performance, and you should practice the stress management techniques in this section to try to bring your test anxiety down to manageable levels.
- **Above 6:** Your level of test anxiety is a serious concern. In addition to practicing the stress management techniques listed in this section, you may want to seek additional, personal help. Call your local high school or community college and ask for the academic counselor. Tell the counselor that you have a level of test anxiety that sometimes keeps you from being able to take the exam. The counselor may be willing to help you or may suggest someone else you should talk to.

ishing just before time is up. Like most visualization techniques, this one works best if you have practiced it ahead of time.

- **Find an easy question.** Skim over the test until you find an easy question, and answer it. Getting even one circle filled in gets you into the test-taking groove.
- **Take a mental break.** Everyone loses concentration once in a while during a long test. This is normal, so you should not worry about it. Instead, accept what has happened. Say to yourself, "Hey, I lost it there for a minute. My brain is taking a break." Put down your pencil, close your eyes, and do some deep breathing for a few seconds. Then you will be ready to go back to work.

Try these techniques ahead of time, and see whether they work for you!

Step 3: Make a Plan

Time to complete: 50 minutes
Activity: Construct a study plan

Maybe the most important thing you can do to get control of yourself and your exam is to make a study plan. Too many people fail to prepare simply because they fail to plan. Spending hours on the day before the exam poring over sample test questions not only raises your level of test anxiety, it is also simply no substitute for careful preparation and practice over time.

Do not fall into the cram trap. Take control of your preparation time by mapping out a study schedule. There are four sample schedules on the following pages, based on the amount of time you have before the exam. If you are the kind of person who needs deadlines and assignments to motivate you for a project, here they are. If you are the kind of person who does not like to follow other people's plans, you can use the suggested schedules here to construct your own.

In constructing your plan, you should take into account how much work you need to do. If your score on the sample test was not what you had hoped, consider taking some of the steps from Schedule A and fitting them into Schedule D, even if you do have only three weeks before the exam.

You can also customize your plan according to the information you gathered in Step 1. If the exam you have to take does not include laboratory procedures, for instance, you can skip Chapter 7 and concentrate instead on some other area that is covered. The following table lists all the chapters you need to study for each exam.

Even more important than making a plan is making a commitment. You cannot improve your skills in reading, writing, and judgment overnight. You have to set aside some time every day for study and practice. Try for at least 20 minutes a day. Twenty minutes daily will do you much more good than two hours crammed into a Saturday.

If you have months before the exam, you are lucky. Do not put off your study until the week before the exam! Start now. Even ten minutes a day, with half an hour or more on weekends, can make a big difference in your score.

Schedule A: The Leisure Plan

This schedule gives you six months to sharpen your skills. If an exam is announced in the middle of your preparation, you can use one of the later schedules to help you compress your study program. Only study the chapters that are relevant to the type of exam you will be taking.

Time Preparation
Exam minus 6 months: Answer the questions in the diagnostic test in Chapter 3. Then study the explanations for the answers until you know you could answer all the questions correctly.
Exam minus 5 months: Read Chapters 4 and 5 and work through the exercises. Start going to the library once every two weeks to read books or magazines about veterinary pharmacology and surgical preparation. Find other people who are preparing for the test and form a study group.
Exam minus 4 months: Read Chapters 6, 7, and 8 and work through the exercises. Use at least one of the additional resources for each chapter. Remember to read up on veterinary dentistry and laboratory procedures.
Exam minus 3 months: Read Chapters 9 and 10 and work through the exercises. You are still doing your reading on animal care and nursing and diagnostic imaging, right?
Exam minus 2 months: Read Chapter 11 and work through the exercises. Do your supplemental reading on anesthesia and analgesia.
Exam minus 1 month: Take the practice test in Chapter 12. Use your score to help you decide where to concentrate your efforts this month. Go back to the relevant chapters and use the additional resources listed there, or get the help of a friend or teacher.
Exam minus 1 week: Take the practice test in Chapter 12. See how much you have learned in the past months. Concentrate on what you have done well and decide not to let any areas where you still feel uncertain bother you.
Exam minus 1 day: Relax. Do something unrelated to veterinary technology exams. Eat a good meal and go to bed at your usual time.

Schedule B: The Just-Enough-Time Plan

If you have three to six months before the exam, that should be enough time to prepare for the written test, especially if you score above 70 on the diagnostic test in Chapter 3. This schedule assumes four months; stretch it out or compress it if you have more or less time, and only study the chapters that are relevant to the type of exam you will be taking.

Time Preparation
Exam minus 4 months: Take the diagnostic test in Chapter 3 to determine where you need the most work. Read Chapters 4, 5, and 6 and work through the exercises. Use at least one of the additional resources listed in each chapter. Start going to the library once every two weeks to read books about veterinary technician topics.
Exam minus 3 months: Read Chapters 7, 8, and 9 and work through the exercises.
Exam minus 2 months: Read Chapter 10 and work through the exercises. You are still doing your reading, right?
Exam minus 1 month: Take the practice test in Chapter 12. Use your score to help you decide where to concentrate your efforts this month. Go back to the relevant chapters and use the extra resources listed there, or get the help of a friend or teacher.
Exam minus 1 month: Take the practice test in Chapter 12. Use your score to help you decide where to concentrate your efforts this month. Go back to the relevant chapters and use the additional resources listed there, or get the help of a friend or teacher.
Exam minus 1 week: Take the practice test in Chapter 12. See how much you have learned in the past months. Concentrate on what you have done well and decide not to let any areas where you still feel uncertain bother you.
Exam minus 1 day: Relax. Do something unrelated to veterinary technology exams. Eat a good meal and go to bed at your usual time.

Schedule C: More Study in Less Time

If you have one to three months before the exam, you still have enough time for some concentrated study that will help you improve your score. This schedule is built around a two-month time frame. If you have only one month, spend an extra couple of hours a week to get all these steps in. If you have three months, take some of the steps from Schedule B and fit them in. Only study the chapters that are relevant to the type of exam you will be taking.

Time Preparation
Exam minus 8 weeks: Take the diagnostic test in Chapter 3 to find one or two areas you are weakest in. Choose the appropriate chapter(s) from among Chapters 4 to 11 to read during these two weeks. Use some of the additional resources listed there. When you get to those chapters in this plan, review them.
Exam minus 6 weeks: Read Chapters 4 to 7 and work through the exercises.
Exam minus 4 weeks: Read Chapters 8 to 11 and work through the exercises.
Exam minus 2 weeks: Take the practice test in Chapter 11. Then score it and read the answer explanations until you are sure you understand them. Review the areas where your score is lowest.
Exam minus 1 week: Take the practice test in Chapter 12, concentrating on the areas where a little work can help the most.
Exam minus 1 day: Relax. Do something unrelated to veterinary technician exams. Eat a good meal and go to bed at your usual time.

Schedule D: The Cram Plan

If you have three weeks or less before the exam, you really have your work cut out for you. Carve half an hour out of your day, every day, for study. This schedule assumes you have the whole three weeks to prepare; if you have less time, you will have to compress the schedule accordingly. Only study the chapters that are relevant to the type of exam you will be taking.

Time Preparation

Exam minus 3 weeks: Take the diagnostic test in Chapter 3. Then read the material in Chapter 4 and work through the exercises.

Exam minus 2 weeks: Read the material in Chapters 5 to 11 and work through the exercises. Take the practice test in Chapter 12, score it, and review your areas of weakness.

Exam minus 1 week: Evaluate your performance on the practice test in Chapter 12. Review the parts of Chapters 4 to 11 that you had the most trouble with. Get a friend or teacher to help you with these sections.

Exam minus 2 days: Review the practice tests in Chapters 3 and 12. Make sure you understand the answer explanations.

Exam minus 1 day: Relax. Do something unrelated to veterinary technician exams. Eat a good meal and go to bed at your usual time.

Step 4: Learn to Manage Your Time

Time to complete: 10 minutes to read; many hours of practice!

Activities: Practice these strategies as you take the practice tests in this book.

Steps 4, 5, and 6 of the LearningExpress Test Preparation System put you in charge of your exam by showing you test-taking strategies that work. Practice these strategies as you work through this book, and then you will be ready to use them on test day.

First, you will take control of your time on the exam. The first step in achieving this control is to find out the format of the exam you are going to take. Veterinary technician exams will vary by state and may have different sections that are each timed separately. If this is true of the exam you will be taking, you will want to practice using your time wisely on the practice exams and trying to avoid mistakes while working quickly. Other types of exams do not have separately timed sections. If this is the case, just practice pacing yourself on the practice exams so you do not spend too much time on difficult questions.

- **Listen carefully to directions.** By the time you get to the exam, you should know how the test works, but be sure to listen just in case something has changed.
- **Pace yourself.** Glance at your watch every few minutes, and compare the time to how far you have gotten in the section. Leave time for review, so that when one-quarter of the time has elapsed, you should be more than a quarter of the way through the section, and so on. If you are falling behind, pick up the pace a bit.
- **Keep moving.** Do not dither around on one question. If you do not know the answer, skip the question and move on. Circle the number of the question in your test booklet in case you have time to come back to it later.
- **Keep track of your place on the answer sheet.** If you skip a question, make sure you skip on the answer sheet, too. Check yourself every five to ten questions to make sure the question number and the answer sheet number are still the same.
- **Do not rush.** Though you should keep moving, rushing will not help. Try to keep calm and work methodically and quickly.

Step 5: Learn to Use the Process of Elimination

Time to complete: 20 minutes
Activity: Complete worksheet on Using the Process of Elimination (pages 14 and 15)

After time management, your next most important tool for taking control of your exam is using the process of elimination wisely. It is standard test-taking wisdom that you should always read all the answer choices before choosing your answer. This helps you find the right answer by eliminating wrong answer choices. And, sure enough, that standard wisdom applies to your exam, too.

Let us say you are facing a vocabulary question that goes like this:

13. "Biology uses a *binomial* system of classification." In this sentence, the word *binomial* most nearly means
    a. understanding the law.
    b. having two names.
    c. scientifically sound.
    d. having a double meaning.

If you happen to know what *binomial* means, you do not need to use the process of elimination, but let us assume that, like many people, you do not. So, you look at the answer choices. *Understanding the law* certainly does not sound very likely for something having to do with biology. So, you eliminate choice a—and now you only have three answer choices to deal with. Mark an **X** next to choice a so you never have to read it again.

Move on to the other answer choices. If you know that the prefix *bi-* means *two*, as in *bicycle*, you will flag answer b as a possible answer. Make a check mark beside it, meaning *good answer; I might use this one.*

Choice c, *scientifically sound*, is a possibility. At least it is about science, not law. It could work here; though, when you think about it, having a scientifically sound classification system in a scientific field is kind of redundant. You remember the *bi-* in *binomial*, and probably continue to like answer b better. But you are not sure, so you put a question mark next to c, meaning *well, maybe.*

Now, look at choice d, *having a double meaning*. You are still keeping in mind that *bi-* means *two*, so this one looks possible at first. But then you look again at the sentence the word belongs in, and you think, *Why would biology want a system of classification that has two meanings? That would not work very well!* If you are really taken with the idea that *bi-* means *two*, you might put a question mark here. But if you are feeling a little more confident, you will put an **X**. You have already got a better answer picked out.

Now, your question looks like this:

13. "Biology uses a *binomial* system of classification." In this sentence, the word *binomial* most nearly means
    X a. understanding the law.
    ✔ b. having two names.
    ? c. scientifically sound.
    ? d. having a double meaning.

You have got just one check mark, for a good answer. If you are pressed for time, you should simply mark answer **b** on your answer sheet. If you have got the time to be extra careful, you could compare your check mark answer to your question mark answers to make sure that it is better. (It is: The *binomial* system in biology is the one that gives a two-part genus and species name, like *homo sapiens*.)

It is good to have a system for marking good, bad, and maybe answers. We recommend this one:

    X = bad
    ✔ = good
    ? = maybe

If you do not like these marks, devise your own system. Just make sure you do it long before test day—while you are working through the practice exams in this book—so you will not have to worry about it during the test.

Even when you think you are absolutely clueless about a question, you can often use process of elimination to get rid of one answer choice. If so, you are better prepared to make an educated guess, as you will see in Step 6. More often, the process of elimination allows you to get down to only two possibly right answers. Then you are in a strong position to guess. And sometimes, even though you do not know the right answer, you find it simply by getting rid of the wrong ones, as you did in the previous example.

Try using your powers of elimination on the questions in the worksheet Using the Process of Elimination beginning on page 14. The answer explanations there show one possible way you might use the process to arrive at the right answer.

The process of elimination is your tool for the next step, which is knowing when to guess.

Use the process of elimination to answer the following questions.

1. Ilsa is as old as Meghan will be in five years. The difference between Ed's age and Meghan's age is twice the difference between Ilsa's age and Meghan's age. Ed is 29. How old is Ilsa?
   a. 4
   b. 10
   c. 19
   d. 24

2. "All drivers of commercial vehicles must carry a valid commercial driver's license whenever operating a commercial vehicle." According to this sentence, which of the following people need NOT carry a commercial driver's license?
   a. a truck driver idling his engine while waiting to be directed to a loading dock
   b. a bus operator backing her bus out of the way of another bus in the bus lot
   c. a taxi driver driving his personal car to the grocery store
   d. a limousine driver taking the limousine to her home after dropping off her last passenger of the evening

3. Smoking tobacco has been linked to
   a. increased risk of stroke and heart attack.
   b. all forms of respiratory disease.
   c. increasing mortality rates over the past ten years.
   d. juvenile delinquency.

4. Which of the following words is spelled correctly?
   a. incorrigible
   b. outragous
   c. domestickated
   d. understandible

Answers

Here are the answers, as well as some suggestions as to how you might have used the process of elimination to find them.

1. **d.** You should have eliminated choice **a** right off the bat. Ilsa cannot be four years old if Meghan is going to be Ilsa's age in five years. The best way to eliminate other answer choices is to try plugging them in to the information given in the problem. For instance, for choice **b**, if Ilsa is 10, then Meghan must be 5. The difference between their ages is 5. The difference between Ed's age, 29, and Meghan's age, 5, is 24. Is 24 two times 5? No. Then choice **b** is wrong.

   You could eliminate choice **c** in the same way and be left with choice **d**.

2. **c.** Note the word NOT in the question, and go through the answers one by one. Is the truck driver in choice **a** operating a commercial vehicle? Yes, idling counts as operating, so he needs to have a commercial driver's license. Likewise, the bus operator in choice **b** is operating a commercial vehicle; the question doesn't say the operator has to be on the street. The limo driver in choice **d** is

operating with a passenger in her vehicle. However, the driver in choice **c** is not operating a commercial vehicle, but his own private car.

3. **a.** You could eliminate choice **b** simply because of the presence of the word all. Such absolutes hardly ever appear in correct answer choices. Choice **c** looks attractive until you think a little about what you know—aren't fewer people smoking these days, rather than more? So how could smoking be responsible for a higher mortality rate? (If you didn't know that mortality rate means the rate at which people die, you might keep this choice as a possibility, but you would still be able to

eliminate two answers and have only two to choose from.) And choice **d** is plain silly, so you could eliminate that one, too. You are left with the correct choice, **a.**

4. **a.** How you used the process of elimination here depends on which words you recognized as being spelled incorrectly. If you knew that the correct spellings were outrageous, domesticated, and understandable, then you were home free. If you knew the correct spelling of one or two of these words, you could improve your chances of guessing correctly by using elimination. Surely you knew that at least one of those words was wrong!

Step 6: Know When to Guess

Time to complete: 20 minutes
Activity: Complete worksheet on Your Guessing Ability (pages 17 and 18)

Armed with the process of elimination, you are ready to take control of one of the big questions in test taking: Should I guess? The first and main answer is Yes. Unless the exam has a so-called *guessing penalty*, you have nothing to lose and everything to gain from guessing. The more complicated answer depends both on the exam and on you—your personality and your intuition.

Most veterinary technology exams do not use a guessing penalty. The number of questions you answer correctly yields your score, and there is no penalty for wrong answers. So most of the time, you need not worry—simply go ahead and guess. But if you find that your exam does have a guessing penalty, you should read the section on page 16 to find out what that means to you.

How the Guessing Penalty Works

A guessing penalty really only works against random guessing—filling in the little circles to make a nice pattern on your answer sheet. If you can eliminate one or more answer choices, as previously outlined, you are better off taking a guess than leaving the answer blank, even on the sections that have a penalty.

Here is how a guessing penalty works: Depending on the number of answer choices in a given exam, some proportion of the number of questions you get wrong is subtracted from the total number of questions you got right. For instance, if there are four answer choices, typically the guessing penalty is one-third of your wrong answers. Suppose you took a test of 100 questions. You answered 88 of them right and 12 wrong.

If there is no guessing penalty, your score is simply 88. But if there is a one-third point guessing penalty, the scorers take your 12 wrong answers and divide by 3 to come up with 4. Then they subtract that 4 from your correct-answer score of 88 to leave you with a score of 84. Thus, you would have been better off if you had simply not answered those 12 questions that you were not sure of. Then your total score would still be 88 because there would not be anything to subtract.

What You Should Do about the Guessing Penalty

You now know how a guessing penalty works. The first thing this means for you is that marking your answer sheet at random does not pay. If you are running out of time on an exam that has a guessing penalty, you should not use your remaining seconds to mark a pretty pattern on your answer sheet. Instead, take those few seconds to try to answer one more question right.

But as soon as you get out of the realm of random guessing, the guessing penalty no longer works against you. If you can use the process of elimination to get rid of even one wrong answer choice, the odds stop being against you and start working in your favor.

Sticking with our example of an exam that has four answer choices, eliminating just one wrong answer makes your odds of choosing the correct answer one in three. That is the same as the one-out-of-three guessing penalty—even odds. If you eliminate two answer choices, your odds are one in two—better than the guessing penalty. In either case, you should go ahead and mark one of the remaining answer choices.

When There Is No Guessing Penalty

As noted previously, most veterinary technology exams do not have a guessing penalty. That means that, all other things being equal, you should always go ahead and guess, even if you have no idea what the question means. Nothing can happen to you if you are wrong. But all other things are not necessarily equal. The other factor in deciding whether or not to guess, besides the guessing penalty, is you. There are two things you need to know about yourself before you go into the exam:

- Are you a risk-taker?
- Are you a good guesser?

Your risk-taking temperament matters most on exams with a guessing penalty. Without a guessing penalty, even if you are a play-it-safe person, guessing is perfectly safe. Overcome your anxieties, and go ahead and mark an answer.

But what if you are not much of a risk-taker, and you think of yourself as the world's worst guesser? Complete the worksheet Your Guessing Ability on the next two pages to get an idea of how good your intuition is.

Step 7: Reach Your Peak Performance Zone

Time to complete: 10 minutes to read; weeks to complete!
Activity: Complete the Physical Preparation Checklist (page 20)

To get ready for a challenge like a big exam, you have to take control of your physical, as well as your mental, state. Exercise, proper diet, and rest will ensure that your body works with, rather than against, your mind on test day, as well as during your preparation.

Exercise

If you do not already have a regular exercise program going, the time during which you are preparing for an exam is actually an excellent time to start one. And if you are already keeping fit—or trying to get that way—do not let the pressure of preparing for an exam fool you into quitting now. Exercise helps reduce stress by pumping wonderful good-feeling hormones called endorphins into your system. It also increases the oxygen supply throughout your body, including your brain, so you will be at peak performance on test day.

A half hour of vigorous activity—enough to raise a sweat—every day should be your aim. If you are really pressed for time, every other day is fine. Choose an activity you like and get out there and do

The following are ten really hard questions. You are not supposed to know the answers. Rather, this is an assessment of your ability to guess when you do not have a clue. Read each question carefully, as if you were expected to answer it. If you have any knowledge at all of the subject of the question, use that knowledge to help you eliminate wrong answer choices. Use this answer grid to fill in your answers to the questions.

1. ⓐ ⓑ ⓒ ⓓ
2. ⓐ ⓑ ⓒ ⓓ
3. ⓐ ⓑ ⓒ ⓓ
4. ⓐ ⓑ ⓒ ⓓ
5. ⓐ ⓑ ⓒ ⓓ
6. ⓐ ⓑ ⓒ ⓓ
7. ⓐ ⓑ ⓒ ⓓ
8. ⓐ ⓑ ⓒ ⓓ
9. ⓐ ⓑ ⓒ ⓓ
10. ⓐ ⓑ ⓒ ⓓ

1. September 7 is Independence Day in
   a. India.
   b. Costa Rica.
   c. Brazil.
   d. Australia.

2. Which of the following is the formula for determining the momentum of an object?
   a. $p = mv$
   b. $F = ma$
   c. $P = IV$
   d. $E = mc^2$

3. Because of the expansion of the universe, the stars and other celestial bodies are all moving away from each other. This phenomenon is known as
   a. Newton's first law.
   b. the big bang.
   c. gravitational collapse.
   d. Hubble flow.

4. American author Gertrude Stein was born in
   a. 1713.
   b. 1830.
   c. 1874.
   d. 1901.

5. Which of the following is NOT one of the Five Classics attributed to Confucius?
   a. the *I Ching*
   b. the *Book of Holiness*
   c. the *Spring and Autumn Annals*
   d. the *Book of History*

6. The religious and philosophical doctrine that holds that the universe is constantly in a struggle between good and evil is known as
   a. Pelagianism.
   b. Manichaeanism.
   c. neo-Hegelianism.
   d. Epicureanism.

7. The third Chief Justice of the U.S. Supreme Court was
   a. John Blair.
   b. William Cushing.
   c. James Wilson.
   d. John Jay.

8. Which of the following is the poisonous portion of a daffodil?
   a. the bulb
   b. the leaves
   c. the stem
   d. the flowers

9. The winner of the Masters golf tournament in 1953 was
   a. Sam Snead.
   b. Cary Middlecoff.
   c. Arnold Palmer.
   d. Ben Hogan.

10. The state with the highest per-capita personal income in 1980 was
    a. Alaska.
    b. Connecticut.
    c. New York.
    d. Texas.

Answers

Check your answers against the correct answers below.

1. c.
2. a.
3. d.
4. c.
5. b.
6. b.
7. b.
8. a.
9. d.
10. a.

How Did You Do?

You may have simply gotten lucky and actually known the answer to one or two questions. In addition, your guessing was more successful if you were able to use the process of elimination on any of the questions. Maybe you did not know who the third Chief Justice was (question 7), but you knew that John Jay was the first. In that case, you would have eliminated answer **d** and, therefore, improved your odds of guessing right from one in four to one in three.

According to probability, you should get two and a half answers correct, so getting either two or three right would be average. If you got four or more right, you may be a really terrific guesser. If you got one or none right, you may be a really bad guesser.

Keep in mind, though, that this is only a small sample. You should continue to keep track of your guessing ability as you work through the sample questions in this book. Circle the number of questions you guessed on as you make your guess; or, if you do not have time while you take the practice tests, go back afterward and try to remember which questions you guessed at. Remember, on a test with four answer choices, your chances of getting a right answer is one in four. So keep a separate guessing score for each exam. How many questions did you guess on? How many did you get right? If the number you got right is at least one-fourth of the number of questions you guessed on, you are at least an average guesser, maybe better—and you should always go ahead and guess on the real exam. If the number you got right is significantly lower than one-fourth of the number you guessed on, you need to improve your guessing skills.

---

it. Jogging with a friend always makes the time go faster, or take your iPod.

But do not overdo it. You do not want to exhaust yourself. Moderation is the key.

Diet

First of all, cut out the junk. Go easy on caffeine and nicotine, and eliminate alcohol and any other drugs from your system at least two weeks before the exam.

What your body needs for peak performance is simply a balanced diet. Eat plenty of fruits and vegetables, along with protein and carbohydrates. Foods that are high in lecithin (an amino acid), such as fish and beans, are especially good brain foods.

The night before the exam, you might carbo-load the way athletes do before a contest. Eat a big plate of spaghetti, rice and beans, or whatever your favorite carbohydrate is.

Rest

You probably know how much sleep you need every night to be at your best, even if you do not always get it. Make sure you do get that much sleep, though, for at least a week before the exam. Moderation is important here, too. Too much sleep will just make you groggy.

If you are not a morning person and your exam will be given in the morning, you should reset your internal clock so that your body does not think you are taking an exam at 3 A.M. You have to start this process well before the exam. The way it works is to get up half an hour earlier each morning, and then go to bed half an hour earlier that night. Do not try it the other way around; you will just toss and turn if you go to bed early without having gotten up early. The next morning, get up another half an hour earlier, and so on. How long you will have to do this depends on how late you are used to getting up. Use the Physical Preparation Checklist on the next page to make sure you are in tip-top form.

Step 8: Get Your Act Together

Time to complete: 10 minutes to read; time to complete will vary
Activity: Complete worksheet on Final Preparations (page 22)

You are in control of your mind and body; you are in charge of test anxiety, your preparation, and your test-taking strategies. Now is the time to take charge of external factors, such as the testing site and the materials you need to take the exam.

Find Out Where the Test Is and Make a Trial Run

The testing agency or your veterinary technology instructor will notify you when and where your exam is being held. Do you know how to get to the testing site? Do you know how long it will take to get there? If not, make a trial run, preferably on the same day of the week at the same time of day. Make note on the Final Preparations worksheet of the amount of time it will take you to get to the exam site. Plan on arriv-ing 10 to 15 minutes early so you can get the lay of the land, use the bathroom, and calm down. Then figure out how early you will have to get up that morning, and make sure you get up that early every day for a week before the exam.

Gather Your Materials

The night before the exam, lay out the clothes you will wear and the materials you need to bring with you to the exam. Plan on dressing in layers; you will not have any control over the temperature of the ex-amination room. Have a sweater or jacket you can take off if it is warm. Use the checklist on the Final Preparations worksheet to help you pull together what you will need.

Do Not Skip Breakfast

Even if you do not usually eat breakfast, do so on exam morning. A cup of coffee does not count. Do not eat doughnuts or other sweet foods, either. A sugar high will leave you with a sugar low in the middle of the exam. A mix of protein and carbohy-drates is best: cereal with milk and just a little sugar, or eggs with toast, will do your body a world of good.

Step 9: Do It!

Time to complete: 10 minutes, plus test-taking time
Activity: Ace the Veterinary Technology Exam!

Fast-forward to exam day. You are ready. You made a study plan and followed through. You practiced your test-taking strategies while working through this book. You are in control of your physical, mental, and emotional state. You know when and where to show up and what to bring with you. In other words, you are better prepared than most of the other people taking the veterinary technology test with you. You are psyched.

PHYSICAL PREPARATION CHECKLIST

For the week before the exam, write down (1) what physical exercise you engaged in and for how long and (2) what you ate for each meal. Remember, you are trying for at least half an hour of exercise every other day (preferably every day) and a balanced diet that is light on junk food.

Exam minus 7 days

Exercise: _____ for _____ minutes

Breakfast: _____

Lunch: _____

Dinner: _____

Snacks: _____

Exam minus 6 days

Exercise: _____ for _____ minutes

Breakfast: _____

Lunch: _____

Dinner: _____

Snacks: _____

Exam minus 5 days

Exercise: _____ for _____ minutes

Breakfast: _____

Lunch: _____

Dinner: _____

Snacks: _____

Exam minus 4 days

Exercise: _____ for _____ minutes

Breakfast: _____

Lunch: _____

Dinner: _____

Snacks: _____

Exam minus 3 days

Exercise: _____ for _____ minutes

Breakfast: _____

Lunch: _____

Dinner: _____

Snacks: _____

Exam minus 2 days

Exercise: _____ for _____ minutes

Breakfast: _____

Lunch: _____

Dinner: _____

Snacks: _____

Exam minus 1 day

Exercise: _____ for _____ minutes

Breakfast: _____

Lunch: _____

Dinner: _____

Snacks: _____

Just one more thing. When you are done with the exam, you will have earned a reward. Plan a celebration. Call up your friends and plan a party, or have a nice dinner for two—whatever your heart desires. Give yourself something to look forward to.

And then do it. Go into the exam, full of confidence, armed with test-taking strategies you have practiced until they have become second nature. You are in control of yourself, your environment, and your performance on the exam. You are ready to succeed. So do it. Go in there and ace the exam. And look forward to your future career as a veterinary technician!

Getting to the Exam Site

Location of exam site: _____

Date: _____

Departure time: _____

Do I know how to get to the exam site?   Yes _____   No _____   (If no, make a trial run.)

Time it will take to get to exam site _____

Things to Lay Out the Night Before

Clothes I will wear   _____

Sweater/jacket   _____

Watch   _____

Photo ID   _____

Four #2 pencils   _____

Other Things to Bring/Remember

_____   _____

_____   _____

_____   _____

_____   _____

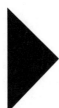 DIAGNOSTIC TEST

CHAPTER OVERVIEW

This diagnostic test is the first of two 100-question tests in this book based on actual Veterinary Technician exams commonly used today. Another practice exam is available online. Of course, none of these questions and answers are reproduced from the actual VTNE, which are kept secret, but this test has been formatted much as the national exam is.

Before taking this test, study Chapter 2, The LearningExpress Test Preparation System, to help you develop skills to succeed on the vet tech exams and any future tests you may take in any field.

Please use the answer sheet on page 25. Once you have completed the test in the allotted time, go to the Answers and Explanations on page 37 and count the number of questions you answered correctly. Make a note of the questions you answered incorrectly; you will want to concentrate your review on those subjects.

1.	a	b	c	d	35.	a	b	c	d	69.	a	b	c	d
2.	a	b	c	d	36.	a	b	c	d	70.	a	b	c	d
3.	a	b	c	d	37.	a	b	c	d	71.	a	b	c	d
4.	a	b	c	d	38.	a	b	c	d	72.	a	b	c	d
5.	a	b	c	d	39.	a	b	c	d	73.	a	b	c	d
6.	a	b	c	d	40.	a	b	c	d	74.	a	b	c	d
7.	a	b	c	d	41.	a	b	c	d	75.	a	b	c	d
8.	a	b	c	d	42.	a	b	c	d	76.	a	b	c	d
9.	a	b	c	d	43.	a	b	c	d	77.	a	b	c	d
10.	a	b	c	d	44.	a	b	c	d	78.	a	b	c	d
11.	a	b	c	d	45.	a	b	c	d	79.	a	b	c	d
12.	a	b	c	d	46.	a	b	c	d	80.	a	b	c	d
13.	a	b	c	d	47.	a	b	c	d	81.	a	b	c	d
14.	a	b	c	d	48.	a	b	c	d	82.	a	b	c	d
15.	a	b	c	d	49.	a	b	c	d	83.	a	b	c	d
16.	a	b	c	d	50.	a	b	c	d	84.	a	b	c	d
17.	a	b	c	d	51.	a	b	c	d	85.	a	b	c	d
18.	a	b	c	d	52.	a	b	c	d	86.	a	b	c	d
19.	a	b	c	d	53.	a	b	c	d	87.	a	b	c	d
20.	a	b	c	d	54.	a	b	c	d	88.	a	b	c	d
21.	a	b	c	d	55.	a	b	c	d	89.	a	b	c	d
22.	a	b	c	d	56.	a	b	c	d	90.	a	b	c	d
23.	a	b	c	d	57.	a	b	c	d	91.	a	b	c	d
24.	a	b	c	d	58.	a	b	c	d	92.	a	b	c	d
25.	a	b	c	d	59.	a	b	c	d	93.	a	b	c	d
26.	a	b	c	d	60.	a	b	c	d	94.	a	b	c	d
27.	a	b	c	d	61.	a	b	c	d	95.	a	b	c	d
28.	a	b	c	d	62.	a	b	c	d	96.	a	b	c	d
29.	a	b	c	d	63.	a	b	c	d	97.	a	b	c	d
30.	a	b	c	d	64.	a	b	c	d	98.	a	b	c	d
31.	a	b	c	d	65.	a	b	c	d	99.	a	b	c	d
32.	a	b	c	d	66.	a	b	c	d	100.	a	b	c	d
33.	a	b	c	d	67.	a	b	c	d					
34.	a	b	c	d	68.	a	b	c	d					

Practice Test

Pharmacology

1. A 35-lb dog comes into the clinic with a pyoderma (skin infection). The veterinarian prescribes cephalexin twice a day for 2 weeks. The dosage is 30 mg/kg. Cephalexin comes in 250-mg and 500-mg capsules. How many capsules should be sent home with the animal?
   a. 7
   b. 14
   c. 21
   d. 28

2. A 12-lb dog comes into the clinic for allergic skin disease. The veterinarian prescribes a decreasing dosage of prednisone with the dose decreasing by half every day. He would like to begin the dosage at 2 mg/kg and decrease until the animal is at 0.5 mg/kg every other day. Total length of therapy should be 10 days. Prednisone comes in 5-mg and 20-mg tablets. How many tablets should be sent home with the animal?
   a. 10
   b. 7
   c. 5
   d. 4

3. The doctor asks you to dispense digoxin for a client's dog. The recommended dose is 0.22 mg/m^2, where m^2 is the number of square meters of body surface area. The dog's body surface area is 0.8 m^2. The digoxin elixir is available in a 0.15-mg/ml concentration. This drug is *very* toxic (has a low therapeutic index). The doctor has asked you to start the dosage at 60% of the normal calculated dose for this patient. Based on this, how many ml should the dog receive at each dose?
   a. 0.1
   b. 0.5
   c. 0.7
   d. 1.0

4. The veterinarian orders 7 mEq of potassium chloride to be added to the IV fluids. The vial is labeled 20 mEq in 10 ml. How many ml will be added to the fluid bag?
   a. 1.3
   b. 3.5
   c. 5
   d. 12

5. Given a 45% solution and sterile diluent, prepare 3 liters of 15% solution. What quantity each of diluent and solution will be needed to make this solution?
   a. diluent 1 L, solution 2 L
   b. diluent 1.5 L, solution 1.5 L
   c. diluent 2 L, solution 1 L
   d. diluent 3 L, solution 1 L

6. Which drug is commonly used as a cough suppressant in dogs?
   a. aminophylline
   b. butorphanol
   c. diazepam
   d. dextromethorphan

7. Which dewormer is effective against pulmonary worms?
   a. pyrantel pamoate (Strongid)
   b. praziquantel (Droncit)
   c. fenbendazole (Panacur)
   d. metronidazole (Flagyl)

8. Which of the following drugs is commonly used to treat ventricular arrhythmias?
   a. lidocaine
   b. digoxin
   c. atenolol/propranolol
   d. enalapril

9. Which of the following fluids can be administered at the same time as a blood transfusion through the same IV catheter?
   a. lactated Ringer's
   b. 2.5% dextrose + half-strength LRS
   c. Normosol–R
   d. 0.9% sodium chloride

10. Which of the following can be used to treat an animal with von Willebrand disease prior to surgery to prevent bleeding?
    a. vasopressin
    b. desmopressin
    c. vitamin K
    d. aspirin

11. Which antibiotic penetrates the blood–brain barrier, making it a good treatment choice for bacterial meningitis?
    a. gentamicin
    b. enrofloxacin
    c. cloxacillin
    d. cephalexin

12. An epileptic dog is started on anticonvulsant therapy (such as phenobarbital or potassium bromide) when
    a. seizures occur every 6 months or less.
    b. each individual seizure lasts less than one minute.
    c. the dog urinates or defecates during the seizure.
    d. the seizures occur in clusters.

13. Which of the following is true regarding ivermectin use?
    a. It is safe to give to collies at miticidal concentrations (200 µg/kg).
    b. It is effective for treatment of adult heartworms.
    c. It may be given orally, subcutaneously, or intravenously for treatment of demodectic mange.
    d. Toxicity causes neurologic signs.

14. What is the topical treatment (dip) for generalized demodecosis in dogs?
    a. rotenone
    b. amitraz
    c. pyrethrin
    d. lyme sulfur

Surgical Preparation and Assisting

15. How should gloved in people pass each other in the surgical suite?
    a. back to back
    b. front to back
    c. side to side
    d. it doesn't matter

16. Which portion of the draped animal is considered sterile?
    a. the scrubbed surface of the animal
    b. the portion underneath the drape
    c. the portion of the animal exposed within the draped field
    d. the portion of the drape not in contact with the animal

17. What is the name of the common procedure performed on horses with anatomical deformities of the vulva that could potentially lead to vaginal contamination with feces?
   a. trephination
   b. Caslick's procedure
   c. onychectomy
   d. episiotomy

18. Which is the most commonly used surgical blade?
   a. #10
   b. #11
   c. #12
   d. #15

19. What do the numbers on a scalpel blade refer to?
   a. the size of the blade
   b. the shape of the blade
   c. the length the cutting edge
   d. the type of blade holder needed

20. To what do the numbers on a suture refer?
   a. the size of the needle
   b. the thickness of the suture
   c. the needle shape
   d. the type of the suture

21. When can a dog be safely extubated?
   a. It can be done when he is paddling.
   b. It can be done when he is sternal unassisted.
   c. It can be done when he is gagging.
   d. It depends on the breed.

22. Which of the following is in the correct order?
   a. gown, glove, mask
   b. mask, gown, glove
   c. mask, glove, gown
   d. gown, mask, glove

23. Which of the following can act as a sterilant?
   a. glutaraldehyde
   b. alcohol
   c. chlorhexidine
   d. quaternary ammonium compounds (such as Roccal-D™)

24. Which of the following is NOT an antiseptic?
   a. povidone iodine
   b. alcohol
   c. chlorhexidine
   d. quaternary ammonium compounds

25. Soap and warm water are used to scrub some surgical instruments. The instruments were soaked in cold water for 10 minutes prior to being scrubbed. Which of the following is true?
   a. The instruments are now ready for the autoclave.
   b. The instruments should now be dried and lubricated with instrument milk.
   c. The instruments should be ultrasonically cleaned with a dental machine.
   d. Cold water should not have been used because it will cause the instruments to rust.

26. How long can muslin-wrapped, steam-sterilized packs be stored on an open shelf?
   a. one week
   b. three to four weeks
   c. seven to eight weeks
   d. three months

27. Which of the following is a valid reason to call the owner prior to or during a surgical procedure?
   a. change in extent of procedure
   b. change in length of procedure
   c. change in cost of procedure
   d. all of the above

28. Which of the following does NOT need to be included on a pack wrap?
   a. the date of sterilization
   b. the name of the person preparing and sterilizing the pack
   c. the hospital name
   d. the pack type (spay, orthopedic, etc.)

29. An endotracheal tube with too large a diameter can cause which of the following?
   a. intubation of one bronchus
   b. tracheal necrosis
   c. increased airway resistance
   d. intubation of the esophagus

30. Which of the following is NOT a characteristic of the ideal suture material?
   a. increased memory
   b. decreased tissue drag
   c. increased knot holding
   d. decreased reactivity

Dentistry

31. What is the hardest substance in the body?
   a. bone
   b. dentin
   c. enamel
   d. cartilage

32. Which part of the tooth is affected when you have a periapical abscess?
   a. the periodontal ligament
   b. the pulp
   c. the gingiva
   d. the enamel

33. Which of the following is the *medical* reason for polishing a tooth?
   a. It provides a smooth surface.
   b. It removes some tooth staining.
   c. It looks pretty.
   d. It removes more bacteria than scaling alone.

34. Which of the following describes canine dentition?
   a. aradicular hypsodont
   b. radicular hypsodont
   c. aradicular brachyodont
   d. radicular brachyodont

35. Which of the following is true of horses?
   a. They only have enamel on the labial surface of their teeth.
   b. They are more likely than cats to develop true dental caries.
   c. Tooth root abscesses are easily treated intraorally.
   d. They do not have canines.

36. Which of the following methods will give the best results when trimming chinchilla incisors?
   a. guillotine nail clippers
   b. scissors
   c. diamond wheel
   d. rasp

37. Which of the following is true of rats?
   a. They have brachyodont premolars and molars.
   b. They may need to have their teeth floated.
   c. They have a palatal ostium.
   d. They are highly prone to cheek tooth impaction.

38. Which of the following are endodontic instruments?
   a. the elevator
   b. the barbed broach
   c. the probe
   d. dental stone

Laboratory Procedures

39. Which of the following is NOT true of phlebotomy for laboratory techniques?
   a. Multiple sticks if the animal is wriggling may cause invalidation of chemistry results.
   b. Use of a vacutainer can minimize artifacts.
   c. Use of a large syringe with a small needle can lead to hemolysis.
   d. Blood should be drawn within three hours of a meal for bile acids testing.

40. Which of the following blood tubes would NOT be used for calcium testing?
   a. purple or lavender top
   b. green top
   c. red top
   d. tiger top

41. Which portion of the blood smear should be examined for microfilaria?
   a. the body
   b. the monolayer
   c. the feathered edge
   d. none of the above

42. Which of the following is correct for the calculation of the mean cell hemoglobin concentration (MCHC)?
   a. PCV/6
   b. (PCV × 10)/Hb
   c. (Hb × 10)/RBC
   d. (Hb × 100)/PCV

43. A poodle comes in with a PCV of 60 and TP of 8 g/dl. Which of the following statements is true?
   a. This animal is anemic.
   b. This animal has polycythemia.
   c. This animal is dehydrated.
   d. This animal is within normal limits.

44. A golden retriever comes into the clinic with pale mucous membranes and bloody diarrhea. Her PCV is 20. She had severe coughing two weeks earlier, but this is now resolved. Which of the following parasites is likely with these clinical signs?
   a. *Ancylostoma caninum*
   b. *Toxascaris leonine*
   c. *Diplydium caninum*
   d. *Paragonimus kellicotti*

45. A horse comes in with staggering and other neurologic symptoms. Which of the following could potentially cause these symptoms in horses?
   a. *Cryptosporidium*
   b. *Eimeria*
   c. *Sarcocystis*
   d. *Isospora*

46. An Abyssinian cat presents with jaundice, a PCV of 15, and hemoglobinuria. Her BUN:creatinine ratio is elevated (>20:1). On a CBC you notice signet ring-shaped inclusions in the RBCs. Which of the following is a probable cause?
   a. *Cytauxzoon felis*
   b. *Mycoplasma haemofelis*
   c. lead poisoning
   d. cholestasis and acute renal failure

47. Which of the following is the *least* accurate test for heartworm disease?
   a. modified Knott's test
   b. heartworm indirect/antibody test
   c. heartworm direct/antigen test
   d. blood smear

48. An animal comes in with BUN of 60 and a creatine level of 4. Which of the following is true?
  a. These are normal levels.
  b. These levels indicate prerenal azotemia.
  c. These levels indicate renal azotemia.
  d. These levels indicate portosystemic shunt disease.

49. A dog comes in with epistaxis. You are asked to run some tests. The BMBT (buccal mucosal bleeding time) is prolonged, the platelet count is 100,000/µl, the PT (prothrombin time) and PTT (partial thromboplastin time) are both increased, and the fibrin split products are elevated. Which of the following is true?
  a. The primary hemostatic mechanisms are compromised.
  b. The secondary hemostatic mechanisms are compromised.
  c. Fibrinolysis is excessive.
  d. all of the above

50. Which of the following is a good reason to perform bone marrow testing?
  a. An animal is on chemotherapy and is severely anemic.
  b. An animal has *Ehrlichia canis*, a platelet count of 20,000, and epistaxis.
  c. An animal has a lymphocyte elevation on CBC and generalized lymphadenopathy. The lymphocytes are predominantly medium to large.
  d. An animal has a PCV of 60 and a TP of 6.5.

51. A fluid sample is on the counter of the laboratory without a label. It has a TP of 2.3, a specific gravity of 1.015, and 2,500 cells/mm³. Which of the following is true?
  a. It is chyle.
  b. It is a transudate.
  c. It is a modified transudate.
  d. It is an exudate.

52. A dog presents with PU/PD of three weeks' duration. Which of the following is NOT a test for diagnosing this problem?
  a. vasopressin test
  b. Na:K ratio
  c. ACTH stimulation test
  d. T3/T4

53. A cat has elevated BUN, creatinine, and phosphorus levels and a low specific gravity. The sediment shows epithelial cell casts. The PCV is decreased and the TP is within normal limits. Which of the following statements is correct?
  a. The cat has tubular disease.
  b. The cat has glomerular disease.
  c. The cat has cystitis.
  d. none of the above

Animal Care and Nursing

54. What is the common name for Aujeszky's disease?
  a. plague
  b. canine infectious tracheobronchitis
  c. pseudorabies
  d. distemper

55. What disease is caused by *Yersinia pestis*?
  a. plague
  b. canine infectious tracheobronchitis
  c. pseudorabies
  d. distemper

56. What is another name for mad itch?
  a. plague
  b. canine infectious tracheobronchitis
  c. pseudorabies
  d. distemper

57. Which of the following is required when handling sheep?
  a. a chute
  b. stanchions
  c. placing them on their backs
  d. care to avoid damaging the wool

58. What is one of the causative agents for kennel cough?
  a. *Yersinia pestis*
  b. *Bordetella bronchiseptica*
  c. *Morbillivirus*
  d. *Ehrlichia canis*

59. Where are the anal sacs located?
  a. at 12:00 and 6:00
  b. at 3:00 and 9:00
  c. at 4:00 and 8:00
  d. at 5:00 and 7:00

60. What is the causative agent for hard pad disease?
  a. plague
  b. canine infectious tracheobronchitis
  c. pseudorabies
  d. canine distemper

61. Hearing protection is always needed when handling which species?
  a. porcine
  b. ovine
  c. canine
  d. equine

62. What type of organism is parvovirus?
  a. a DNA virus with envelope
  b. a DNA virus without envelope
  c. an RNA virus
  d. a prion

63. What is the maximum time that urinary catheters on closed-collection systems should be maintained?
  a. 5 hours
  b. 12 hours
  c. 24 hours
  d. 48 hours

64. What type of organism causes distemper?
  a. a DNA virus with envelope
  b. a DNA virus without envelope
  c. an RNA virus
  d. a prion

65. Which of the following is NOT a means of parenteral administration?
  a. PO
  b. IV
  c. IO
  d. IP

66. Which species requires vitamin C supplementation in their food?
  a. guinea pigs
  b. canines
  c. equines
  d. bovines

67. Which types of enemas should never be given to cats?
  a. osmotic
  b. phosphate
  c. glycerine
  d. petroleum jelly

68. Which of the following is NOT a good method of cat restraint?
  a. lying on top of the cat
  b. cat bag
  c. cat stretch
  d. net

69. Which of the following is true regarding bird restraint?
  a. Passerine birds will die if held in dorsal recumbency.
  b. The wings should be restrained to prevent injury.
  c. The sternum should be free to ensure adequate breathing.
  d. Typically, bird restraint requires one hand.

70. Buster is a 5-year-old unneutered unvaccinated M Catahoula Leopard Hound. According to his owner, he is a great hog dog, but after his last hunt the dog developed severe itching around the head and neck. The owner said that he had fed Buster a bit of the raw meat after the boar was dressed, because he had done such a great job. What does Buster probably have?
  a. distemper virus
  b. pseudorabies
  c. rabies
  d. erysipelas

71. Which of the following test combinations is in the correct order in an ocular exam?
  a. Tono-Pen, Schirmer, culture and sensitivity, funduscopic exam
  b. Schirmer, Tono-Pen, culture and sensitivity, funduscopic exam
  c. Schirmer, Tono-Pen, funduscopic exam, culture and sensitivity
  d. funduscopic exam, Tono-Pen, Schirmer, culture and sensitivity

72. Which of the following is true regarding rabbit restraint?
  a. They should be carried by the ears.
  b. They should be flipped onto their back for every procedure.
  c. They should be carried like a football with their head tucked into your elbow.
  d. Aggressive rabbits should be declawed to prevent scratching.

73. Which of the following fluid administration methods should NOT be used in a patient in shock?
  a. IP
  b. SQ
  c. IV
  d. IO

74. Sadsack is a 4-month-old unvaccinated Basset Hound puppy that was just purchased from a backyard breeder in Georgia. He has yellow mucus coming from his eyes and nose and is coughing. There are yellow spots on his teeth and he has very thick and rigid foot and nasal pads. He also has a rash on his abdomen. What does Sadsack probably have?
  a. canine distemper
  b. kennel cough
  c. canine influenza
  d. hypothyroidism

75. In food animals, where is the ideal location for IM injections?
  a. epaxial muscles
  b. hamstrings
  c. neck muscles
  d. quadriceps group

76. Fred is a 6-year-old unvaccinated M/N Jack Russell terrier. He presents with rear limb paralysis and odd behaviors of 3 to 4 days' duration. Puncture wounds are present on physical exam. The owner says Fred always has injuries because he is an avid hunter and likes to run through the woods. What is the most likely cause of Fred's problem?
  a. canine distemper
  b. rabies
  c. pseudorabies
  d. leptospirosis

77. Run for Gold is an unneutered male 2-year-old Greyhound from the track. He has had a dry, hacking cough of 1 week's duration. The cough is worse on tracheal palpation. A kennel mate died 1 week earlier after a 3-day course of cough followed by a very high fever (104 degrees) and epistaxis. What does Run for Gold probably have?
   a. canine distemper
   b. *Bordetella bronchiseptica*
   c. canine influenza
   d. canine hepatitis

Diagnostic Imaging

78. A Thoroughbred presents with right foreleg lameness. The veterinarian suspects a slab fracture of the cranial aspect of the carpus. Which of the following views would be the *least* likely to show a slab fracture of the anterior carpus?
   a. dorsoproximal 60-degree dorsodistal oblique carpus
   b. flexed lateromedial carpus
   c. lateromedial carpus
   d. dorsopalmar carpus

79. Which subatomic particle makes x-rays when it strikes the anode?
   a. neutron
   b. electron
   c. proton
   d. gamma ray

80. Which of the following allows adjustment of the number of x-rays produced by the tube?
   a. kVp
   b. mA
   c. mAs
   d. time

81. Which of the following does NOT affect the amount of heat produced by an x-ray tube?
   a. time
   b. stationary vs. rotating anode
   c. oil
   d. kVp

82. Which of the following may be thrown into the trash or down the drain without special treatment according to the EPA (Environmental Protection Agency)?
   a. lead backing
   b. old radiographic film
   c. developer
   d. fixer

83. Your digital x-ray is being repaired and you have to take routine radiographs and use a dip tank for processing. Your developer temperature is 60 degrees. How long should your film be in the developer prior to being placed in the water bath?
   a. 7 minutes
   b. 5 minutes
   c. 1 minute
   d. 6 minutes

84. Which of the following organs will have the *least* potential for somatic damage from scatter radiation?
   a. the thyroid gland
   b. the skin
   c. the liver
   d. the cornea and lens of the eye

85. If a radiograph has small black half-moon shapes on it after developing, which of the following is likely?
   a. They are from handling the radiograph prior to developing.
   b. They are from dirty cassettes.
   c. They are from scratches after developing.
   d. They are from dirt or contrast media on the animal's coat.

Anesthesia and Analgesia

86. How many pins does an oxygen tank have?
   a. 1
   b. 2
   c. 3
   d. 4

87. Which of the following is true of oxygen?
   a. It has a low volatility.
   b. It is not flammable.
   c. Common tank sizes are E and H.
   d. It is in both liquid and gas states in the canister.

88. Which of the following is the *maximum* gas pressure that may be used during intermittent positive-pressure ventilation (*IPPV*, or assisted ventilation)?
   a. 4 cm H_2O
   b. 8 cm H_2O
   c. 12 cm H_2O
   d. 20 cm H_2O

89. Which of the following drugs is a dissociative anesthetic?
   a. zolazepam
   b. thiopental
   c. tiletamine
   d. morphine

90. A dog is waking up out of anesthesia midway through a procedure. Which of the following is NOT a potential cause of this change in anesthetic plane?
   a. The anesthetist is hitting the oxygen flush valve too often during assisted ventilation.
   b. The anesthetic is ineffective.
   c. The vaporizer for the anesthetic gas is empty.
   d. The animal was disconnected from the anesthesia machine.

91. Which of the following is *false* for precision out-of-circle vaporizers and nonprecision in-circle vaporizers?
   a. Units on in-circle vaporizers are not in percent.
   b. Temperature will affect in-circle vaporizers.
   c. Nonprecision vaporizers are usually used for methoxyflurane.
   d. The amount of gas that the animal gets is different depending on conditions with both types of vaporizers.

92. Which of the following is *false* for rebreathing systems?
   a. Hypercapnia is possible.
   b. Lower levels of gas anesthetic may be used.
   c. There is increased resistance.
   d. Hyperventilation may occur, resulting in apnea.

93. What is the appropriate size reservoir bag for a 20-lb Jack Russell Terrier cross?
   a. half liter
   b. 1 liter
   c. 3 liter
   d. 5 liter

94. What are the benefits of giving an assisted/sigh breath to an animal under anesthesia?
  a. It prevents atelectasis.
  b. It improves breathing rates.
  c. It prevents hypercapnia.
  d. all of the above

95. Which of the following is *false* about soda lime CO_2 absorbent?
  a. Old soda lime crumbles easily.
  b. Old soda lime may turn blue or purple if it is saturated with CO_2.
  c. Soda lime should be changed a minimum of once a month.
  d. The reaction of CO_2 with soda lime is exothermic.

96. A 12-pound patient is receiving oxygen at a rate of 40 ml/minute. What sort of system is he on?
  a. a rebreathing open-circuit system
  b. a rebreathing semiclosed-circuit system
  c. a rebreathing closed-circuit system
  d. a nonrebreathing system

97. Which of the following patients would do best on a nonrebreathing system?
  a. a 600-g African Grey parrot
  b. a 60-lb Rottweiler
  c. a 14-lb cat
  d. a 200-lb calf

98. Of the following anesthetic gases, which is the most toxic to humans?
  a. methoxyflurane
  b. halothane
  c. isoflurane
  d. sevoflurane

99. Which of the following has the highest MAC?
  a. halothane
  b. isoflurane
  c. sevoflurane
  d. methoxyflurane

100. A St. Bernard under anesthesia has a heart rate of 100 bpm on propofol and isoflurane. Which of the following is TRUE?
  a. This is an okay heart rate because propofol causes tachycardia.
  b. This animal may be going into shock.
  c. This is a normal heart rate in this breed.
  d. This animal is in stage III plane I anesthesia.

Answers and Explanations

Pharmacology

1. d. 35 lb = 16 kg, so 16 kg × 30 mg/kg × 1 capsule/500 mg × 2 × 14 days = 28 500 mg capsules.

2. b. The dosage at day 1 is 10 mg, day 2 is 5 mg, day 3 is 2.5 mg, then 2.5 mg eod, so a total of 7 tablets of the 5-mg form is required.

3. c. 0.8 × 0.22 × 1 ml/0.15 mg = 1.17 ml regular dose. 1.17 × 0.6 = 0.7 ml.

4. b. 20mEq/10 ml = 2 mEq/ml. 7 mEq × 1 ml/2 mEq = 3.5 ml.

5. c. $C_1 \times V_1 = C_2 \times V_2$. $V_1 = (C_2 \times V_2)/C_1 = 15\% \times 3 L/45\% = 1 L$ of solution and 2 L of diluent.

6. b. Butorphanol is commonly used as a cough suppressant. Aminophylline is a bronchodilator, diazepam is a sedative, and dextromethorphan is not used in veterinary medicine.

7. c. Fenbendazole is the drug of choice for lungworms. Pyrantel works well for hookworms and roundworms, praziquantel works well for tapeworms and flukes, and metronidazole works best for protozoa.

8. a. Lidocaine works well for ventricular arrhythmias. Digoxin is used to increase cardiac contractility, atenolol is generally used for supraventricular arrhythmias, and enalapril is used as a venovasodilator and a blood-pressure modifier.

9. d. Sodium chloride is the only fluid that may be administered in the line along with whole blood.

10. b. Desmopressin can be used to pretreat animals with von Willebrand disease (VWD). Vasopressin is used to test for and treat diabetes insipidus, vitamin K is used to treat secondary hemostatic disorders, and aspirin is an anticoagulant and would increase bleeding.

11. b. Enrofloxacin penetrates the blood–brain barrier and is frequently used for treatment of bacterial meningitis.

12. d. Isolated or infrequent seizures can often go without treatment. Most seizures involve loss of consciousness and urination and/or defecation.

13. d. Ivermectin toxicity causes neurologic dysfunction. Ivermectin can be given orally, subcutaneously, or as a pour-on, but not intravenously, is effective for the treatment of microfilarial, but not adult, heartworm disease, and is not safe to give to collies at high concentrations.

14. b. Amitraz is the topical dip treatment for generalized demodecosis. Rotenone may be used for localized lesions, but pyrethrins and lyme sulfur are ineffective for demodecosis.

Surgical Preparation and Assisting

15. a. Back to back is the correct way to pass each other in surgery because it prevents contamination of the area that will be in close proximity to the surgical field.

16. d. The portion of the drape not in contact with the animal, the table, or the surgeon is considered sterile. Remember, the animal can be *aseptic* or *antiseptic*, but not *sterile* (because it cannot be placed in an autoclave).

17. b. The Caslick's procedure is a common procedure performed on horses with incompetent vulvas that would otherwise allow contamination of the vaginal tract. Trephination is relieving pressure on the brain by boring a hole in the skull. Onychectomy is declawing. An episiotomy is extending the vulvar opening to enable removal of the fetus during parturition.

18. a. The most commonly used surgical blade is #10. This has a broader, rounded blade edge. The #11 blade is shaped like half of an arrow and is often used to make stab incisions or for onychectomy procedures. The #12 blade is curved with the blade edge on the inside of the curve. It is also used for onychectomy procedures. The #15 blade has a similar blade to the #10, but covers a much smaller area. It may be used for procedures where fine control is needed.

19. b. The number on the scalpel blade refers to the shape of the blade. The size of the blade and the size of the cutting edge are determined by the blade's shape. The type of blade holder needed will also depend on this property. Beaver blades require special holders and are often used in ophthalmic procedures, for instance.

20. b. The number on the suture refers to the thickness of the suture material. The smaller the number, the thicker the suture (for example, 5-0 is thinner than 2-0 suture). The appropriate size and shape of the needle are given on the package. Reverse cutting means that the cutting edge of the needle is on the inside of the curve, for example. The type of suture is written in large letters on the label.

21. d. A dog can generally be safely extubated when he is swallowing, but some breeds, such as brachycephalic animals, should be kept intubated until they are chewing. Movement of extremities is not an indication of swallowing capability. If an animal cannot swallow, he cannot prevent aspiration of vomit during recovery and therefore should be kept intubated. Gag reflex, likewise, is not a good indication for extubation.

22. b. The correct order is to put on your mask, booties, and scrubs prior to scrubbing, then your gown, then your gloves after you are scrubbed.

23. a. Glutaraldehyde acts as a sterilant for cold sterilization as well as a disinfectant. Chlorhexidine and alcohol are antiseptics. Chlorhexidine and quaternary ammonium compounds are disinfectants.

24. d. Quaternary ammonium compounds are disinfectants. Povidone iodine, alcohol, and chlorhexidine may all act as antiseptics on living tissue.

25. b. The instruments should be dried and lubricated with instrument milk. They are then ready for the autoclave. If ultrasonic cleaners (*not* ultrasonic scalers or dental machines) are available, they can be used prior to drying and lubricating the instruments. Cold water will help to loosen blood and prevent corrosion of instruments.

26. b. Muslin-wrapped, steam-sterilized packs may be stored on an open shelf for up to 4 weeks and in a closed cabinet for up to 8 weeks.

27. d. Any change in plan during surgery should prompt a call to the owner. This will prevent miscommunication and will enable you to get adequate permission prior to continuing. Remember to write everything in the record. This will prevent potential legal issues. If something is not in the record it did not officially get done.

28. c. The hospital name does not need to be on the outside of the pack. The date of sterilization and the name of the person who wrapped the pack are mandatory. The pack type is also mandatory if the clinic performs different types of surgery (orthopedic pack, soft-tissue pack, ophthalmic pack, etc.). If the clinic only performs spays and neuters, it may not be critical to show pack type on the label.

29. b. Large-diameter endotracheal tubes can cause tracheal necrosis. Too long a tube can result in intubation of only one bronchus. Too small a diameter tube can result in increased airway resistance. Intubation of the esophagus may occur with either faulty technique or inadequate visualization of the glottis.

30. a. Increased memory can cause problems with suture handling. The ideal suture should have minimal tissue drag and excellent knot holding capability and cause minimal tissue reaction.

Dentistry

31. c. Enamel is the hardest substance in the body. Bone and dentin are next, but cartilage is relatively soft.

32. b. The pulp is infected, so the route of least resistance is the apical delta, so that is where the abscess forms. The periodontal ligament and the gingiva are affected with periodontal abscesses. The enamel is only affected by FORLs (feline odontoclastic resorptive lesions) and cavity lesions.

33. a. The medical reason for polishing is to smooth out the microscopic abrasions that are formed by scaling. A smoother surface makes it more difficult for bacteria to get a purchase on the tooth. Polishing does not really remove tartar or bacteria, but it does make the tooth shinier.

34. d. Canines have radicular brachyodont teeth, which have a closed root and do not continue to grow throughout the dog's life.

35. b. Horses develop dental caries on the unenameled surface of the tooth. Rabbits have enamel only on the labial surface, but not equines. Tooth root abscesses are often removed extraorally. Horses do have canine teeth.

36. c. The diamond wheel should be used for tooth trimming in rodents. The other methods can cause the tooth to shatter.

37. a. Rats have brachyodont premolars and molars, so their teeth do not need to be floated and they rarely get tooth impactions. Palatal ostiua are found in guinea pigs and chinchillas.

38. b. The barbed broach is used to remove the pulp from the pulp cavity during an endodontic procedure. The elevator is used for exodontics, the probe is used for tooth assessment, and the dental stone is used to create a model of the teeth for orthodontic appliances or restorative dentistry.

Laboratory Procedures

39. d. Blood should be drawn preprandially (before eating) and again three hours after a meal for bile acid testing. Traumatic venipuncture technique and use of a small needle with a large syringe can both lead to hemolysis. Vacutainers will minimize hemolysis and ensure adequate blood mixing in the blood tubes.

40. a. EDTA, the anticoagulant in purple-top tubes, acts as a chelating agent that forms an irreversible binding with calcium. Heparin works on thrombin and does not affect calcium. Red- and tiger-top tubes are fine because the clot does not affect albumin which carries calcium.

41. c. Microfilaria are brought to the feathered edge because they are relatively large compared to the blood cells. The monolayer is the area that should be examined for blood cell morphology.

42. d. MCHC = (Hb × 100)/ PCV. Choice **a** is the formula for the estimated red blood cell count; choice **b** is not a formula for an RBC (red blood cell) index, and choice **c** is the formula for MCH (mean corpuscular hemoglobin).

43. c. The animal is dehydrated, so the PCV increase is related to decreased dilution, not to polycythemia (RBC overgrowth).

44. a. Hookworms. She has anemia and bloody diarrhea because *A. caninum* sucks blood into the intestines. The cough is from larval migration through the lungs. *D. caninum* does not suck blood or cause anemia, *T. leonine* has a longer prepatent period, and *P. kellicotti* would not have affected the intestines.

45. c. *Sarcocystis* is the causative agent of equine protozoal myelitis. *Cryptosporidium* causes diarrhea, *Eimeria* does not migrate to the central nervous system (CNS), and *Isospora* is not found in horses.

46. a. *Cytauxzoon* will cause liver failure along with extravascular hemolysis in domestic cats. *Mycoplasma haemofelis* causes milder disease and is usually only seen in FeLV or FIV positive cats. Lead poisoning can cause anemia, but will not show parasitic inclusions in the RBC. Cholestasis and acute renal failure are unlikely in this case.

47. d. Because of the small sample size, the blood smear is the least accurate of all the tests listed.

48. b. This is prerenal azotemia because the BUN:Cr ratio is >20:1. It would be <5:1 in portosystemic shunt disease and 5–20:1 for renal azotemia.

49. d. Primary hemostasis (BMBT tests this), secondary hemostasis (PT and PTT), and fibrinolysis (FSP) are all affected.

50. c. Findings are suspicious for lymphoma/lymphoid leukemia and should be evaluated further.

51. b. The definition of a transudate is TP < 2.5, cellularity <5,000 and specific gravity <1.018.

52. d. PU/PD is common with diabetes insipidus (vasopressin test), hyperadrenocorticism (ACTH), or hypoadrenocorticism (ACTH and Na:K ratio), and uncommon with hypothyroidism in dogs.

53. a. Tubular disease will cause increased BUN and Cr levels, phosphorus elevations, and low specific gravity. Tubular disease also has casts. If it were glomerular in origin, the protein level in the urine would be increased. Cystitis would cause none of these symptoms.

Animal Care and Nursing

54. c. Mad itch and pseudorabies are both common names for Aujeszky's disease.

55. a. Bubonic plague is caused by the bacterium *Yersinia pestis*.

56. c. Mad itch is also known as pseudorabies.

57. d. Sheep handling requires care to avoid damaging the wool. Sheep are cast by grabbing them by the scruff and placing them on their rear ends with the feet facing away from you and the back leaning against your legs.

58. b. *Bordetella bronchiseptica* has been isolated from many animals with kennel cough.

59. c. The anal sacs are located at 4:00 and 8:00 on an imaginary watch face if looking at the anus. They are either expressed by digital pressure externally or by gentle insertion of the finger into the anus and expressing from the interior of the rectum.

60. d. Canine distemper is the causative agent for hard pad disease.

61. a. Hearing protection is always needed when handling swine and many species of avians.

62. b. Parvovirus is a naked DNA virus, which means that it is resistant to many disinfectants and to UV (ultraviolet) light.

63. d. Urinary catheters should be maintained for less than 48 hours to prevent secondary infections.

64. c. Distemper is an RNA virus similar to measles in people.

65. a. Parenteral administration means via a needle, so PO (per os), or by mouth, is not parenteral. All the other methods are.

66. a. Guinea pigs and primates are the only species that require vitamin C supplementation in their food to prevent scurvy.

67. b. Phosphate enemas should not be given to cats because they cause toxicities. Osmotic, glycerine, and petroleum jelly enemas provide lubrication or draw water into the tract and ease passage of stool.

68. a. Generally, cats respond better to minimal manual restraint. Remote restraint devices such as the cat bag and the net make handling easier.

69. c. Birds do not have a diaphragm, so the chest muscles are responsible for breathing. Restraint of the wings and feet is a two-handed operation.

70. b. Buster could have gotten pseudorabies from the raw boar meat. Erysipelas would just have caused a rash or abscess. Rabies is improbable and distemper must be transmitted by another dog and would have a different symptom picture.

71. b. The Schirmer tear test should be performed prior to all other tests, then a drop of numbing agent should be added and the intraocular pressure and C and S can be performed. Finally, a mydriatic is introduced, and the fundus is examined.

72. c. Rabbits should always be transported like a football. They should *never* be carried by their ears or declawed. Flipping them on their backs for hypnosis should only be done for painful or stressful procedures if needed.

73. b. Animals in shock have decreased blood pressure, so the ability for the fluids to leave the subcutaneous space is decreased. Intraperitoneal fluids can be administered to neonates when veins are difficult to access, but intraosseous and intravenous administration are preferred.

74. a. Canine distemper is the most likely cause of these symptoms. He has thickened foot and nasal pads, typical respiratory symptoms, and a rash. The only symptom missing is diarrhea.

75. c. In food animals, the neck muscles are used for injections because all the other sites potentially become cuts of meat.

76. b. Ascending paralysis and behavior changes are typical of rabies, especially in conjunction with the wound history. This is reportable to the county health department.

77. c. This is likely canine influenza. Distemper and *B. bronchiseptica* do not generally cause hemorrhagic pneumonia, although they do cause the cough on tracheal palpation. Canine influenza is highly contagious in Greyhounds and has a high morbidity and moderate mortality rate.

Diagnostic Imaging

78. d. The dorsopalmar (AP) carpus would not show a slab fracture of the anterior surface of the carpal bone. The other views would be more likely to reveal a slab fracture of 79 area.

79. b. Electrons are produced by the cathode, travel across the space, and strike the anode under the influence of a strong electromagnet. This produces x-rays. Neutrons and protons are too heavy to travel, and gamma rays are pure energy, not particles.

80. b. The number of x-rays produced is determined by the mA, while the speed of the x-rays is determined by the kVP. Time is also involved to a certain extent.

81. b. The kVp does not affect the heat production as much as the mA. The amount of time and the mA determine how hot the tube gets. Stationary anodes are much more likely to overheat than rotating anodes. The oil allows heat dispersion.

82. c. The developer can be thrown down the drain because the silver has not dissociated from the film. Fixer and radiographic film both contain elemental silver, and the lead backing from nonscreen film should also be disposed of properly in accordance with state law.

83. a. Normal developing time at 68 degrees is 5 minutes. The developer is 8 degrees cooler than the recommended temperature; $\frac{8}{2} \times 30 = 120$ seconds or an additional 2 minutes in the developer.

84. c. The liver is contained relatively deep within the body. The thyroid gland, skin, and eye are relatively superficial.

85. a. Small black crescents come from fingertip or fingernail bending the film prior to developing. Dirty cassettes, scratches, and dirt would show up as white areas on the radiograph.

Anesthesia and Analgesia

86. c. Oxygen tanks have three pins. Other gases cannot be placed on oxygen yokes because the pins will not match.

87. **c.** Oxygen comes in green E and H tanks in most clinics. The tanks are filled with pressurized gas. Oxygen is highly volatile and flammable, but not explosive.

88. **d.** The maximum gas pressure that should be given to an airway is 20 cm H_2O. Anything higher than that could cause alveolar rupture. To be safe, 12–14 cm H_2O is a good goal during IPPV.

89. **c.** Like ketamine, tiletamine is a dissociative anesthetic. Zolazepam is a premedication, morphine is an opiate, and thiopental is a barbiturate.

90. **b.** The anesthetic is effective because the animal was anesthetized before she started waking up. The other three reasons all relate to a decreased amount of anesthetic getting to the patient (none left in the vaporizer, dilution by hitting the oxygen flush valve too often, or animal disconnected).

91. **d.** Precision vaporizers deliver the same concentration of gas no matter what the environmental conditions. Nonprecision vaporizers are usually used for methoxyflurane and will be affected by temperature and humidity.

92. **d.** Hyperventilation rarely occurs on rebreathers, but CO_2 increases and increased airway resistance can occur because part of the inspired gases contain CO_2. Lower concentrations of gas anesthetics may be used with rebreathers.

93. **b.** 20 lb = 9 kg; the size of the reservoir should be 6×10 ml/kg = 540 ml bag. The larger bag should be used if the animal is slightly over the smaller size, so 1 liter is perfect.

94. **d.** Assisted breathing prevents atelectasis, improves breathing rates, and prevents hypercapnia.

95. **a.** Old soda lime is hard and unable to be crumbled. It will turn purple while the CO_2 is reacting, should be changed monthly, and has an exothermic (heat-producing) reaction with CO_2.

96. **c.** The patient is on a closed-circuit system because his oxygen flow rate is the same as his requirements. The other systems would require a higher flow rate of oxygen.

97. **a.** Smaller patients do better on nonrebreathing systems because they have lower airway resistance.

98. **a.** Methoxyflurane has been implicated in abortions, liver failure, and other health problems. Halothane has also been implicated in abortions in humans. Isoflurane and sevoflurane are less likely to cause human complications, but should be treated with caution and scavenger systems to prevent exposure.

99. **c.** Sevoflurane has the highest MAC (minimum alveolar concentration) so it requires a higher percentage to cause effect.

100. **b.** Saint Bernards generally have low heart rates and propofol generally also causes bradycardia, so an elevated heart rate is of concern. Stage III anesthesia is also associated with decreased heart rate.

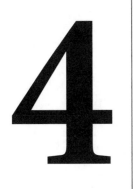

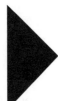

PHARMACOLOGY

CHAPTER OVERVIEW

Understanding the common drug categories and products used to prevent or treat animal diseases is crucial for success in a veterinary practice or other related employment situation. With the inherent responsibilities of the veterinary technician for patient care, recognition of the effects of drugs on animals is equally important, particularly if the patient experiences side effects. Also important for the veterinary technician student is correctly answering the pharmacology questions on the VTNE, which represent 14% of the exam. With the move on the VTNE to allow calculator usage during the examination, the need for the veterinary technician student to be able to complete dosage calculations successfully and to convert between several systems of drug measurement has increased.

The development and availability of veterinary drugs is ever increasing, requiring the technician to strive to stay current on newer products. Additionally, veterinary technicians are often the appropriate staff member in a veterinary clinic to supervise drug inventories as well as to order and maintain the veterinary pharmacy.

Learning all there is to know about all of the veterinary pharmaceuticals is challenging. Full appreciation of the actions of drugs is often not possible until one sees the drugs in action. However, some of the specific strategies listed here may help increase your retention of knowledge. First, it is helpful to appreciate the mechanism of actions of drugs by reviewing physiology. As an example, a simple model could be used to understand how antihistamines work in a patient with an allergic reaction. Many allergens cause the release of histamine from mast cells. Histamine can be responsible for a number of clinical signs including nasal discharge, chemosis, and pruritis. Antihistamines such as diphenhydramine (Benadryl®) work because they interfere with mast cell release of histamine. Reviewing the mechanisms of drug action will increase your understanding and retention knowledge about drugs.

Additional ideas for learning about drugs include case study reports that can help with understanding. Worksheet assignments, or surveys of specific drugs used at local veterinary clinics while students are on internships, can also help. Rewriting drug names and actions on flash cards helps some students; it is said that repetition is the mother of learning—repeat, repeat, and repeat! Lastly, it is helpful to divide the items to be learned into blocks of no more than seven. Breaking things down into bite-sized chunks makes the information easier to retain. In this chapter we break drugs down into smaller categories.

Key Terms

absorption
agonism
analgesic
antagonism
anthelmintic
anti-inflammatory
antimicrobial
antipyretic
antitussive
biotransformation
contraindication
decongestant

distribution
diuretic
efficacy
emetic
excretion
expectorant
generic drug
half-life
inotropic
legend drug
metabolism
pharmacodynamics
pharmacokinetics
proprietary drug
regimen
therapeutic index
therapeutic range
withdrawal time

Concepts and Skills

The enormous field of veterinary pharmacology can be divided into four topics.

- pharmacology principles
- drug categories
- measurement systems
- dosage calculations

Pharmacology Principles

Pharmacology is the study of the chemistry, effects, and uses of drugs. **Pharmacodynamics** is the resultant action of drugs on living beings. **Pharmacokinetics** essentially means the motion of drugs in a body. This motion or movement of drugs includes the absorption, distribution, metabolism, and excretion of drugs or how the drug gets into the body, how the drug reaches its action site, how the drug works at the action site, and how it is removed from the body. Sometimes, the mnemonic ADME can be helpful for students to remember the four actions (*absorption, distribution, metabolism,* and *excretion*) associated with pharmacokinetics.

Absorption is the uptake of the drug into or across body tissues or cells. There are a number of mechanisms of absorption; most drugs must cross several different cell layers to arrive at the target area for the drug. The correct route of administration is crucial for proper absorption. Drugs can be administered via many routes either enteral or parenteral. **Distribution** is the movement of the drugs to the intended target tissues. Among the factors that affect distribution are blood perfusion of the target tissue and the characteristics of the drug itself. The receptor or target tissue or organ is the place within the body where the drug exerts its effect. When drugs reach the intended target, several actions can occur: molecules bind to receptors and cause (**agonism**) a reaction or

prevent (**antagonism**) a reaction; the drugs then physically facilitate a response within cells or tissues, or facilitate a chemical reaction.

Drug **metabolism** is necessary for drugs to be excreted from the body. Drugs either are excreted unchanged or are modified so that the drug is no longer active. Modification of the drug by living organisms is called **biotransformation**; most of the modification of drugs occurs in the liver. Biotransformation may lead to inactive drug metabolites or, in some situations, to drug metabolites that have specific effects on the body. Some drugs are administered in an inactive form and must undergo biotransformation to exert the intended drug action. Most drugs are excreted from the body through either the kidneys or the digestive tract. Normal kidney function is very important to the **excretion** of many drugs. (See Figure 4.1.)

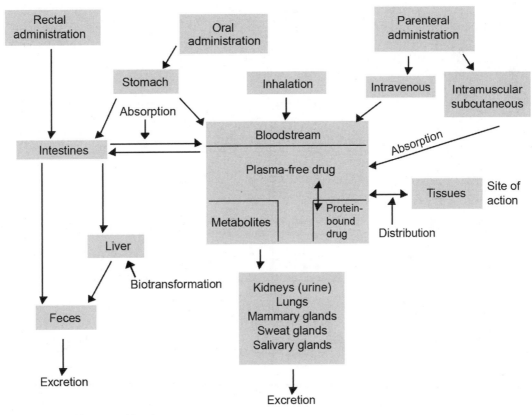

Figure 4.1 *Pharmacokinetics*

Any drug in any animal can create a wide range of responses from no effect to a toxic effect. The intended activity or response of a drug is the drug's **efficacy**. The **therapeutic range** or therapeutic dose of a drug is the amount of a drug needed to impact target tissues and safely create the desired drug action. (See Figure 4.2.) The **therapeutic index** is the difference between a safe and therapeutic dose of a drug and its toxic dose. A drug that has a wide therapeutic index is considered much safer to use than a drug with a narrow therapeutic index. **Half-life** is the length of time needed for a drug to decrease in its active form within the body by half. The correct dose and correct frequency are important considerations that impact on therapeutic range and half-life.

Proper administration of any drug is crucial for the patient. Proper drug usage to achieve an anticipated outcome is called the drug **regimen**. The correct dose of any drug, the correct frequency of administration, and the correct route of administration have already been mentioned. Most teachers and clinicians recommend that students recall the five rights of drug administration or a drug regimen. I emphasize that there are in fact *six* rights: right patient, right drug, right route of administration, right frequency of administration, right time of administration, and right withdrawal time. **Withdrawal time** is the critical time during which a drug must not be administered to an animal intended for food consumption or an animal from which milk will be used for human consumption. It is the responsibility of all members of the veterinary medical team to be aware of the importance of all six of these rights both for the patient and for consumers.

Drug Categories

A number of drug categories are important for the veterinary technician to know. Though not inclusive of all drugs, 12 categories are used in this text, from anti-infective drugs through fluid therapy products. There are many products and many combination drug products used in veterinary medicine especially

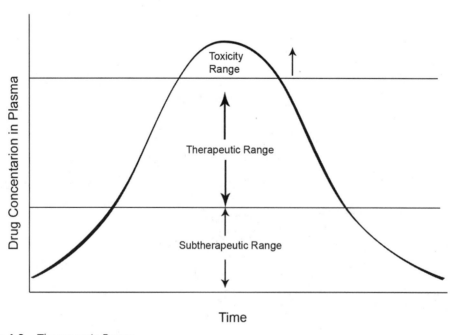

Figure 4.2 *Therapeutic Range*

otics, ophthalmics, and topical products. Combination drug products are often used to gain the benefit of each drug or more importantly to increase the effects of each product synergistically. In this text, we have listed the major drug categories with explanation of how they work, major indications of the usage, and significant side effects. Not all drugs in each category have been listed.

Drug names can be confusing for students because there are chemical names, generic names, and brand, trade, or **proprietary** names. The chemical name of a drug is usually derived from its chemical structure and the **generic** name is often a shortened version of the chemical name. Brand names are also known as trade or proprietary names. Generic names are best used in a veterinary hospital setting but the reality is that many brand names are universally used for routinely used drugs. Students need to be aware of the most common brand names.

An example of a chemical name is dexamethasone sodium phosphate. Most members of the veterinary team might refer to this drug either by its generic name, dexamethasone, or by its most common brand name, Azium®. Both would be correct, but often there are other brand names. In human medicine, this same drug might be called Decadron®. In this chapter the generic name will be used for most drugs, but when use of a brand name is quite universal, the brand name will also be used. Adding to the confusion is the fact that some drugs can also

be referred to either as prescription or **legend** drugs or as *over-the-counter (OTC)* drugs. These terms refer to the regulation of the drug from a prescribing standpoint. Legend drugs are those drugs that are deemed by regulating agencies to have potential for misuse or abuse and therefore are considered to be prescription drugs. These drugs are identified by their legend: *This drug is for use by or under the direction of a licensed veterinarian.* OTC drugs are thought to be safe enough for any consumer to use properly.

Antimicrobials

Antimicrobial, or anti-infective, drugs are those that work to either kill (cidal action) or inhibit the reproduction or growth (static action) of microorganisms including bacteria, fungi, or viruses. This group of drugs is divided into antibiotics, antifungals, and antivirals. There are many antimicrobial products on the veterinary market. There are also numerous combination products that blend various antimicrobials, sometimes with corticosteroid or other medications. Combination products are particularly common for otics, ophthalmics, and topical medications.

Antibiotics

Antibiotics are those drugs that work either to kill or to inhibit bacteria. This group of drugs is probably the largest used in veterinary medicine. Terminology

MECHANISMS OF ACTION OF ANTIBIOTICS		
ACTION	RESULT	EXAMPLES
Inhibit cell wall synthesis	bactericidal	penicillins, cephalosporins
Inhibit protein synthesis	bactericidal or bacteriostatic	aminoglycosides, tetracyclines, macrolides, lincomycins, chloramphenicol
Interfere with metabolism	bacteriostatic	sulfonamides
Impair nucleic acids	bactericidal	quinolones
Alter cell membrane permeability	bactericidal or bacteriostatic	polymyxins

used for antibiotics include bactericidal (kill bacteria) or bacteriostatic (inhibit growth or reproduction), spectrum of action or activity (narrow vs. broad), and minimum inhibitory concentration (MIC). Minimum inhibitory concentration (Figure 4.3) is the dose of an antibiotic needed to inhibit the growth of bacteria.

Antibiotics work through five well-recognized mechanisms of action. These mechanisms can often help students remember the differences between the numerous antibiotics in the veterinary market. (See Figure 4.4.)

Antibiotics covered here will concentrate on common veterinary products or those with specific indications. As mentioned, antibiotics are probably one of the largest groups of drugs used in veterinary medicine and there are many additional products other than the ones that will be mentioned here.

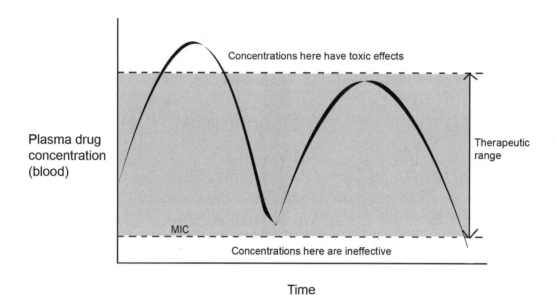

Figure 4.3 *Minimum Inhibitory Concentration*

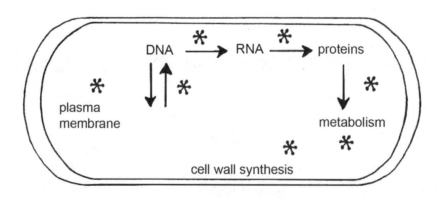

Figure 4.4 *Antibiotic Targets*

Penicillins

Penicillins are one of the most common antibiotic groups of drugs used in veterinary medicine. Often they can be recognized by the suffix *cillin* in the generic name. (See Figure 4.5.) They are also referred to as beta-lactams. Penicillins are bactericidal and interfere with bacterial cell-wall synthesis. The spectrum of activity is predominantly against gram-positive and some gram-negative organisms. Penicillins are well absorbed by injection but some penicillins (such as Penicillin G) are inactivated by stomach acid. Certain bacteria, particularly *Staphylococci*, develop resistance to penicillins due to the production of enzymes (penicillinases). Penicillins are relatively safe, although occasional patients exhibit a range of hypersensitivity reactions including (rarely) anaphylaxis.

PENICILLINS		
GENERIC NAME	**BRAND NAME**	**COMMENTS**
Penicillin G	Flocillin®	usually administered by injection; usage especially on large animals, narrow spectrum to mostly gram-positives; often combined with procaine
Penicillin V	various	acid resistant so given orally, narrow-spectrum to gram-positives
Ampicillin	Polyflex®	broad-spectrum, oral or parenteral forms
Amoxicillin	Amoxitabs®, Amoxiject®	broad-spectrum but absorbed better orally than Ampicillin
Cloxicillin, oxacillin	Dri-Clox®	penicillinase-resistant; includes intramammary usage
Ticarcillin, carbenicillin	Ticar®	extended spectrum; intrauterine usage in mares
Amoxicillin with clavulanic acid	Clavamox®*	very popular, potentiated amoxicillin with wide spectrum of activity to include many gram-negatives

*Clavulanic acid or clavulanate potassium is a penicillinase inhibitor. Addition of this drug, which has no antibiotic activity itself, to Amoxicillin significantly extends the spectrum of activity.

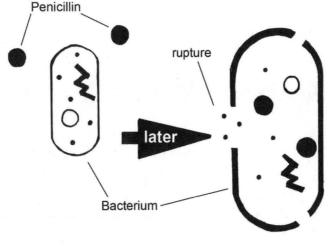

Figure 4.5 *How Penicillin Works*

Cephalosporins

Cephalosporins are chemically similar to penicillins but with a broader spectrum of activity. Like penicillins, they interfere with cell-wall synthesis and are considered quite safe for usage. They are often recognized by the prefix -*ceph* or -*cef* in the generic name. Cephalosporins are classified by generations, which usually relate to when they were developed. The oldest cephalosporins are first- and second-generation products and are generally given orally. Newer cephalosporins are third-, fourth-, and recently fifth-generation products, which are usually given by injection to resistant bacterial organisms. Newer-generation products are expensive and are not used as commonly in veterinary medicine as in human medicine. Cephalosporins are primarily used in small-animal medicine, though some newer generation products are used by injection on large animals.

CEPHALOSPORINS		
GENERIC NAME	BRAND NAME	COMMENTS
Cephalexin	Keflex®	first-generation, oral usage common
Cefadroxil	Cefa-tabs®, Cefa-drops®	first-generation, oral usage common
Cephapirin	Cefa-lak®	first-generation, intramammary preparations
Cefaclor	Ceclor®	second-generation, oral usage common
Ceftiofur	Naxcel®, Excenel®	third-generation injectable used in large animals
Cefpodoxime	Simplicef®	third-generation oral product with once-daily dosing in dogs
Cefovecin	Convenia®	advanced-generation product given SQ with efficacy up to 14 days in dogs and cats

Aminoglycosides

Aminoglycosides are commonly used broad-spectrum antibiotics that work by inhibiting protein synthesis which impedes bacterial cell division. They are considered bactericidal. Most are administered parenterally because of poor gastrointestinal absorption. Aminoglycosides are often used in topical preparations, including ophthalmic and otics. Most are excreted via the kidneys and can cause nephrotoxicity. Ototoxicity can also occur. Aminoglycosides are often recognized by the suffixes -*micin*, -*mycin*, or -*cin*. They are not effective against anaerobes so they are often used synergistically with penicillins.

AMINOGLYCOSIDES		
GENERIC NAME	BRAND NAME	COMMENTS
Gentamycin	Gentocin®	parenteral and topical preparations, intrauterine usage; nephrotoxic and ototoxic
Neomycin	Biosol®	primarily used in topical preparations; nephrotoxic
Tobramycin	Tobrex®	primarily used in ophthalmic preparations
Kanamycin	Kantrim®	not as active as some aminoglycosides
Amikacin	Amiglyde®	intrauterine usage in horses; nephrotoxic

Tetracyclines

Tetracyclines are commonly used antibiotics that are considered bacteriostatic but may be bactericidal at higher doses. They work similarly to aminoglycosides by inhibiting bacterial protein synthesis. Tetracyclines are popularly used in large-animal medicine, including medicated feed formulations, and are also specifically used for the treatment of rickettsial and bacterial diseases such as Lyme disease. Tetracylines are usually recognized by the suffix *-cycline*. Tetracyclines may affect young animal bone and tooth development and may cause fever to occur in some cats. Oral preparations are common but clients should be warned not to administer the antibiotic with milk, milk products such as cheese, or antacids because this may inactivate the drug. Injectable products must be stored in dark bottles or they become inactivated. Outdated injectable products become toxic and should be discarded.

TETRACYCLINES		
GENERIC NAME	**BRAND NAME**	**COMMENTS**
Tetracycline	Panamycin®, Duramycin® powder	topical and oral preparations primarily used
Oxytetracycline	Liquamycin®, Terramycin®, Oxytet®	injectable and oral preparations, administer slowly intravenously
Chlorotetracycline	Aureomycin®	oral products used as feed preparations for large animals
Doxycycline	Vibramycin®	common usage for rickettsia and some protozoa

Macrolides

Macrolides are considered bacteriostatic; they work to inhibit protein synthesis primarily against gram-positive bacteria. The drugs may be recognized by the suffix *-cin* or *-mycin* but must not be confused with aminoglycosides. There are species-specific sensitivities and contraindications with macrolides. Care should be used with some of these products as they may be harmful or even fatal in humans.

MACROLIDES		
GENERIC NAME	**BRAND NAME**	**COMMENTS**
Erythromycin	Erythro-100®, Gallimycin 100®	primarily used in food animals, oral preparations
Tylosin	Tylan®	popular usage in swine, occasional in dogs
Tilmicosin	Micotil®	subcutaneous usage for respiratory diseases in cattle, dangerous if injected accidentally in humans
Azithromycin	Zithromax®	long half-life with oral administration in many species

Lincosamides

Some books include lincosamides with macrolides because of their similar mechanisms of action to inhibit protein synthesis. However, lincosamides can be bacteriostatic or bactericidal depending on tissue concentration. Also, importantly, lincosamides can be quite effective against anaerobic bacteria and therefore against bite wounds, oral infections, pyodermas, and osteomyelitis. Again, as with macrolides, there are species-specific contraindications particularly for rabbits, horses, ruminants, guinea pigs, and hamsters.

LINCOSAMIDES		
GENERIC NAME	BRAND NAME	COMMENTS
Lincomycin	Lincocin®, Lincomix®	dogs, cats, and swine; oral food preparations
Clindamycin	Antirobe®	dogs and cats, but caution with high doses for cats

Chloramphenicol and Florfenical

Choramphenicol is a bacteriostatic drug that may be bactericidal at high dosages. It inhibits bacteria by inhibiting protein synthesis. This drug is chosen for its ability to penetrate specific tissues including CNS, respiratory, eye, and prostate. Caution must be used by humans handling chloramphenicols, especially capsule or powder formulations that can be inhaled or topical formulations that can be absorbed. Use with lactating animals should be avoided due to offspring ingestion and subsequent hepatic toxicosis.

CHLORAMPHENICOLS		
GENERIC NAME	BRAND NAME	COMMENTS
Chloramphenicol	Chloromycetin®, Chloramphenicol ophthalmic®	this drug is banned for use in food animals; to be used with care in cats; oral powders or capsules to be used with extreme care by humans to avoid aplastic anemia
Florfenical	Nuflor®	approved for use in cattle for respiratory diseases, not known to cause aplastic anemia in humans

Sulfonamides

Sulfonamides, also known as sulfa drugs, are among the oldest antibacterials used. They have a broad spectrum of activity including against some protozoa, especially coccidia and toxoplasma organisms. Sulfa drugs work by interfering with folic acid synthesis. Folic acid is needed by bacteria for metabolism. Numerous bacteria have developed resistance to sulfonamides. Some sulfonamides are not absorbed from the gastrointestinal tract but exert the effect within the bowel lumen. The major side effect of sulfa drugs is crystal formation in the kidneys if the patient is not adequately hydrated or if the urine is acidic. Dogs may have more drug sensitivities to sulfas than other species; these sensitivities include skin reactions, liver conditions, and anemia. Another negative side effect is decreased tear production, seen primarily in dogs, especially in certain breeds. Decreased tearing may lead to keratoconjunctivitis sicca (KCS).

Sulfonamides are often mixed with other bacteriostatic compounds including trimethoprim, pyrimethamine, and ormetoprim that interfere with folic acid conversion by bacteria. These compounds are rarely used individually (with the exception of pyrimethamine for protozoa). The combination of these compounds with sulfonamides potentiates the efficacy, thus potentiated sulfonamides are considered bactericidal. All sulfonamides must be used cautiously in food animals due to milk and long-term tissue residues.

SULFONAMIDES		
GENERIC NAME	**BRAND NAME**	**COMMENTS**
Sulfadimethoxine	Albon®	common usage for treatment of coccidia
Sulfasalazine	Azulfidine®	used in dogs for inflammatory bowel disease
Sulfachlorpyridazine	Vetisulid®	used in calves and young pigs for enteritis
Sulfadiazine, sulfamethazole, and sulfadimethoxine	various; often referred to as triple sulfa	may have increased spectrum of activity when mixed
Potentiated sulfas: any of the above mixed with trimethoprim, etc.	Tribrissen®, Primor®, Uniprim®, and others	sulfas commonly mixed with other agents to create potentiation for bactericidal efficacy

Quinolones

Quinolones are also known as fluoroquinolones. All are considered bactericidal because they impair DNA within bacteria. This impairment is caused by interference with an enzyme (DNA gyrase) needed to coil DNA within the bacteria. Quinolones have a wide spectrum of activity against gram-positive and gram-negative organisms but may not be efficacious against anaerobes and some *Streptococcus* organisms. These drugs are used commonly for skin, urinary, and respiratory infections. Penetration with the quinolones includes bone, joints, eyes, and prostate tissues. These drugs may be recognized by the suffix -*xacin*.

The major **contraindication** of quinolones is usage in young growing animals because of the effect these drugs have on cartilage formation. Enrofloxacin may cause blindness in cats. Adequate water consumption is important to minimize crystalluria. Usage in animals with seizure conditions may be contraindicated. Off-label use in food animals is highly regulated due to tissue and milk residues and subsequent concerns for development of resistant bacteria in humans.

QUINOLONES		
GENERIC NAME	**BRAND NAME**	**COMMENTS**
Enrofloxacin	Baytril®	commonly used with parenteral, topical, and oral preparations in dogs, cats, horses, cattle
Orbifloxacin	Orbax®	prohibited for use in food animals; oral preparations for use in dogs, cats, horses
Marbofloxacin	Zeniquin®	prohibited for use in food animals; oral preparations for use in dogs, cats, horses
Difloxacin	Dicral®	prohibited for use in food animals; used in dogs and horses
Moxifloxacin	Avelox®	prohibited for use in food animals; oral and ophthalmic preparations

Polymyxin B

Polymyxin B is an antibiotic in a category by itself due to its action of altering cell membrane permeability. This impact on membranes means that polymyxin B can be considered either bacteriostatic or bactericidal. Polymyxin B is effective only against gram-negative bacteria and is not absorbed when administered orally. Its major use is with the antibiotic bacitracin and the aminoglycoside neomycin, where it is topically applied as an ointment and is also included in ophthalmic preparations for broader-spectrum activity. Polymyxin B can cause toxicities because it affects membranes in animal cells as it does bacterial membranes.

Miscellaneous Antibiotics

Bacitracin is similar to the penicillins in its ability to disrupt cell walls. However, the mechanism is different from that of penicillins, and it is not affected by penicillinase-producing bacteria. Bacitracin is commonly used topically and is often combined with polymyxin B and neomycin.

Rifampin is an antimicrobial that can be bactericidal or bacteriostatic in action and works by inhibiting RNA synthesis in certain bacteria. It is used in equine foals with *Rhodococcus* pneumonia and can be used to treat some fungi in dogs when used with other antifungal drugs. Rifampin is noteworthy for causing orange coloration in urine, saliva, and other bodily discharges.

Metronidazole is an antimicrobial with primary activity against certain intestinal protozoa, especially Giardia. The trade name Flagyl® is commonly used even though it is a human drug. Its action is bactericidal and protozoacidal because it disrupts DNA synthesis within the organism. Metronidazole is commonly used for anaerobic infections in many species. Side effects can include birth defects and occasional neurologic effects. Dosages should be carefully calculated to minimize the neurological effects.

Antifungals

Antifungals are those drugs that kill or inhibit fungal infections. Fungal infections are called mycoses and are usually identified as superficial/topical such as ringworm or deep/systemic such as cryptococcus or blastomycosis. Antifungal drugs have numerous side effects and must be dosed correctly and handled properly, and patient response must be monitored. The three major antifungal drug groups are imidazoles, polyene antifungals, and griseofulvin.

Imidazoles

All of the imidazoles are considered fungicidal and work by disrupting fungal cell membrane, which causes cell leakage. These drugs often have only human labels and may cause hepatic problems and possible teratogenic effects in pregnant animals. Imidazoles are recognized by the suffix *-zole*. The drugs used in veterinary medicine include ketoconazole, miconazole, itraconazole, and fluconazole.

Polyene Antifungals

Polyene antifungals are considered fungicidal and also work by disrupting the fungal cell membrane causing leakage that leads to fungal death. Amphotericin B and nystatin are both toxic, especially amphoterin B which can cause gastrointestinal disturbance, nephrotoxicity, and even cardiac problems. It is used for systemic mycoses. Because it is poorly absorbed, nystatin is used topically, primarily for the treatment of candida.

Griseofulvin

Griseofulvin is considered fungistatic and works by interfering with fungal cell division. Griseofulvin is used only for superficial mycoses. To maximize absorption and metabolism, it is best given with a fatty meal. Griseofulvin is used in dogs, cats, and horses and is considered relatively safe, though teratogenic effects are reported in pregnant cats. Griseofulvin can cause severe bone marrow suppression in FeLV/FIV infected cats.

Antivirals

Antiviral drugs are relatively new to use in veterinary medicine. Drugs available are human-label and cost can be prohibitive. The principal antiviral drugs used include acyclovir and interferon. The drugs are relatively safe, although anemia is reported in cats treated with acyclovir.

Antiparasite Drugs

Antiparasite drugs work to inhibit or kill internal parasites (endoparasites) or external parasites (ectoparasites). These products are either drugs taken enterally or applied topically or chemicals applied topically. Rather than attempting to describe all of the mechanisms of action of these drugs, the emphasis here is on learning which parasite families are affected by a drug or drug family. An example would be to remember which drugs work against cestodes and which ones work against nematodes. Numerous products and combination products in the veterinary market cross parasite families.

Endoparasite Drugs

Internal parasite drugs are usually divided into those drugs that kill or inhibit families of parasites. Those drugs that kill worms, or helminths, are known as **anthelmintics**. Anthelmintics are divided into those drugs that are antinematodal, anticestodal, or antitrematodal in action. Remembering which drugs work against which parasite group (nematodes, cestodes, trematodes) is one effective strategy for remembering these drugs. Endoparasite drugs include those that kill protozoa (antiprotozoal) and those that inhibit coccidia (coccidiostats). The most common coccidiostats are the sulfonamides or potentiated sulfa drugs mentioned under antimicrobials.

Endoparasite drugs are usually administered enterally to animals or applied topically. There are numerous brand names and combination products on the veterinary market for control or prevention of internal parasites or even both internal and external parasites. In general, these drugs are quite safe, with some exceptions of which the veterinary technician should be aware.

ANTINEMATODAL DRUGS			
DRUG FAMILY	**GENERIC NAME**	**BRAND NAME**	**COMMENTS**
Benzimidazoles	thiabendazole, fenbendazole* albendazole† mebendazole	Omnizole® Panacur® Valbazen® Telmintic®	wide safety range, poorly effective against larval stages of development—repeated administration necessary
Tetrahydropyrimidines	pyrantel pamoate pyrantel tartrate morantel tartrate	Strongid®, Nemex® Banminth® Rumatel®	wide safety range, repeat administration; may affect some tapeworms also
Piperazines	piperazine	Pipa-tabs®	effective only for ascarids
Avermectins	ivermectin doramectin	Ivomec® and others Dectomax®	safe but may cause rapid parasite death, effect against some external parasites, heartworm prevention, enteral, injectable, and topical preparations; must be used with care in collies and herding breeds
Milbemycins	moxidectin milbemycin oxime	Proheart®, Quest®, Cydectin® Interceptor®	heartworm prevention and nematodes in horses and cattle; do not use in young dogs or horses

(continued)

ANTINEMATODAL DRUGS (continued)

DRUG FAMILY	GENERIC NAME	BRAND NAME	COMMENTS
Organophosphates	tricholofon dichlorvos coumaphos haloxon	Combot® and others Atgard® and others Baymix® and others Loxon®	narrow margin of safety, effective against some external parasites

*Fenbendazole is effective against some tapeworms (Taenia) and giardia.
†Albendazole is effective also against liver flukes and some tapeworms

ANTICESTODAL DRUGS

GENERIC NAME	BRAND NAME	COMMENTS
Praziqunatel*	Droncit®	popular product, tablets, and combination with febantel, injectable, equine paste combination products, approved to treat many species
Epsiprantel	Cestex®	may see whole tapeworms passed in feces, not effective against *Echinococcus*
Bunamidine	Scolaban®	dogs and cats only, avoid use in young animals, do not break tablets or feed patient for three hours after administering

*Praziquantel may also be used for lung flukes in dogs.

ANTITREMATODAL DRUGS

GENERIC NAME	BRAND NAME	COMMENTS
Clorsulon	Curatrem®	cattle and sheep liver flukes, relatively safe, not recommended for lactating cows
Albendazole	Valbazen®	a benzimidazole used for trematodes in cattle and sheep as well as nematodes, not recommended for lactating cows

ANTIPROTOZOAL DRUGS

GENERIC NAME	BRAND NAME	COMMENTS
Amprolium	Corid®	coccidia in cattle and poultry
Diclazuril	Clincox®	feed additive for coccidia in poultry; can be used for *Sarcocystis* protozoa in horses
Ponazuril	Marquis®	*Sarcocystis* protozoa in horses; preferred over diclazuril in horses

Note: Additionally, sulfa antibiotics and potentiated sulfas are used as coccidiostatic drugs. Metronidazole, the antimicrobial mentioned earlier, is used to treat giardia.

OTHER DRUGS		
GENERIC NAME	BRAND NAME	COMMENTS
Emodepside with praziquantel	Profender®	topical solution for roundworms, hookworms, and tapeworms in cats

HEARTWORM TREATMENT AND PREVENTION DRUGS—PRIMARILY FOR USE IN DOGS		
GENERIC NAME	BRAND NAME	COMMENTS
Melarsomine	Immiticide®	arsenical compound used to treat adult heartworm infections; muscle soreness noted at injection sites
Ivermectin	Heartgard®, Iverheart®	monthly preventive, ivermectin solutions used to treat microfilaria, cat preventive
Milbemycin oxime	Interceptor®, Sentinel®	monthly preventive, also treats many nematodes; Sentinel® also contains lufenuron for flea control
Imidacloprid, moxidectin	Advantage Multi®	topical applied monthly as preventive for heartworm, treatment for fleas and nematodes in dogs and cats
Selamectin	Revolution®	topical applied monthly as preventive for heartworm, fleas, ear mites, and sarcoptic mange. Also control roundworms and hookworms in cats.
Diethylcarbamazine	Nemacide®, Filaribits®	daily heartworm preventive for dogs

Ectoparasite Drugs

Ectoparasite drugs are those that kill or inhibit families of external parasites. The most common families of external parasites are fleas, lice, mites, ticks, and biting insects (flies). An important distinction of drugs that treat ectoparasites is whether the parasite feeds or ingests blood or merely lives on the host's epithelial tissues. Those that feed on blood are often easier to kill with systemic-acting ectoparasitic drugs. Control or death of external parasites that spread diseases such as Rocky Mountain Spotted Fever helps reduce the incidence of these diseases.

Ectoparasite drugs may be applied by sprays, baths, pour-ons, powders, collars, applicators such as livestock-rubbing devices, spot-on applicators; some are even administered enterally. In general, many of the drugs used to treat or prevent ectoparasites are insecticides and must be used and disposed of with care. Some insecticides are potentially very toxic. Some ectoparasite drugs work by interfering with the maturation of insects and are used to disrupt life-cycle maturation. These drugs are called insect growth regulators (IGRs). Some drugs used for ectoparasites are merely repellents or are added with other drugs or insecticides to promote synergistic or increased efficacy.

INSECTICIDES

DRUG FAMILY	GENERIC NAME	BRAND NAME	COMMENTS
Pyrethrins	pyrethrin	Mycodex®	derived from chrysanthemum flowers, generally safe, often mixed with other insecticides
Pyrethroids	allethrin, resmethrine, permethrine, tetramethrin	many names and products	synthetic pyrethrins, generally safe, often mixed with other insecticides. Toxic to cats.
Carbamates	carbaryl bendiocarb propoxur	Sevin® and other names many products many products	similar to organophosphates in action; work by inhibiting cholinesterase
Organophosphates	chlorpyrifos dichlorvos cythioate diasinon fenthion	many products Vapona® Proban® Escort® Spotton®	all are cholinesterase inhibitors and must be used carefully and not with other cholinesterase-inhibiting insecticides. Highly toxic.
Chlorinated hydrocarbons	lindane methoxychlor	Kennel Dip® Cattle Dust®	environmental contamination concerns (may be removed from market)
Formamidines	amitraz	Mitaban® and others	not a cholinesterase inhibitor, used primarily as a dip for demodectic mange in dog
Neonicotinoids	nitenpyram	Capstar®	oral tablets used to kill adult fleas

REPELLENTS, INSECT GROWTH REGULATORS, AND OTHER

DRUG FAMILY	GENERIC NAME	BRAND NAME	COMMENTS
Insect growth regulators	methoprene fenoxycarb	many products	found in various products for flea control
Repellents	DEET, Butox PPG, MGK 11, MGK326	many products and many combinations with pyrethrins or pyrethroids	repels mosquitoes and flies, some caution using DEET in young animals and cats: use dilute concentrations
Rotenone	rotenone	lotions and shampoos	natural plant-origin insecticide that may be in combination products
D-Limonene	limonene	many products	some activity for fleas and other insects but only slight residual effect
Metaflumizone	metaflumizone with amitraz	ProMeris®	spot-on application for fleas and ticks
Avermectins	ivermectin	Ivomec®	systemic treatment for canine sarcoptic mange and local for ear mites in cats and dogs

FLEA AND TICK MONTHLY PREVENTION		
GENERIC NAME	BRAND NAME	COMMENTS
Fipronil	Frontline®	Spot-on application in dogs and cats; tick prevention for only 30 days, up to 90 for fleas
Imidacloprid	Advantage®	flea control for up to 4 weeks
Imidacloprid and permethrin	K9 advantix®	flea and tick control for up to 30 days Toxic to cats.
Lufenuron (chitin inhibitor for fleas)	Program® Sentinel®	oral monthly flea control; product with milbemcin for additional control of some nematodes

Anti-Inflammatory Drugs

Anti-inflammatory drugs are divided into two general classes: corticosteroid or steroidal anti-inflammatory drugs and nonsteroidal anti-inflammatory drugs (NSAIDs). Damaged or inflamed cells release arachidonic acid. Arachidonic acid is acted on by either cyclooxygenase or lipoxygenase enzymes to produce the inflammatory mediators prostaglandins, thromboxanes, or leukotrienes. These mediators are primary contributors responsible for the cardinal signs of inflammation. The drugs work by blocking the inflammatory process or inhibiting the release of the inflammatory mediators (see Figures 4.6 and 4.7). The two classes of anti-inflammatory drugs are distinct. These drugs are very commonly used for both acute and chronic inflammatory conditions in many species. As well as the classes corticosteroids and NSAIDs, there are a variety of miscellaneous drugs used in veterinary medicine as anti-inflammatories.

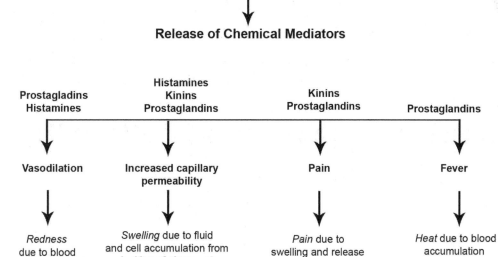

Figure 4.6 *Tissue Injury*

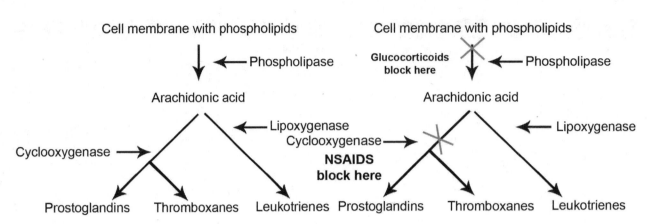

Figure 4.7 *Anti-Inflammatory Pathway*

Corticosteroids

Corticosteroids are also known as steroids, glucocorticoids, or cortisones and mimic the action of the body's natural corticosteroid, cortisol. Corticosteroids are classified by their duration of activity and formulation. They are potent anti-inflammatories, stabilize cell membranes to minimize cell breakdown, and are used for allergic reactions; they can also inhibit scar tissue formation and limit transplant rejection. These drugs are particularly effective in reducing edema. Reduction of pain with corticosteroids is secondary to the reduction of inflammation. There are a number of potentially deleterious side effects of corticosteroids including immune system depression, delayed healing, protein breakown, and potential gastrointestinal ulceration. Also, overuse of these drugs can lead to ia-

trogenic hyperadrenocorticism or Cushing's syndrome. The most common side effects of corticosteroids are polyuria, polydipsia, and polyphagia. Corticosteroids are also reported to cause abortions in ruminants, especially in cattle and horses. It is incumbent on the veterinary team to advise clients of common side effects and to use these drugs prudently to minimize these deleterious effects.

Corticosteroids are available in tablets, injectables, lotions, ointments, and boluses for large animals. These drugs are used in combination with antibiotics in a variety of veterinary preparations for topical use. There are water-soluble products for rapid intravenous administration and repository products for long-term effects. Most corticosteroids can be recognized by the suffix *-sone* or *-lone.*

CORTICOSTEROIDS		
GENERIC NAME	**BRAND NAME**	**COMMENTS**
Prednisone/prednisolone	many products	intermediate-acting
Dexamethasone	Azium® tablets, injectables, boluses	long-acting, more potent action than prednisone
Methylprednisolone	Medrol® tablets, Depo-medrol® injection (repository)	intermediate-acting but more potent action than prednisone
Triamcinolone	Vetalog®	intermediate-acting but more potent than prednisone
Betamethasone	Betasone®	long-acting and more potent than prednisone

Nonsteroidal Anti-Inflammatory Drugs

Nonsteroidal anti-inflammatory drugs (NSAIDs) are among the most commonly used categories of drugs in veterinary medicine because there are fewer side effects than are seen with corticosteroids. Additionally, NSAIDs provide analgesia by impacting on pain receptors (see Chapter 5). Some NSAIDs are potent **antipyretics** also. The major side effects of NSAIDs arise from the reduction of normal or good prostaglandins and primarily involve the gastrointestinal tract and kidneys. There is wide variation in the tolerance and efficacy of these drugs between species. Cats in particular do not tolerate NSAIDs well and caution must be exercised for use in this species. NSAIDs are the most commonly used drug in veterinary patients for chronic pain such as that associated with degenerative joint disease (DJD). A number of products have been developed recently for chronic pain in dogs. These products are considered cyclooxygenase (COX)-2 inhibitors and are intended to reduce the side effects caused by the reduction of good prostaglandins (see Chapter 5).

NONSTEROIDAL ANTI-INFLAMMATORY DRUGS (NSAIDs)		
GENERIC NAME	**BRAND NAME**	**COMMENTS**
Aspirin (acetylsalicylic acid)	many products and strengths (enteric-coated products)	also known for reduction of platelet aggregation, often measured in grains
Phenylbutazone	many products and formulations, especially for horses	primarily used in horses, injectable must be given IV only
Flunixin	Banamine® and others; many formulations	potent antipyretic, used in many species but labeled for horses and cattle
Carprofen	Rimadyl® (injectable and oral products)	approved for use in dogs
Ketoprofen	Ketofen®	injectable for horses
Etodolac	EtoGesic® (oral product only)	labeled for chronic pain in dogs
Deracoxib	Deramaxx® (oral product only)	labeled for both acute and chronic pain in dogs
Firocoxib	Previcox® (oral product only)	labeled for chronic pain in dogs
Meloxicam	Metacam® (injectable and oral products)	labeled for acute and chronic pain in dogs and one-time SQ injection in cats
Tepoxalin	Zubrin® (oral product only; rapid-release product)	labeled for chronic pain in dogs

MISCELLANEOUS ANTI-INFLAMMATORY DRUGS

GENERIC NAME	BRAND NAME	COMMENTS
Acetaminophen	Tylenol® and others	not really an NSAID but has analgesic and antipyretic actions; toxic to cats at all doses
Polysulfated glycosaminoglycan	Adequan® (used IM or intra-articularly especially in horses)	derived from bovine cartilage, used for degenerative joint disease in horses and dogs
Hyaloronate	Hylavet® (intra-articular) Legend® (IV or intra-articular)	used for degenerative joint disease in horses
Glycosamines and Chondrotin sulfate	many products	administered orally to maintain cartilage and reduce degenerative joint disease in many species
Meclofenamic acid	Arquel®	miscellaneous NSAID for inflammation in horses
DMSO (dimethyl sulfoxide)	Dimoso® and other gels and solutions, Synotic® (otic solution with steroids)	solvent with anti-inflammatory activity used topically; administered orally or IV for neurological diseases
Dipyrone	Novin® and others	used to reduce smooth-muscle spasms and pain in horses primarily
Gold salts	human formulations	used for treatment of immune-mediated dermatitis
Cyclosporine A	Atopica®	immunosuppressive used in dogs for atopic dermatitis

Cardiovascular Drugs

Cardiovascular drugs are those that work on the heart and blood vessels. This group of drugs includes vasodilators, diuretics, anti-arrhythmics, catecholamines, and positive **inotropic** drugs. Vasodilators affect the dilation of blood vessels either directly or by preventing the formation of potent vasoconstrictor enzymes known as ACE (angiotensin-converting enzyme) inhibitors. **Diuretics** decrease the workload of the heart by removing water via the kidneys. Anti-arrhythmics restore normal electrical activity to the heart muscle by regulating electrolytes used by cardiac muscle or by blocking automaticity of cardiac tissues (beta blockers). Catecholamines act by mimicking the sympathetic nervous system to increase contractility of the heart. Positive **inotropic** drugs affect contractility of the heart. Often these drugs are used together to achieve patient improvement depending on the condition and severity of disease. One of the more common diseases, seen especially in older dogs, is congestive heart failure (CHF). Also, both dilatory and hypertropic forms of cardiomyopathy are seen in animals.

CARDIOVASCULAR DRUGS

DRUG FAMILY	GENERIC NAME	BRAND NAME	COMMENTS
Vasodilators	nitroglycerine	human drug	applied topically to hairless skin
	hydralazine	Apresoline® (human drug)	often used with diuretics as arteriolar vasodilator
	prazosin	Minipress® (human drug)	combined vasodilator used for treatment of CHF and dilated cardiomyopathy in dogs
ACE inhibitor	enalapril	Enacard®	commonly used for CHF in dogs

CARDIOVASCULAR DRUGS *(continued)*			
DRUG FAMILY	**GENERIC NAME**	**BRAND NAME**	**COMMENTS**
Diuretics	furosemide chlorothiazide	Lasix® Diuril®	common use and potent loop diuretic occasional use as thiazide diuretic; may cause hypokalemia
Anti-arrhythmics	quinidine lidocaine	usually generic usually generic	used for atrial fibrillation in horses local anesthetic, given IV for emergency arrhythmia treatment
Calcium channel blockers	diltiazem verapmil	Cardizem® human products	control of supraventricular arrhythmias and hypertension
Beta blockers	propranolol atenolol sotalol metoprolol	Inderal® (human product) Tenormin® Betapace® Lopressor® (tablets and injectable)	used to treat hypertrophic cardiomyopathy in dogs used to slow cardiac rates, especially in cats with cardiomyopathy used for ventricular arrhythmias used to control tacharrhythmias
Catecholamines	epinephrine dopamine	usually generic usually generic	stimulates contractions of the heart when cardiac arrest occurs increases heart rate and blood pressure
Positive inotropic drugs	pimobendan digitalis	Vetmedin® Cardoxin®, Lanoxin® (tablets and elixirs)	ACE positive inotropic drug and vasodilator labeled for dogs for CHF narrow margin of safety: must be careful with weight-related doses

Respiratory Drugs

There are a number of indications for respiratory drugs in veterinary medicine in both large and small animal species. Many of the diseases are secondary to respiratory tract infections, including pneumonia, or secondary to cardiovascular diseases such as congestive heart failure. There are primary respiratory tract conditions such as allergy and asthmatic-like conditions. Drugs used for respiratory diseases include expectorants, mucolytics, antitussives, bronchodilators, antihistamines, decongestants, respiratory stimulants, and several miscellaneous drug categories.

Expectorants are drugs that dilute and liquefy respiratory tract secretions to facilitate removal of the secretions primarily from the lungs. Mucolytics decrease the viscosity of respiratory tract secretions, also in order to facilitate the removal of secretions from the lungs. Most **antitussives** in veterinary medicine work centrally at the midbrain level to suppress the cough center. Bronchodilators are used to reduce the spasmodic contractions of bronchioles and bronchi. Several different types of drugs are used as bronchodilators, including antihistamines. Antihistamines are those drugs that either suppress or block the release of histamine from mast cells during allergic reactions. The action is to cause bronchodilation and prevent mast cell degranulation. **Decongestants** reduce swelling of nasal tissues and are more commonly used in human medicine. Respiratory stimulants are used to stimulate breathing and principally work by stimulating the midbrain respiratory center. Of the miscellaneous drugs used to treat respiratory conditions, the most common are corticosteroids, diuretics, and antimicrobials, listed earlier in this chapter.

RESPIRATORY DRUGS			
DRUG FAMILY	GENERIC NAME	BRAND NAME	COMMENTS
Expectorants	guaifenesin	Mucinex®	smooth-muscle relaxant used for large-animal anesthesia, found in many human preparations for expectorant action
Mucolytics	aceylcysteine	Mucomyst® (human preparations) Sputlosin®	often used by nebulization equine oral formulation
Antitussives	butorphanol	Torbutrol®	synthetic narcotic used via injection or tablets especially for kennel cough
	hydrocodone	Hycodan® (human products)	narcotic agonist
	codeine	Codeine (human preparations)	narcotic agonist
	dextromethorphan	human products	nonnarcotic with similar effects to codeine and hydrocodone
Bronchodilators: cholinergic blockers	glycopyrrolate, atropine	various forms	primarily used as preanesthetic drugs or as organophosphate toxicity antidote
Brochodilators: beta-adrenergic agonists	epinephrine albuterol	usually generic Proventil®	emergency or rescue bronchodilator human preparation used for bronchodilation
	clenbuterol terbutaline	Ventipulmin® Brethine®	veterinary label for use in horses human preparation used for bronchodilation
Bronchodilators: methylxanthines	aminophylline	usually generic	human label, bronchodilation and mild cardiac stimulation; similar effect from caffeine and theobromine found in chocolate
Antihistamines	diphenhydramine pyrilamine hydroxyzine	Benadryl® Histavet® Atarax®	used for skin and respiratory allergies used for skin and respiratory allergies used for skin and respiratory allergies
Decongestants	ephedrine pseudoephedrine	human preparations human preparations	can be used orally or nasally can be used orally or nasally
Respiratory stimulants	doxapram	Dopram®	works at midbrain to stimulate breathing in neonates and anesthesia patients

Gastrointestinal Drugs

There are numerous drugs that affect the gastrointestinal tract. The gastrointestinal tract performs many functions and there is great variation in anatomy and function of the GI tract in veterinary species. There are drugs that cause vomiting (emetics) and drugs that minimize or stop vomiting (antiemetics). There are antidiarrheal drugs and there are laxative drugs or agents. The gastrointestinal tract, especially the liver, is involved in the metabolism of drugs. Therefore, consideration must be given to liver function as well as to the ability to absorb drugs from the gastrointestinal tract, particularly when the drugs are being given enterally. Lastly, many conditions and even other drugs (especially NSAIDs) can impact gut function and potentially cause gastrointestinal irritation or even ulceration. This is why there are drugs that protect the gastrointestinal tract.

Emetics can work at the brain level or at the stomach level to stimulate emesis. Antiemetics also work at the stomach level or systemically to reduce vomiting. Antidiarrheal drugs work at the intestinal tract level or can impact on nervous input to gut function. There are substances that are protective to the gastrointestinal tract and those that minimize the absorption of various substances or toxins from the gut. Because animals can have a variety of constipation or impaction issues affecting feces passage, there are a number of agents that can lubricate the intestinal tract facilitating feces passage, as well as agents that promote peristalsis and those that bring more fluid into the intestines to promote gut movement. There are a number of different mechanisms for protecting the gastrointestinal tract as well as a variety of antiulcer medications.

GASTROINTESTINAL DRUGS

DRUG FAMILY	GENERIC NAME	COMMON NAME OR BRAND	COMMENTS
Emetic	apomorphine	usually generic	controlled substance that works at central brain level
	syrup of ipecac	usually generic	stomach irritant—do not use outdated product or extract products
	hydrogen peroxide	usually generic	dilute with water, H_2O_2 releases oxygen, distends and irritates stomach
Antiemetic	chlorpromazine	Thorazine®	phenothiazine tranquilizer used as antiemetic in dogs and cats
	metoclopramide	Reglan®	works at both brain and stomach level to increase contractions and emptying
	dimenhydrinate	Dramamine®	antihistamine for motion sickness in dogs and cats
	diphenhydramine	Benadryl®	antihistamine
	trimethobenzamide	Tigan®	antihistamine for use in dogs only
	maropitant citrate	Cerenia®	NK-1 receptor antagonist suppresses vomiting in dogs; injectable and oral
Antiemetic, antidiarrheal	aminopentamide	Centrine®	anticholinergic reduces GI spasms in dogs and cats
Antidiarrheal	diphenoxylate	Lomotil®	synthetic narcotic analgesic
	loperamide	Imodium®	synthetic narcotic analgesic
	propantheline	Pro-Banthine®	anticholinergic for dogs and cats
Protectants	bismuth subsalicylate	Pepto-Bismol® (corrective mixture)	used in small and large animals; use carefully because subsalicylate converts to aspirin
	kaolin/pectin	bismuth Kaopectolin®	used in small and large animals
Adsorbent	activated charcoal	Toxiban® and charcoal products	primarily used to minimize absorption of toxins
Enema	sodium phosphate	Fleet® and other	hyperosmotic agent used for enemas; not for use in cats

(continued)

GASTROINTESTINAL DRUGS (continued)			
DRUG FAMILY	**GENERIC NAME**	**COMMON NAME OR BRAND**	**COMMENTS**
Laxative	magnesium hydroxide	Milk of Magnesia® Carmilax® (bovine products)	hyperosmotic agent that holds water in GI tract
	magnesium sulfate	Epsom Salts®	hyperosmotic agent used in large animals
	psyllium	Metamucil® and numerous others	plant fiber products for constipation and impactions in horses
	wheat bran	wheat bran	fed to horses for impactions
	mineral oil	mineral oil—heavy or light	lubricants used in horses for colic and impactions
	petrolatum	Laxatone® and others	oral products used in cats for hairball and constipation
	docusate calcium docusate sodium	Surfak® Colase®	surfactant stool softener used for constipation, impaction in numerous species; may be used as an enema
Antiulcer, H₂ receptor antagonists	cimetidine ranitidine famotidine	Tagamet® Zantac® Pepcid®	human products used for treatment and prevention of GI ulcers in many species
Antiulcer, proton pump inhibitor	omeprazole	Prilosec® Gastrogard® (equine)	used for treatment and prevention of gastric ulcers in horses
Antiulcer, antacids	aluminum/magnesium hydroxide magnesium hydroxide	Mylanta® Amphojel® Magnalax®	used for treatment of ulcers in small animals and rumen bloat in ruminants
Antiulcer, protectants	sucralfate	Carafate®	gastric mucosal protectant used in many species, especially horses
Antiulcer, prostaglandin E-analogs	misoprostol	Cytotec®	used primarily to treat ulcers secondary to NSAIDs

Urinary Drugs

Many drugs are excreted via the urinary tract so there are a number of drugs that are contraindicated in renal diseases. Some drugs can be used with renal diseases but must have altered dosages so that renal function is not compromised. A number of drugs exert that effect or have secondary effects on the renal system. Drugs with a specific effect on the kidneys include diuretics, cholinergic agonists used to increase bladder tone, and urinary tract acidifiers or alkalizers. Diuretics have been listed previously under cardiovascular drugs and all work at the kidney level for the removal of extra fluids from the body via urine. Osmotic diuretics, which work to draw water into renal excretions, will also be included in this section. Osmotic diuretics are used for reducing edema, especially that associated with cranial trauma, and to treat acute renal failure. (See Figure 4.8.) The cholinergic agonist, bethanechol, is used to stimulate urinary bladder emptying by increasing muscle tone. Urinary acidifiers work to promote a more acidic urine filtrate and help dissolve or prevent sturvite urinary crystals. Urinary alkalizers are used to promote more alkaline urine and to minimize calcium oxalate and cystine urinary crystals.

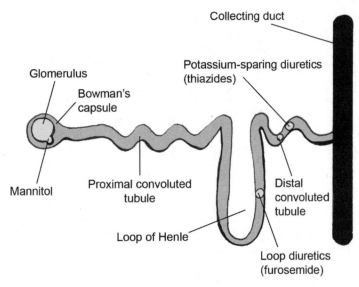

Figure 4.8 *Diuretics in the Urinary Tract*

URINARY DRUGS			
DRUG FAMILY	**GENERIC NAME**	**BRAND NAME**	**COMMENTS**
Diuretic—loop	furosemide	Lasix®	used in CHF, acute renal failure and other disorders
Diuretic—thiazide	chlorothiazide	Diuril®	used in CHF
Diuretic—osmotic	mannitol	Mannitol® 20%	used in cranial trauma and glaucoma
Cholinergic agonist	bethanechol	Urecholine® (human product)	used to stimulate bladder emptying
Urinary acidifier	methionine ammonium chloride	Methioform® Uroeze®	aid in dissolution of struvite crystals
Urinary alkalizer	potassium citrate	Urocit® (human product)	aid in dissolution of calcium oxalate and cystine crystals

Hormones

There are numerous hormones or hormonal drugs, both naturally occurring and synthetic. These drugs are used to correct hormonal deficiencies, control overproduction of hormones, or obtain a desired effect by giving additional hormones. An example of achieving a desired effect is through the use of hormonal substances to synchronize estrous cycles to facilitate artificial insemination in farm animals. A number of hormonal deficiencies are treated with replacement hormones. Examples of these deficiencies include hypothyroidism and diabetes mellitus. Some animals, especially cats, can have excesses of thyroid hormone that are treated by blocking hormone production. Hormones work through either positive or negative feedback mechanisms. If too little thyroid hormone is produced by the thyroid gland, thyroid-stimulating hormone (TSH) is produced at the pituitary level to try to increase production from the thyroid. Replacement therapy will lower the TSH levels being produced. (See Figure 4.9.)

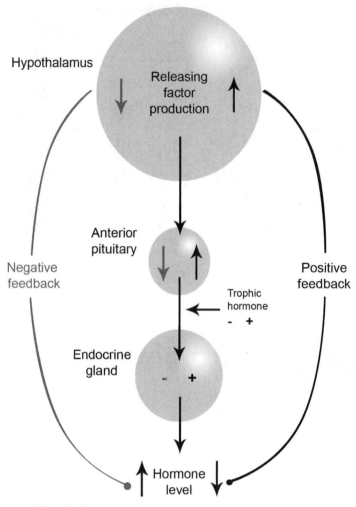

Hypothalamus

Releasing factor production

Anterior pituitary

Negative feedback

Positive feedback

Trophic hormone
-   +

Endocrine gland

-   +

Hormone level

Figure 4.9   *Hormone Feedback*

The greatest number of hormones used in veterinary medicine are those that affect reproduction. These are often called gonadotropins. Gonadotropins are substances that target the gonads to act like either follicle-stimulating hormone (FSH) or luteinizing hormone (LH). Another name for hormones that affect reproduction is gonadal hormones. Gonadal hormones are usually divided into estrogens, progestins, and androgens. Some gonadal hormones are used to stimulate estrus behaviors or the estrous cycle whereas others are used to suppress reproductive behaviors. Prostaglandins are fatty acid substances that cause numerous mechanisms to occur in the body. The principal prostaglandin produced in the body that is used for reproduction is prostaglandin F_2alpha. It is used to cause lysis of corpus luteum tissue. Some prostaglandins and other gonadal hormones are used to terminate pregnancy; these are called abortifacient drugs. Many of these drugs are also used in treatment regimens associated with embryo transfer in cattle and horses. Lastly, some of the hormones that are used for reproduction purposes cause uterine contraction.

GONADAL, GONADOTROPIN, AND OTHER REPRODUCTION HORMONES

DRUG FAMILY	GENERIC NAME	BRAND NAME	COMMENTS
Estrogens	estradiol cypionate	ECP® injection	used to treat numerous species; abortifacient
	diethylstilbestrol	DES® oral products	used primarily in small animals, including for urinary incontinence
Progestins	megestrol	Ovaban®	used in dogs and cats, including feline skin and behavior problems
	altrenogest	Regumate®	horse product to synchronize or suppress estrus or maintain pregnancy
	norgestomet	Syncro-Mate-B®	cattle product to synchronize estrus
Androgens	testosterone cypionate	Danazol® (human product)	used in dogs for urinary incontinence
	mibolerone	Cheque® drops	used in dogs for prevention of estrus
Gonadotropins	gonadorelin	Cystorelin®	used in cattle to treat cystic ovaries
	chorionic gonadotropin	hCG generic injection	used for various conditions in cattle and horses of both sexes
	follicle stimulating hormone (FSH)	FSH-P injection	used in many species to stimulate estrous cycles and increase ovulation
Prostaglandins	dinoprost, tromthamine	Lutalyse® ProstaMate®	used in many species for estrus synchronization; abortifacient
	fenprostalene	Bovilene	used in cattle for estrus synchronization
	fluprostenol cloprostenol	Equimate® Estrumate®	used in horses for estrus synchronization
Uterine contractility	oxytocin	many products	promotes uterine contractions and milk letdown
Miscellaneous reproduction hormones	bromocriptine mesylate	Parlodel® (human product)	used with prostaglandins as abortifacient

OTHER HORMONES

DRUG FAMILY	GENERIC NAME	BRAND NAME	COMMENTS
Thyroid hormones	levothyroxine or T_4 liothyroxine or T_3 thyroid stimulating hormone (TSH)	Soloxine® and others Cytobin® and others Dermathycin®	hypothyroid treatment used in dogs for hypothyroid treatment
Antithyroid drugs	methimazole carbimazole	Tapazole® Neomercazole®	used in cats for hyperthyroidism
Pancreatic hormones	regular insulin	numerous products, usually human	short-acting insulin used to initiate acute diabetes therapy
	NPH, PZI, Lente insulin	numerous products, human and veterinary	intermediate-acting insulin for long-term control of diabetes
	glargine, detemir	Lantus® Levemir®	long-acting insulin used for long-term control of diabetes

(continued)

OTHER HORMONES (continued)			
DRUG FAMILY	GENERIC NAME	BRAND NAME	COMMENTS
Growth promotion hormones	estradiol, progesterone, testosterone, and combination products used as implants	Synovet® Compudose® Ralgro® others	implants used in cattle to stimulate rapid growth; not for use in dairy cattle
Growth hormone	bovine somatotropin (BST)	Posilac®	injection product for dairy cows to stimulate milk production
Anabolic steroids	stanozolol	Winstrol®	tissue-building effect is used for general debilitation and to stimulate appetite; most of these drugs are controlled substances
	boldenone undecylenate	Equipoise®	horse product for treatment of general debilitation

Behavior Modification Drugs

Behavior modification drugs cause changes because of their effect on brain neurotransmitters. These drugs are primarily used in dogs, cats, and to a lesser extent horses to impact behaviors. The most common drugs used are antidepressants, antianxiety drugs, and hormones. Antidepressants work by preventing the reuptake of the neurotransmitters norepinephrine and serotonin. Antianxiety drugs work by promoting GABA (gamma-Aminobutyric acid), a neurotransmitter that is considered to inhibit behaviors. Hormonal therapy is principally through the use of progesterone substances (progestins) that impact other hormone levels or affect the cerebral cortex.

BEHAVIOR MODIFICATION DRUGS			
DRUG FAMILY	GENERIC NAME	BRAND NAME	COMMENTS
Antidepressants	clomipramine	Clomicalm®	considered a tricyclic antidepressant but works by preventing serotonin reuptake; approved for use in dogs
	fluoxetine	Reconcile®	serotonin reuptake inhibitor approved for use in dogs
Antianxiety drugs	diazepam, lorazepam, alprazolam	Valium®, Ativan®, Xanax®	benzodiazepines are the major human-label antianxiety drugs used in veterinary medicine, mostly in dogs
Progestins	megestrol acetate	Ovaban®	used in dogs and cats for aggression and feline urine spraying
	altrernogest	Regu-Mate®	used in horses, mostly for estrus synchronization, but used to suppress estrus in mares behaviorally; humans must use with caution to prevent absorption through the skin

Fluid Therapy Products

Fluid therapy is a lifesaving technique. Veterinary technicians must be familiar with the different products that are used, as well as be comfortable with fluid therapy calculations and monitoring patients receiving fluids. Fluids can be administered in a variety of methods, either enteral or parenteral, with intravenous administration being the most common route for urgent-care situations. In large animals, many products with electrolytes and other additives are available for oral administration to correct the diarrhea associated with young animal scours. Many of the products or solutions used may contain numerous additives. The most common fluids used in veterinary medicine are the crystalloids, which are best described as electrolyte-rich solutions. The most common crystalloid, and that to which most fluids are compared, is normal saline. Normal saline, also called physiologic saline, is a very isotonic solution of 0.9% sodium chloride and water. Depending on their electrolyte composition, crystalloids are also classified as either replacement or maintenance solutions.

The other major type of fluid products are the colloids, which are large molecular weight substances that stay within the blood vessels. Colloids are used to expand plasma volumes and are often administered as constant rate infusions (CRI). Colloids include various blood transfusion products (whole blood, plasma, etc.) and there are commercially available products also. Hypertonic solutions are used by some veterinarians in emergencies, especially in severe hemorrhage to expand intravascular fluid volumes. These solutions must be used with great care to avoid electrolyte imbalances. Additives are those products that are added to fluids to achieve specific outcomes (additional potassium added to help correct hypokalemia associated with severe diarrhea). The most common additives are electrolytes, substances to balance blood pH, to provide energy (calories), or to supplement vitamins.

FLUID THERAPY PRODUCTS			
FLUID TYPE	GENERIC NAME	BRAND NAME	COMMENTS
Crystalloids	saline	many products	used especially in alkalotic patients and for irrigation; use with caution in congestive heart failure
	Lactated Ringer's Solution (LRS)	many products	contains lactate, which converts in the liver to bicarbonate; used for acidosis patients
	Ringer's Solution	many products	no lactate is added; can be used in alkalotic patients
	dextrose: 5% or $2\frac{1}{2}$% solutions with or without electrolytes	generic products, Normosol R®, Normosol M®	dextrose is added to products as an energy source; numerous products available; solutions of greater than 5% dextrose are not considered isotonic
Colloids	dextran	Dextran 70®	used primarily for shock treatment; must be used with caution due to potential adverse reactions
	hetastarch	Hespan®	expensive human product used to expand intravascular fluid volume
Hypertonic solutions	hypertonic saline is available in 3% to 23% solutions	many products, with 5% being the most commonly used	must be administered IV only, due to hypertonicity

(continued)

FLUID THERAPY PRODUCTS (continued)			
FLUID TYPE	GENERIC NAME	BRAND NAME	COMMENTS
Additives	potassium chloride	many products	additive used for correction of hypokalemia; administer dilute only
	sodium bicarbonate	many products, with 5% and 8% solutions available	used to correct metabolic acidosis; measured in millieqivalents of bicarbonate per milliliter of solution
	50% dextrose	many products	added for energy supplementation; do not use without dilution
	calcium gluconate, calcium chloride	various products, including electrolyte combinations such as CalDextro®	used primarily for treatment of milk fever and other hypocalcemias; administer slowly IV to avoid cardiac arrhythmias
	water soluble vitamins	many products	use care to verify that products are approved for IV administration

Measurement Systems

Three measurement systems are still used for drugs and drug dosages. It is important for the veterinary technician to be able to work between the three systems. The most common system used and the easiest to work with is the metric system. Most of the measurements within the metric system for drugs revolve around volume (milliliters/liters) and weight (milligrams/grams/kilograms). Veterinary technicians must be able to work with different decimals easily within the metric system. The other two systems are the household and apothecary systems. The household system is still used to dispense medications to clients so that they can understand the dispensing directions, and it is often used for calculating and administering medications for large animals. The household system relies on the familiar teaspoons, cups, quarts, gallons, and so on for volume and on pounds for weight measures. The oldest system still used is the apothecary system, which uses drams, ounces, and grains. Some medications are still measured using these two systems.

A simple mnemonic will help you remember some of the conversions in the household system: *Our Cats Play Quietly in Groups.* You just need to remember the cats playing and the numbers 8,2,2,4.

O is for ounces and there are 8 ounces in a cup

C is for cup and there are 2 cups in a pint

P is for pint and there are 2 pints in a quart

Q is for quart and there are 4 quarts in a gallon (**G** is for gallon)

CONVERSIONS COMMONLY USED IN VETERINARY MEDICINE
1 grain (g) = 65 mg
1 teaspoon = 5 milliliters
1 tablespoon = 15 milliliters
1 ounce = 30 milliliters
1 cup = 8 ounces = 240 milliliters
1 dram = 4 milliliters
2.2 pounds = 1 kilogram
2 cups of water = 1 pint = approximately 1 pound

Dosage Calculations

There are three basic calculations that every veterinary technician should be able to perform. There may be other calculations, but these three are the most important and common calculations: determining the amount in a single dose, the percent concentration of a solution, and the drip rate for fluid therapy administration. Now that students are allowed to use calculators when taking the VTNE, the questions can be challenging. It is important to go through the calculations carefully, complete all steps, keep units of measure correct, and most importantly, use common sense. If a dosage answer seems unreasonable, most likely there has been a mistake in the steps taken to reach it. Backtrack to correct the answer. For example, if the answer for a dosage for a 30-pound dog comes out to 30 milliliters of medication to be administered intramuscularly, that is probably not the correct answer. Logically, we know that we would not give a 30-pound dog that much medication intramuscularly.

Single-Dose Calculations

There are three steps to most single-dose calculations. The mnemonic is *DAD* where the first *D* is the *d*osage, which is multiplied by the *a*nimal's weight, and that product is divided by the *d*rug concentration.

Example 1. If you are administering amoxicillin at 10 mg/kg to a 25 kilogram dog and you have 250 mg amoxicillin capsules in your pharmacy, how many capsules are required for each dose?

The formula using the mnemonic is:

Dose (10 mg)
×
Animal's weight (25 kg)
= 250 mg
÷
Drug concentration (250 mg/capsule)
= 1 capsule

It is crucial to remember the three steps and keep track of the correct units. This same three-step process can be used for injectable dosages also.

Example 2. If a horse is to be given 20,000 IU of penicillin G/kg, the horse weighs 1100 pounds, and the penicillin concentration is

300,000 IU per milliliter, how much is administered each dose?

In this situation, you need to convert pounds to kilograms. Remember that the weight conversion calculation is to be done first and then fit into the *DAD* mnemonic. One kilogram = 2.2 pounds, so this horse weighs 500 kilograms.

Dose (20,000 IU)
×
Animal's Weight (500 kg)
= 10,000,000 IU
÷
Drug concentration (300,000 IU/ml)
= 33.3 milliliters

Percent-Concentration Calculations

In order to dilute a concentrated solution to prepare a weaker solution, you must calculate the percent of the concentration. This type of calculation is important in order to create solutions that may be safe enough to administer into the body or even to create appropriate concentrations of tissue fixatives. For example, if you need to take a stock solution of formaldehyde and dilute it to make a 10% buffered formalin solution, you would use a percent-concentration calculation. Another example that occurs quite commonly in a veterinary practice is to create a 5% dextrose solution from a 50% stock dextrose solution for administration to a patient who is deemed to need some calories along with other supportive fluids. Here, the formula to remember is $V_1 \times C_1 = V_2 \times C_2$:

(V_1) Volume of solution one multiplied by (C_1) the Concentration of solution one =
(V_2) Volume of solution two multiplied by (C_2) the Concentration of solution two

Example 1. If you want to prepare 100 milliliters of a 5% dextrose solution to administer to an animal intravenously and you only have a 50% stock solution of dextrose available for dilution with sterile water, you would want to dilute the stock solution. A 50% dextrose solution should not normally be administered without some dilution. You can use the $V_1 \times C_1 = V_2 \times C_2$ formula to calculate how much of the stock solution to add to make this solution safe for intravenous administration.

$100 \times 5 =$ unknown $V_2 \times 50$
V_1 is 100 milliliters multiplied by C_1 which is 5% = 500
$500 = V_2$ which is the unknown multiplied by 50%
$500 \div 50 = 10$ milliliters

Therefore, you will take 10 milliliters of the 50% stock solution and add it to 90 milliliters of sterile water to create a new solution of 100 milliliters of 5% dextrose which would be safe enough for administration.

Example 2. If you need to give an isopropyl alcohol dip or bath to a heat-stroke animal and you want to use a 10% alcohol solution, but all you have in the veterinary clinic is 90% alcohol, available in gallon bottles, how much of the 90% solution is needed to make one gallon of the dilute solution? Remember that one gallon contains 128 ounces of fluid.

128 ounces $\times$ 10% = unknown $V_2 \times$ 90%
$1,280 = V_2 \times 90\%$
$1,280 \div 90 = 14.2$ ounces

Therefore, you will take 14.2 ounces of the 90% alcohol and dilute it with approximately 114 ounces of water to make a gallon of the 10% solution. The easiest way to do this is to pour the 14.2 ounces, or a little less than 2 cups, of the 90% alcohol into an empty gallon bottle and then q.s. with tap water until you have about one gallon total. (The abbreviation *q.s.* means *as much as is sufficient.*)

Drip-Rate Calculations

Fluid therapy can be lifesaving. Amounts to give over a period of time can be calculated using several methods. Many charts or calculation wheels are available to help the clinician or the veterinary technician determine how much to give. Fluid amounts for sick and dehydrated patients are totaled using the amounts needed to rehydrate the patient, the amounts needed for maintenance, and the amount needed to make up for ongoing losses such as bleeding or diarrhea. Often, the veterinarian prescribes the amount of fluids to give to a patient over a specific period of time and the veterinary technician must calculate the amount of fluid to give per minute (this is known as the drip rate).

Fluids are administered to veterinary patients using three commonly available primary IV administration sets. These sets deliver either 10, 15, or 60 drops per milliliter (ggt/ml) of fluids. Drip-rate calculations are quite easy with a shortcut method using a drop factor technique. The drop factor is easily calculated by taking the number of minutes in one hour (60) and dividing it by the number of drops per milliliter that the administration set delivers. Therefore, a veterinary fluid administration set that delivers 15 drops per milliliter would have a drop factor of 4 (60 minutes $\div$ 15 drops per ml = 4). The administration set that delivers 10 drops per milliliter is sometimes referred to as a *macro* drip because of the large size of the drop. The administration set that delivers 15 drops per milliliter is often referred to as the *standard* drip set, and the set that delivers 60 drops per milliliter is often referred to as a *pediatric* or *microdrip* set. Therefore, the drop factors will always be either 6, 4, or 1.

60 minutes $\div$ 10 ggt/ml = 6
60 minutes $\div$ 15 ggt/ml = 4
60 minutes $\div$ 60 ggt/ml = 1

Because this method of drip-rate calculation uses what is considered a factor rather than an equals sign (=), it is more appropriate to use the *almost equal* sign (≈) when determining the final answer.

Remember that there are three steps to fluid drip rate calculations: Determine the amount of fluids to give per hour and then divide that by the drop factor to determine the amount of fluids to give per minute (the drip rate).

Example 1. If you need to administer 2,400 ml of fluids to a larger dog over 24 hours and will use a standard veterinary fluid administration set that delivers 15 drops per milliliter, what is the drip rate?

Step 1. Calculate the amount to give per hour:
2,400 milliliters of fluids ÷ 24 hours =
        100 ml/hour
Step 2. Determine the drop factor:
60 minutes per hour ÷ 15 ggt/ml = 4
Step 3. Divide the amount to give per hour by the drop factor to calculate the drip rate:
100 ml/hour ÷ drop factor of 4 = 25 ggt/min

Example 2. If you need to administer 240 milliliters of fluids to a dehydrated cat using a pediatric administration set for the next 8 hours, what is the drip rate per hour?

Step 1. 240 ml ÷ 8 hours = 30 ml/hour
Step 2. 60 minutes ÷ 60 ggt/ml = 1 for the drop factor
Step 3. 30 ml/hour ÷ drop factor of 1 = 30 ggt/min

From a simple administration standpoint, this is in essence one drip every 2 seconds for the next 8 hours. Using pediatric or microdrip primary administration sets makes for easy drip rate calculations since the drop factor is always = 1.

Practice Questions

1. Sucralfate and omeprazole are both used in the treatment of gastric ulcers. Which statement is true regarding the mode of action of these drugs?
    a. Sucralfate works much like antacids by neutralizing stomach acid to increase gastric pH, while omeprazole adheres to damaged mucosa and creates a protective, bandage-like barrier.
    b. Sucralfate adheres to damaged mucosa and creates a protective, bandagelike barrier while omeprazole works much like antacids by neutralizing stomach acid to increase gastric pH.
    c. Sucralfate adheres to damaged mucosa and creates a protective, bandagelike barrier while omeprazole acts on parietal cells to directly inhibit gastric acid secretion.
    d. Sucralfate acts on parietal cells to directly inhibit gastric acid secretion while omeprazole adheres to damaged mucosa and creates a protective, bandagelike barrier.

2. If 480 ml of 0.9% sodium chloride solution is to be given IV over 24 hours, what is the correct drip rate if the primary administration set delivers 60 drops/ml?
    a. 10 ggt/min
    b. 20 ggt/min
    c. 200 ggt/min
    d. 480 ggt/min

3. Which of the following drugs is classified as an antibiotic?
 a. melarsomine
 b. praziquantel
 c. dexamethasone
 d. cephalexin

4. The drug carprofen belongs to which category of drugs?
 a. corticosteroids
 b. antitussives
 c. NSAIDs
 d. antifungals

5. A 44-pound dog is to receive furosemide at 1 mg/kg. Furosemide has a concentration of 40 mg/ml. How much should be drawn up for one dose?
 a. 0.5 ml
 b. 1 ml
 c. 2 ml
 d. 4 ml

6. Which of the following statements is most accurate about corticosteroids?
 a. may suppress the immune system
 b. may cause anorexia and anuria
 c. may be administered with NSAIDs concurrently
 d. may contribute to bacterial resistance development

7. You need to mix up a 4% solution of thiopental. You have one 5-gram vial. How much water is needed to prepare the solution?
 a. 40 ml
 b. 100 ml
 c. 125 ml
 d. 400 ml

8. The dosage of amoxicillin is 10mg/kg BID. You have 250 mg and 500 mg capsules available in the pharmacy. How much should be dispensed to a 55-pound dog for one week of treatment?
 a. 7 capsules of the 500 mg strength
 b. 10 capsules of the 500 mg strength
 c. 14 capsules of the 250 mg strength
 d. 20 capsules of the 250 mg strength

9. Which of the following antibiotics should not be administered with dairy products?
 a. tetracycline
 b. amoxicillin
 c. enrofloxacin
 d. cephalexin

10. Which of the following statements is true with regard to a drug with a narrow therapeutic index?
 a. It only takes a small amount of the drug to become toxic.
 b. It will become toxic to the kidneys only at high doses.
 c. The minimal effective dose is close to the toxic dose.
 d. The toxic dose will kill 50% of animals treated.

11. If you are monitoring an animal for signs of toxicity including anorexia, vomiting, and diarrhea, which of the following drug was most likely administered?
 a. digitalis
 b. fenbendazole
 c. metronidazole
 d. furosemide

12. A 30-kg dog is going to receive 40 ml/kg of IV fluids over the next 24 hours. If you use a primary administration set that delivers 15 ggt/ml, what is the drip rate?
   a. 7 ggt/min
   b. 13 ggt/min
   c. 20 ggt/min
   d. 30 ggt/min

13. What two organs are most involved in drug metabolism and excretion?
   a. liver and lung
   b. stomach and kidneys
   c. small intestine and spleen
   d. kidneys and liver

14. NSAIDs
   a. increase blood pressure.
   b. decrease pain and fever.
   c. lower the seizure threshold.
   d. decrease stomach acid secretion.

15. A 1,050-pound horse is to be given 10,000 IU/pound of penicillin G by injection. The penicillin available has a concentration of 300,000 IU per ml. What is the amount of each injection to be given?
   a. 20 ml
   b. 25 ml
   c. 35 ml
   d. 50 ml

16. Toxicities can occur rarely when which of the following drugs is given to collies?
   a. pyrantel
   b. milbemycin
   c. fenbendazole
   d. ivermectin

17. Antiemetics
   a. decrease coughing.
   b. decrease vomiting.
   c. increase blood pressure.
   d. induce vomiting.

18. Which of the following drugs is used as a monthly heartworm preventive and which is used as an adulticide for dogs being treated for heartworm disease?
   a. ivermectin and milbemycin
   b. melarsomine and diethylcarbamazine
   c. pyrantel and ivermectin
   d. milbemycin and melarsomine

19. The most toxic of the following ectoparasite drugs are
   a. pyrethroids such as allethrin.
   b. organophosphates such as dichlorovos.
   c. ivermectins such as ivomec.
   d. insect growth regulators such as methoprene.

20. Tapeworm treatment medications include
   a. pyrantel and ivermectin.
   b. epsiprantel and praziquantel.
   c. amprolium and albendazole.
   d. ponazuril and milbemycin.

21. Which of the following cardiac drugs is applied topically to nonhaired skin on dogs?
   a. nitroglycerine
   b. pimobendan
   c. enalapril
   d. digitalis

22. Which of the following drugs is a bronchodilator used in horses for the treatment of heaves?
   a. hydrocodone
   b. clenbuterol
   c. diphenhydramine
   d. doxapram

23. Which of the following gastroenteritis treatments contains aspirinlike compounds and may contribute to gastrointestinal ulcers?
    a. psyllium
    b. kaolin and pectin
    c. cimetidine
    d. bismuth subsalicylate

24. How many milliliters in an ounce of medication?
    a. 5
    b. 10
    c. 15
    d. 30

25. Medications that have a caution sign on the label and that are considered to be safe for use by a licensed veterinarian are called
    a. controlled substances.
    b. legend drugs.
    c. compounded drugs.
    d. illicit substances.

26. Which statement about antimicrobial drugs is most accurate?
    a. Each antimicrobial is only effective against one family of bacteria.
    b. Improper dosing may lead to bacterial resistance.
    c. Almost all antimicrobials have zero withdrawal times.
    d. All penicillin antimicrobials must be given parenterally.

27. Which of the following insecticides is derived from flowers and is known for its safety?
    a. pyrethrins
    b. carbamates
    c. ivermectins
    d. enrofloxacins

28. Which of the following drugs is used for the synchronization of estrus in cows?
    a. oxytocin
    b. diethylstilbestrol
    c. norgestomet
    d. estradiol cyprionate

29. Fluids routinely used to correct acidosis include
    a. saline.
    b. lactated Ringer's solution.
    c. hypertonic saline.
    d. 50% dextrose.

30. Drugs used to correct hyperthyroidism in cats include
    a. levothyroxine.
    b. methimazole.
    c. liothyroxine.
    d. estradiol.

31. The process of modifying drugs in the liver to either inactive or active metabolites is called
    a. excretion.
    b. biotransformation.
    c. absorption.
    d. distribution.

32. Minimum inhibitory concentration is the amount of a drug needed to inhibit the growth of
    a. bacteria.
    b. viruses.
    c. internal parasites.
    d. external parasites.

33. Penicillin antibiotics are often inactivated by staphylococcus bacteria due to the production of
    a. acid in the stomach.
    b. potentiation of the antibiotic with other drugs.
    c. a narrow spectrum of activity of most penicillins.
    d. penicillinase enzyme.

34. Clomipramine, lorazepam, and fluoxetine are examples of drugs that are considered
    a. behavior medication drugs for dogs.
    b. diuretics for use in numerous species.
    c. common antimicrobials.
    d. prostaglandin inhibitor drugs.

35. Drugs that can cause abortions in farm animals include
    a. corticosteroids such as dexamethasone.
    b. progestins such as altrenogest and norgestomet.
    c. diuretics such as chlorothiazide.
    d. antihistamines such as diphenhydramine.

36. Antihistamines are used for respiratory conditions and work due to the
    a. reduction of bronchial spasms.
    b. decrease in the viscosity of secretions.
    c. prevention of mast cell degranulation.
    d. suppression of coughing.

37. The group of drugs that has the most potent antipyretic action are the
    a. corticosteroids.
    b. antihistamines.
    c. nonsteroidals.
    d. antimicrobials.

38. The most common side effects of NSAIDs include
    a. polydipsia and polyurea.
    b. gastrointestinal irritation and ulceration.
    c. mydriasis, antiemesis, and diarrhea.
    d. suppression of mast cell degranulation.

39. Glycosamines and chondroitin sulfates are commonly used for veterinary patients with
    a. congestive heart failure.
    b. degenerative joint disease.
    c. chronic renal failure.
    d. chronic respiratory diseases.

40. A 550-kilogram horse is to receive IV fluids at a rate of 20 ml/pound of body weight per 24 hours. How much fluid should this horse receive in the first 24 hours?
    a. 11 liters
    b. 22 liters
    c. 33 liters
    d. 44 liters

41. If a goat is to receive 30 milliliters of medication BID for 8 days, how much medication will be dispensed?
    a. 240 milliliters
    b. one cup
    c. one pint
    d. one liter

42. Guifenesin is a smooth muscle relaxant used for
    a. nembulization to reduce respiratory mucous secretion viscosity.
    b. large animal anesthesia and expectoration of respiratory secretions.
    c. control of arrhythmias caused by anticholinergics.
    d. positive inotropic effects on the heart.

43. Why would aminoglycoside antibiotics probably not be a good choice for treatment of a deep puncture wound?
   a. Aminoglycosides are ineffective against gram-negative bacteria found in a puncture wound.
   b. Aminoglycosides are ineffective against most anaerobes found in a deep puncture wound.
   c. Aminoglycosides are very effective against many gram-negative bacteria.
   d. Aminoglycosides are very effective when administered orally.

44. In which of the following animals is enrofloxacin (Baytril®) contraindicated?
   a. a 14-week-old puppy with diarrhea
   b. a 6-year-old dog with a puncture into a joint
   c. a 12-year-old cat with a dental abscess
   d. an 11-month-old cat with a bite wound

45. A drug used for its gastrointestinal antiprotozoal and anaerobic effects in dogs is
   a. amoxicillin with clavulanic acid (Clavamox®).
   b. cefpodoxime (Simplicef®).
   c. doxycycline (Vibramycin®).
   d. metronidazole (Flagyl®).

46. Enrofloxacin, orbifloxacin, and marbofloxacin are examples of what family of antibiotics?
   a. aminoglycosides
   b. quinolones
   c. sulfonamides
   d. tetracyclines

47. An example of a drug used for its antiprotozoal effect is
   a. ponazuril in horses with sarcocystis.
   b. albendazole in sheep with haemonchus.
   c. epsiprantel in dogs with echinococcus.
   d. fipronil in dogs with ixodes.

48. When two antimicrobials are mixed together to create a bactericidal effect, the term used to describe the improved efficacy is
   a. potentiation
   b. biotransformation
   c. pharmacodynamics
   d. inotropism

49. Of the following, which is a potential side effect of chronic corticosteroid administration?
   a. hyperthyroidism
   b. hyperadrenocorticism
   c. hypothyroidism
   d. hypoinsulinism

50. In which species is the use of sodium phosphate enemas contraindicated?
   a. felines
   b. equines
   c. canines
   d. bovines

Answers and Explanations

1. c. Sucralfate works by creating a bandagelike protection on the stomach wall and omeprazole is an antiulcer drug that works by the inhibition of the proton pump to lower gastric acid secretion.

2. b. 480 ml ÷ 24 hours = 20 ml/hour, the drop factor is 60 minutes/hour ÷ 60 ggt/min ≈ 1, so then 20 mlml/hour ÷ drop factor of 1 = 20 ggt/min.

3. d. Cephalexin is a cephalosporin antibiotic.

4. c. Carprofen is a nonsteroidal anti-inflammatory drug.

5. a. 44 pounds = 20 kilograms, 20 kilograms × 1 mg/kg = 20 mgs, 20 mgs ÷ 40 mg/ml = 0.5 ml.

6. a. Corticosteroid anti-inflammatory drugs have side effects of polydipsia, polyurea, polyphagia, immune system depression, and delayed healing times.

7. c. The knowns are 5-gram vial contains 5,000 mg of thiopental and 4% = 40 mg/ml, using $V_1 \times C_1 = V_2 \times C_2$ where $1 \times 5{,}000$ mg = Unknown $\times 40$ mg/ml = 125 ml.

8. c. 55 pounds = 25 kilograms, 25 kilograms × 10 mg/kg = 250 mg capsules given two times daily for 7 days = 14 capsules of the 250 mg strength.

9. a. Tetracyclines should not be given with dairy products due to calcium binding.

10. c. Narrow therapeutic index drugs do not have a wide margin of safety so the minimal effective dosage is close to the toxic dose. Therefore, dosage calculations with narrow index drugs must be very accurate.

11. a. Digitalis has a very narrow therapeutic index and patients must be monitored for signs of toxicity which include emesis, diarrhea, and anorexia. The other choices are relatively safe drugs without these side effects.

12. b. 30 kg × 40ml/kg = 1,200 ml, 1,200 ml ÷ 24 hours = 50 ml/hour, the drop factor is 15 ggt/ml ÷ 60 minutes/hour ≈ 4, so then 50 ml/hour ÷ 4 drop factor = 12.5 ggt/min which must be rounded to 13 ggt/min.

13. d. The two organs of drug metabolism and excretion are the kidneys and liver.

14. b. The effects of NSAIDs are analgesia and antipyresis.

15. c. 1,050 lbs × 10,000 IU/lb = 10,500,000 IU. 10,500,000 ÷ 300,000 IU/ml = 35 ml.

16. d. Collies and shelties are occasionally susceptible to ivermectin toxicity.

17. b. By definition, antiemetic drugs decrease vomiting.

18. d. Milbemycin is approved as a monthly heartworm preventive and melarsomine is the only approved drug for treating adult heartworms in dogs.

19. b. Organophosphates are the most toxic ectoparasite drugs commonly used.

20. b. The two most common anticestode drugs on the veterinary market are praziquantel and epsiprantel.

21. a. Nitroglycerine must be applied topically in nonhaired portions of the dog's skin. The other drugs are given orally.

22. b. Clenbuterol is a common bronchodilator drug used in horses for the chronic respiratory condition known as heaves.

23. d. Bismuth subsalicylate contains salicylates which are aspirin compounds that may cause gastrointestinal ulcers.

24. d. There are 30 milliliters in an ounce of medication.

25. b. Legend drugs are those prescription drugs that contain the legend *This drug is for use by or under the direction of a licensed veterinarian.*

26. b. One of the major problems with inappropriate dosing of antibiotics is the potential of increased bacterial resistance.

27. a. Pyrethrins are developed from flowers and are likely some of the most safe ectoparasite drugs on the market, including careful use on puppies and kittens.

28. c. Norgestomet is a progestin hormonal product specifically indicated for estrus synchronization in cattle.

29. b. Lactated Ringer's solution contains lactate, which is converted in the liver to increase blood pH in clinical cases of metabolic acidosis.

30. b. Methimazole and carbimazole are the only two approved drugs for the treatment of cats with hyperthyroidism.

31. b. Biotransformation is the process of modifying drugs in the liver into active or inactive metabolites.

32. a. Minimum inhibitory concentration (MIC) is a common term used for determining the dose of antibiotics needed to inhibit bacterial growth.

33. d. Certain bacteria but particularly the staphlococci produce the enzyme penicillinase, which can inactivate many penicillin antibiotics.

34. a. Clomipramine, lorazepam, and fluoxetine are common behavior modification drugs used in dogs.

35. a. Dexamethasone and other corticosteroids must be used with extreme caution in pregnant ruminants and horses due to the induction of abortion.

36. c. By action, antihistamines work to reduce histamine release from degranulated mast cells.

37. c. NSAIDs are the most effective fever-reducing drugs on the veterinary market.

38. b. NSAIDs are notorious for contributing to the formation of gastrointestinal irritation and ulceration due to the effect of the drugs on the suppression of good or needed prostaglandins.

39. b. Some of the most common nutraceuticals used include glycosamines and chondroitins for degenerative joint diseases in many species.

40. b. 550 kilograms = 1,100 pounds, a 1,100-pound horse is given fluids at 20 ml/pound = 22,000 ml or 22 liters/24 hours.

41. c. 30 milliliters × two times daily for 8 days = 480 milliliters or 16 ounces. One pint = 16 ounces.

42. b. Guifenesin is used IV as a muscle relaxant for anesthesia in horses and cattle and is found in a number of respiratory drug combinations for its expectorant effect.

43. b. Aminoglycosides are a poor choice for an anaerobic infection because they require oxygen for their effect of inhibiting protein synthesis.

44. a. Enrofloxacin is contraindicated in young animals with developing cartilage due to its effect on cartilage formation.

45. d. Metronidazole is commonly used in dogs for treatment of giardia and for other anaerobic infections.

46. b. Enrofloxacin, orbifloxacin, and marbofloxacin are quinolones, also known as fluoroquinolone antibiotics.

47. a. The only answer choice referring to a protozoal disease is a horse with sarcocystis, also known as equine protozoal myelitis. The drug of choice for this disease is ponazuril.

48. a. When two antibiotics are mixed together to improve efficacy synergistically, the two drugs potentiate each other.

49. b. One of the potential side effects of corticosteroid administration is the potential for iatrogenic Cushing's syndrome or hyperadrenocorticism.

50. a. Phosphate enemas are contraindicated in cats due to the potential for hyperphosphatemia.

5 ▶ SURGICAL PREPARATION AND ASSISTING

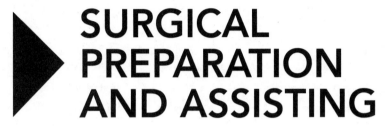

CHAPTER OVERVIEW

The ability to properly prepare the animal, surgical suite, and surgical personnel for a procedure is very important in veterinary medicine. Proper surgical preparation increases surgical survival rates and decreases complications by decreasing the number of pathogenic organisms that may contaminate the surgical field, providing a routine that minimizes possible errors before, during, and after the procedure and providing adequate record keeping for following potentially harmful trends in the animal's vital signs during the anesthetic period.

K nowledge of appropriate instrumentation and procedures for common veterinary surgeries allows the technician to be better prepared for surgery. Proper patient and pack preparation save anesthetic time and also increase survival rates for the animal. The watchword for veterinary surgery is *preparedness*. The better prepared the technician is prior to beginning the surgical procedure, the lower the likelihood of complications for the patient.

Key Terms

absorbable
antisepsis
aponeurosis
asepsis
Caslick's procedure
caudectomy
chlorhexidine
cleanliness
closed gloving
cryptorchidectomy
dehiscence
disinfection
elective surgery
ethylene oxide
extubation
fenestrated
indicator strips
intraoperative
intubation
iodorphors
laparotomy
nonabsorbable
nonelective surgery
onychectomy
open gloving
orchidectomy
ovariohysterectomy
pack
postoperative
preoperative
sterility
surgeon
zoonotic

Concepts and Skills

Surgical preparation and assisting can be broken down into four main topics:

- preoperative preparation
- intraoperative procedures
- postoperative procedures
- common surgical procedures

Preoperative Preparation

Proper **preoperative** preparation of the patient, instruments, and surgical suite will reduce the infection rate (morbidity) and increase the success of any surgical procedure. Before the 1900s, disinfection, sterile instruments, and hand washing prior to surgery (whether of animals or people) were not commonly used. Even anesthesia was a rarity. The anesthetic usually used was either ether, liquor, or chloroform, all of which caused liver problems. As a result, many patients died from infection and/or shock. Since the institution of good nursing protocols including asepsis (without germs), patient survival rate has increased in both humans and animals and there have been fewer postoperative complications.

Cleanliness, Disinfection, Antisepsis, Asepsis, Sterility

These five words should be blazed into the minds of everyone in the veterinary clinic. Not only do animals need to be protected from nosocomial infections (infections coming from the hospital) when they come in for surgery, but equally important, the human population must be protected from **zoonotic** diseases (animal diseases that may be infectious to humans). In order to achieve these goals, maintaining a clean, clutter-free facility with a minimum of dust-collecting surfaces is necessary. All surfaces should be able to be wiped down or laundered. Veterinary technicians are often in charge of clinic maintenance, which includes providing a clean and polished facility. Not only does a clean, clutter-free facility help to reduce infection rate and minimize odors, it also demonstrates that the clinic is professional. Clients notice stains, dust, feces in the driveway, urine puddles, and odors. Impressions are important, and the clinic should strive to make good ones every day.

Cleanliness is the removal of dirt and debris from a surface. This may be performed with soap and water and does not require disinfection.

Disinfection is the removal of living organisms from a surface to an acceptable level that will not cause/transmit infection. This is performed with a disinfectant. Disinfection can only be performed on nonliving objects because the process kills living organisms (including the patient's cells). Contact time, or the amount of time the product is in contact with the surface, is important. Follow label directions for the product. Disinfectants do not necessarily clean, so cleaning should be performed prior to disinfection. Higher concentrations of disinfectants do not mean that the mixture will be stronger. In many cases, in fact, a concentration that is too high will make a product less effective.

Antisepsis is the removal of infectious organisms from a living surface to an acceptable level. This is performed with an antiseptic. Antiseptics work best at the correct dilution, and contact time is important. Be sure to follow label directions. Remember that it is only possible to disinfect nonliving surfaces.

Asepsis is the condition of lacking infectious organisms. This is what preoperative preparation hopes to achieve. By proper antisepsis and disinfection and the use of sterile instruments, drapes, and technique, the surgical field can be kept free of infectious organisms that could cause problems with healing.

Products

Various products can be used as disinfectants, antiseptics, or both. The category depends on the amount of tissue damage or toxicity that the product causes. Clean surfaces without visible soil, oils, or dirt are easier to disinfect than dirty surfaces and will require shorter contact times. It is important to mix disinfectants and antiseptics according to label directions.

Antiseptics

The two most commonly used antiseptics are **povidone-iodine** (an antimicrobial) and **chlorhexi-**

dine (an antibacterial). They are commonly used as surgical scrubs, superficial disinfectants, and wound flushes. Iodine will kill tissues in high concentrations, but is a very effective bactericide. Most of the iodines used in clinical practice are iodophors. **Iodophors** are iodine molecules complexed with a surfactant (soap) that allows the iodine to be released slowly. Iodophors such as povidone-iodine tend to stain less and are less toxic to cells and tissues. Iodine will provide residual antiseptic activity for several hours after scrubbing. Alcohol will destroy the residual benefits of iodine and should not be used as the alternating scrub. Saline or water should be used instead. Some animals (and people) are sensitive to iodine compounds and will develop rashes. Long-term use can lead to absorption of the iodine through the skin, which can cause thyroid problems.

Chlorhexidine is effective against bacteria, viruses, and fungi. The residual antisepsis is not affected by alcohol and it may be used on relatively dirty areas (iodine should only be used on precleaned tissue). It is superior to iodine as a surgical scrub and a hand scrub because of the spectrum of organisms that it is effective against and its quick onset of action. Chlorhexidine is a rapid antiseptic that requires a short contact time. Very dilute chlorhexidine (1:40 dilution with water or saline) may be used as a flush. Higher concentrations will destroy cells and tissues.

Alcohols and phenols have both been used as antiseptics and disinfectants. The phenols have been phased out because of the high potential for toxicity (especially in cats). Alcohols (ethyl and isopropyl) should only be used on intact skin because they will cause pain and cell death in subcutaneous tissues. Alcohols have no residual effect and are not effective against fungus and bacterial spores. Most of the time, alcohol scrubs are alternated with chlorhexidine scrubs to help cleanse, degrease, and scrub an area for surgery.

Disinfectants

Disinfectants are generally not used on living tissue because they cause cell death at effective concentrations. They are usually excellent bactericides, but the virucidal and fungicidal properties vary depending on the product.

Quaternary ammonium compounds are actually soaps or detergents. They have very little effect on naked viruses or spores (which do not have a fat coating), but have some cleaning activity along with disinfection. Viruses with a lipid coating and gram-negative bacteria are particularly susceptible to quaternary ammonium compounds because these compounds destroy the lipids in the cell walls. Benzalkonium chloride is the most common. If hard water (water that contains a high level of calcium salts) is used, the solution may be inactivated by the chemical reaction with the salts. Quaternary ammonium compounds should not be used to clean items containing cotton (surgical drapes or gowns) because cotton, a natural fiber, also inactivates the compound.

Sodium hypochlorite, or bleach, is an excellent disinfectant. It is particularly good for the elimination of bacteria and viruses and some fungi (dermatophytes). It will kill any living tissue and should not be used on skin or in open wounds.

Formaldehyde and glutaraldehyde are toxic and irritating to tissues. They should never be used for antisepsis, but are effective disinfectants if given enough contact time as stated on the labels.

Instrumentation

The instrumentation for sterilization varies with the type of hospital, the type of equipment, and the surgeon's preference. Some sterilization procedures are dangerous for the operator. Prior to a surgical procedure, technicians should always familiarize themselves with the operation of equipment as well as the safety protocols. Untrained personnel should not operate sterilization equipment.

Most prepackaged items, such as suture material, injectable medications and vaccines, gloves, and single-use drapes and gowns, come in presterilized packaging. Sterilization occurs in the factory and may be either by irradiation (used for heat-sensitive items such as latex gloves and paper) or filtration (used for liquids such as injectables).

Steam Autoclave

Steam is the most commonly used method of sterilization. In general, heat will destroy bacteria by destroying protein. Boiling water by itself is not a good sterilant. Steam that is generated by boiling water at increased pressures has better penetration and will destroy all organisms including spore-forming bacteria. Steam should be at 121° Celsius (250° Fahrenheit) for a minimum of 15 minutes in order to sterilize an item completely. In other words, the 15 minutes of contact time is counted not from the time the autoclave is turned on but from the time the pressure and temperature reach the proper level. Instruments may become dulled with steam, so delicate instruments should be processed with gas or plasma sterilization. Steam should not be used on rubber or plastic. Burns and explosions can occur if the autoclave is not properly maintained and operated. Untrained personnel should not operate autoclaves.

Autoclaves range from kitchen pressure cookers to large, walk-in autoclaves at research facilities. Pressure cookers are not good autoclaves because it is impossible to measure the temperature and pressure in the interior. True autoclaves have pressure and temperature gauges that allow better quality control. Most autoclaves in practice are small, countertop, gravity-displacement autoclaves that allow the air to escape from the bottom of the autoclave as the steam rises to the correct pressure in the interior.

After the cycle is completed, the autoclave door should be cracked open slightly to allow the escape of residual steam. Opening the door completely will actually cause condensation to form on the pack. If the pack becomes wet, it is no longer considered sterile and the process must be repeated. The packs should be removed from the autoclave after 20 minutes.

Plasma

Plasma uses hydrogen peroxide gas to sterilize instruments. It may be used for most of the same materials as steam. Wood, paper, plastics, and liquids cannot be sterilized with plasma.

Plasma sterilizers are really vacuum chambers. The chamber is evacuated (placed in a vacuum) and hydrogen peroxide is injected and vaporized. The vapor is bombarded with radio waves, which makes plasma. The peroxide molecules in the plasma are actually free radicals, which means that they have unpaired electrons in their outer shell and are highly reactive. These electrons attack bacteria and viruses and change the protein and nucleic acid structures, destroying them.

Indicator strips are available to indicate the presence of hydrogen gas but they do not indicate the presence of free radicals. Biological indicators, available from distribution companies, must be used. Biological indicators contain resistant bacteria that will be killed by the sterilization process. Failure of the bacteria to grow indicates adequate sterilization.

Gas Sterilization

Gas sterilization uses **ethylene oxide** gas to sterilize materials. The benefit of ethylene oxide sterilization is that it can be used to sterilize materials that will melt or be damaged by steam or plasma, such as drills, cords, tubing, rubber, and fine-tipped ophthalmic instruments. Ethylene oxide will destroy bacteria, fungi, and viruses by causing alkylation of the DNA.

Ethylene oxide is very dangerous and should never be used by untrained personnel. It is flammable, explosive, and highly toxic. Gas sterilizers should be vented to the outside to prevent intoxication of personnel. Packs sterilized with ethylene oxide should be aerated for a minimum of seven days prior to use to prevent intoxication of surgical personnel on opening the pack. Toxicity reactions include fetal mutations, miscarriage, cancer, convulsions, respiratory edema, and death.

Packs for ethylene oxide sterilization should be packaged in plastic and paper packs (steripouches) and sealed before being placed in the chamber. The gas penetrates plastic and paper. Chemical indicators are available, but, as with other methods, biological indicators are the best for evaluation of **sterility**.

Ethylene oxide chambers are operated by breaking the vial of chemical in a pouch and closing the

door of the chamber. Humidity must also be present to enhance killing, but it does not need to be steam under pressure. The higher the temperature, the faster the ethylene oxide will sterilize, but 12 hours at room temperature will be adequate, so heating is not necessary.

Dry Heat

Dry heat is used to sterilize items that cannot tolerate moisture, including powder, dirt, bedding, and so on. An advantage of dry heat is that it will not cause corrosion and dulling of blade edges as steam does. The disadvantage is that it takes more time and higher temperatures than steam. Dry heat must be applied at either 320° Fahrenheit for 2 hours or 340° Fahrenheit for 1 hour. Dry heat should be in a convection oven that moves the heated air over the instruments. Regular ovens should not be used because they heat unevenly.

Cold Sterilization

Cold sterilization typically uses glutaraldehyde. Contact time for cold sterile is a minimum of 3 hours in solution. This process should only be used for nonsterile procedures because of the possibility of contamination when instruments are removed with a contaminated tool. The instruments must be cleaned thoroughly and dried prior to being placed in the bath to ensure the proper concentration of glutaraldehyde and the proper penetration of the solution. Instruments must be rinsed prior to use because glutaraldehyde is toxic to tissues.

Chlorhexidine may also be used, but it tends to crystallize and may cause corrosion of instruments over time. With any cold sterilization, cleaning an instrument that has fallen on the floor and putting it into the cold sterile bath for 5 minutes (which is common in many veterinary practices), is not sufficient. A minimum of 3 hours contact time is essential.

Preoperative Preparation of the Surgical Suite

The cleanliness and level of disinfection should be highest in the surgical suite. The surgical suite should be swept, dusted, and mopped prior to the rest of the clinic in order to keep it as clean as possible. All cleaning equipment should be specific for the surgical suite and not used for the rest of the hospital. Dirty mops and mop buckets may have contaminants that can reduce the asepsis of the surgical suite. Mop heads should be laundered regularly. All surfaces in the surgical suite should be nonporous, and there should be nothing in the surgical suite that cannot undergo disinfection. If delicate instruments that cannot be disinfected or cleaned easily must be in the surgical suite, they should be covered with a drape between procedures to decrease dust collection. Even if the surgical suite is not used on a particular day, it should still be on the cleaning rotation to maintain disinfection.

All surfaces, whether they are visible or not, should be cleaned. Surgical tables (including the sides and undersides) and lights should be cleaned after each procedure because they are closest to the surgical site. Anesthesia machine hoses and surfaces should be cleaned frequently for the same reason.

Surgical packs should not be stored in the surgery room itself, because of the possibility of dust collection and contamination. A pass-through door or window should be available to pass the instruments into the surgery from the prep room to minimize contamination and reduce clutter.

If possible, the airflow should be higher in the surgical suite than in the rest of the hospital to reduce the possibility of contaminated air from the rest of the hospital getting into the aseptic atmosphere of the surgery. The doors should be able to be pushed open and swing closed. This will decrease the necessity of opening and closing doors with the hands and enable asepsis to be maintained.

Preoperative Preparation of the Surgical Pack

Surgical packs consist of instruments and other items necessary for a particular surgical procedure. Every veterinarian and every hospital is different with re-

spect to the items that are chosen for the pack. Choices of instruments, numbers of gauze sponges, and other items are all variable. The important things to remember are:

- the packs must remain sterile until opened,
- the packs should be able to be opened easily, and
- the packs should be consistent in numbers of items within a given clinic.

If the pack cannot be opened easily, accidents may occur that can affect sterility of the instruments, rendering the pack useless. If the technician makes five different spay packs with varying numbers of hemostats and gauze sponges, it will be impossible to tell whether or not an item was left inside the animal. Instruments and gauze sponges should be counted before and after every procedure.

Proper pack preparation means that the pack should be made the same way every time. Generally, packs are double-wrapped in paper or cloth or in plastic envelopes. Indicator strips sensitive to the type of sterilization used (steam or gas) should be placed inside the pack along with the instruments to ensure that proper sterilization has occurred. Steam sterilization tape is not adequate for assessing proper penetration of the pack with steam if used alone.

Instruments should also be placed in the pack or on the tray in a specific order to make instrument selection easier for the veterinarian or veterinary assistant during surgery. This will save the surgeon time and will increase the surgeon's ability to focus on the task at hand.

Cleaning Instruments

Prior to inclusion in a pack, instruments should be clean, lubricated, and dry and must be checked for functionality. They should open and close properly, the box locks should lock the instrument, the tines should not be bent, and the tips should meet properly. Improperly operating instruments should either be discarded or sent back to the factory for repair or replacement. Scissors, osteotomes, and elevators should be sharpened and assessed for chips and bent shafts prior to inclusion in a pack. See Postoperative Instrument and Equipment Care on page 100 for a more complete discussion of instrument care.

Packing the Pack

There should be a basic pack inventory for every type of **pack** in the hospital. This inventory should include:

- the number and type of each instrument,
- the number of gauze sponges, towels, and drapes included in the pack, and
- any additional instruments that may need to be added per procedure; these should be made available in separate packs.

Use of an instrument tray will keep the items organized and easily accessible by the surgeon. Pack wraps (whether cloth or paper) should be inspected for holes or wear and discarded when appropriate. Any holes or thin spots are opportunities for contamination of the pack and prevent asepsis from being achieved.

Air circulation within the pack is necessary for adequate steam and gas penetration. Wrapping a pack too tightly (overstuffing) can decrease the ability to sterilize instruments. For the same reason, putting too many packs in the autoclave can also decrease the ability to achieve sterilization. Instruments within the pack should be in the open position (lock boxes should be open, not closed) to enable even heating.

Packs should be wrapped tightly enough and sturdily enough to prevent accidental opening. Wrapping with an envelope closure is the best method. Tabs enable the technician to open the packs without contaminating the interior.

Packs should be labeled with the pack type, the date of sterilization, and the technician's name or initials. They should then be sealed with tape.

Storage of Packs and Longevity

Packs should be stored in a closed cabinet to prevent dust formation. Packs should be inspected frequently. If a pack gets wet, is dropped, or the tape seal is broken, it is no longer considered sterile and must be re-cleaned and resterilized prior to use. Water will wick contaminants and bacteria into the sterile environment, so packs that become wet or are not completely dried after removal from the autoclave must be resterilized. Double-wrapped muslin or paper packs will remain sterile for 7 to 8 weeks if stored in a clean, closed cabinet. Storage in an open cabinet or on a shelf will decrease the effectiveness of sterilization by about half.

Preoperative Preparation of the Patient

The patient is the most important consideration for the technician. Proper preparation of the patient, the operating room, and the surgeon will reduce the risk of intra- and postoperative complications, including infection. All equipment (packs, gowns, gloves, possible suture material, and monitoring equipment) should be gathered and available prior to the surgery to minimize setup time and enable continuous patient monitoring. Anesthesia machines, monitoring equipment, and heat sources should be checked for proper function prior to beginning a procedure. A checklist will ensure consistency. Anesthetics should be prepared in labeled syringes (patient's name, drug, concentration, and dose). A crash cart containing emergency drugs and equipment should be available. Endotracheal tubes should be selected and a laryngoscope with a working light should be available.

Preoperative Laboratory Work

A minimum database is recommended prior to any surgical procedure. The definition of minimum database will vary with the veterinarian and the practice, but generally includes at least a physical examination, PCV (packed cell volume), and TP (total protein). Many practices may recommend a CBC (complete blood count) and chemistry panel as well. In susceptible breeds, or prior to surgeries with potential for excessive hemorrhage, such as ear crops, a von Willebrand test or BMBT (buccal mucosal bleeding time) may be recommended to rule out bleeding tendencies.

The physical examination is especially important to ensure the right animal, right sex, right body part, and right procedure. Never rely on the receptionist or the owner for all the information on a particular animal. It is not uncommon for owners to misidentify the sex of a cat or a rabbit coming in for a neutering procedure, for example. Animals should be identified with their full name and surgical procedure on a cage card and an identification collar to prevent mistakes. Special instructions such as NPO (nil per os, or nothing by mouth) should also be on the cage card as well. Physical exam findings should be in the record in SOAP (subjective, objective, assessment, and plan) format for the veterinarian to review prior to the procedure. All blood should be drawn and the results ready prior to induction (placing the animal under anesthesia).

Owners should be informed by phone of any deviation from the plan. For this reason, it is important to go over an estimate of potential costs and get the owner's contact information (including cell phone and e-mail) prior to admission. Owners should also sign a consent form and possibly a resuscitation consent form in case of anesthetic complications. The technician should discuss the risks of anesthesia with the owner prior to surgery. This will not only inform the owner, but may protect the hospital from potential legal action in case of a surgical or anesthetic complication.

Induction

Modern anesthetic techniques usually involve multiple drugs giving a smoother anesthetic experience. It is important for the technician to be familiar with the specific combination of drugs used by each veterinarian in the practice, including dosages, routes of administration, and order of administration. Anesthetic protocols usually include preanesthetic, anesthesia induction, maintenance, and pain control agents. All medications and induction equipment should be prepared prior to induction and labeled as stated in the section on Preoperative Preparation of the Patient on page 91. This will save time, smooth the induction process, and reduce distraction of the technician from patient monitoring.

Surgical patients should have an indwelling catheter placed prior to surgery to enable anesthetic, fluid, and emergency drug administration. Fluid administration is important during surgery because anesthesia reduces blood pressure and renal blood flow and can lead to shock syndromes. Shock is an emergency condition characterized by a decrease in systemic blood pressure or cardiac output. Warm fluid therapy is a means of increasing body temperature, which also tends to drop several degrees during surgery. Maintaining blood pressure and body temperature will decrease recovery times and intra- and postoperative complications.

Given a few minutes prior to induction, the preanesthetic agent is generally a sedative that reduces the anxiety of the animal during induction and can reduce the amount of induction/maintenance anesthesia needed, thereby increasing the safety of the anesthesia. It may also smooth the recovery process by slowing this process, allowing the animal to adjust to the altered state of consciousness. This step may be omitted with certain anesthetic induction agents. Time of preanesthetic administration should be recorded on the anesthesia record along with the dose and concentration. Some pain control agents (NSAIDs) are given prior to surgery, while some are used as preanesthetics or intraoperatively. Check with the veterinarian for administration times.

Anesthetic induction is the administration of the induction agent. This is usually an injectable anesthetic agent followed by gas anesthesia. All equipment that may be needed during induction should be available. This may include anesthetic masks, induction chambers for cats and some exotic animals (but never for dogs), endotracheal tubes, ties (used to anchor the endotracheal tube to the animal), an empty syringe to inflate the endotracheal tube cuff, a working laryngoscope (with a light), and sterile lube (lubricant). The induction agent is administered and the animal is watched for relaxation and decreased jaw tone. Once this occurs, the animal is intubated.

Intubation is the process of placing the endotracheal tube into the trachea. The tube should be premeasured both for diameter and length. The diameter of the tube should be large enough to have the maximum gas flow, but narrow enough to fit into the trachea comfortably. Too large a diameter may cause necrosis (tissue death) of the trachea. Too small a tube will have increased resistance of flow and may interfere with gas exchange at the alveolus. The length of the tube should be measured by placing the tube externally on the animal from the tip of the nose to the thoracic inlet (beginning of the shoulder blade). If a tube is too long, it may enter a single bronchus and only ventilate one lung. If it is too short, it may not stay in the trachea.

Once jaw tone is decreased, an assistant should hold the maxilla behind the upper canines and extend the neck to straighten out the larynx and trachea. The technician performing the intubation will open the mouth by inserting the finger between the incisors and grabbing the tongue. The tongue is extended to bring the larynx further forward, because the hyoid apparatus that holds the larynx is connected to the base of the tongue. The epiglottis is identified. If it is in normal placement, the tip will be hooked over the soft palate and make visualization of the glottis (the opening in the larynx leading to the trachea defined by the vocal cords and arytenoid cartilage) impossible. If it is in this location, it may be dislodged with the tip of the endotracheal tube and the glottis will be visualized over the leaf-shaped epiglottis. The tube is advanced between the vocal cords and tied in place. The animal is connected to the anesthesia machine (with oxygen and gas anesthetic turned on) and the cuff is inflated. The inflated cuff should prevent gas leakage around the tube and help to prevent aspiration of oral and pharyngeal contents. Overinflation of the cuff may cause pressure necrosis and should be avoided. Cuffs should be avoided completely in animals with complete tracheal rings, such as birds and reptiles. Mammals have a trachealis dorsalis muscle connecting the c-shaped rings of the trachea, and this provides the ability to stretch when the cuff is inflated. Care must be taken inflating cuffs when dealing with cats, as overinflation can lead to tracheal rupture.

The technician should then check whether the endotracheal tube is lodged in the esophagus or the trachea by checking for breathing through the tube. Another method is to palpate the throat area. The trachea should be palpable in nonintubated animals because of the cartilage rings. In intubated animals, if only one cylindrical tube is palpable, the endotracheal tube is correctly placed in the trachea. If two tubes are palpable, the endotracheal tube is in the esophagus and should be removed prior to attempting intubation again.

The gas anesthesia and oxygen flow are then turned on and the machine is connected to the tube. A surgical plane of anesthesia is attained when the animal's eye has rolled to the ventromedial position and there is a loss of the palpebral reflex and jaw tone.

Once a surgical plane of anesthesia is reached, the animal may be prepped for surgery. The anesthetist should note the induction time on the anesthetic record and begin monitoring.

Anesthetic drugs and planes of anesthesia will be more thoroughly discussed in Chapter 11.

Preoperative Shaving and Scrubbing

Proper preoperative preparation decreases the chances of postoperative infection and breaks in intraoperative asepsis. A routine for this preparation is important. If the same steps are followed prior to each surgery, there are fewer opportunities for costly mistakes. Knowing the theory behind the procedures will help you understand their importance.

Shaving

Hair acts as a wick, drawing moisture, bacteria, and dirt into a sterile field. Asepsis cannot be achieved on a hairy animal so the patient must be shaved prior to the procedure. Typically, the boundary of the shaved area should be a minimum of 2 to 4 cm from the edge of the incision, depending on the veterinarian's preference. Some veterinarians like a very broad surgical field, others prefer a small field. Some veterinarians also prefer a smaller incision. In general, if the hair on the animal's sides is long enough to get into the sterile field, it should be clipped. If an orthopedic procedure is being performed, the entire circumference of the limb should be shaved and prepped.

The shaving should be done with a #40 clipper blade, initially in the direction of the hair growth then against the hair growth. The removed hair should be vacuumed from the animal. A lint roller may be used to remove smaller hair fragments from the animal. Some veterinarians prefer a close shave with a double-edged razor after the clip. The area should be scrubbed with surgical scrub to make a lather, then shaved in the direction of hair growth. Hair and dead skin cells may then be removed with a wet sponge.

It is important to prevent irritation of the skin (clipper burn) during the surgical prep. Clipper burn causes irritation similar to small cuts (like paper cuts) that can increase postoperative self-mutilation by the animal. It will also increase the tendency for postoperative infection and possible **dehiscence** of the wound (opening of the wound prior to healing). Excessive pressure during clipping should be avoided and the blade should be held so that the face is as close to parallel to the skin as possible. The skin should be pulled taut to prevent catching the skin in the tines of the blade. Failure to tighten the skin causes chatter marks, which look like railroad tracks. These recommendations are even more important in thin-skinned animals such as cats and rabbits because of the danger of skin tears.

Dull clippers increase the chances of clipper burn, so proper maintenance is important. Clipper blades should be cleaned thoroughly after every use to decrease the potential for disease and parasite transmission. Clippers should be stored in a disinfectant/lubrication bath between uses.

Scrubbing

To scrub means to remove contaminants such as bacteria from the animal's body prior to surgery. It consists of two steps. The first, or preliminary, scrub occurs in the induction area. Alternating scrubs are performed with an antiseptic surgical scrub such as povidone-iodine or chlorhexidine on gauze sponges. If chlorhexidine is used, the second scrub should be alcohol. If povidone-iodine is used, the second scrub should be saline because alcohol removes the long-acting antiseptic properties of iodine. Exam gloves should be worn when performing a preliminary scrub to minimize contamination of the field with bacteria and fungi that may be on the hands.

The technique for the preliminary scrub should be to start with the surgical scrub over the proposed incision site. A spiral pattern should make increasing circles toward the edge of the shaved area. Once a sponge has traveled over an area, it should not touch that area again. The alcohol or saline sponge is then placed over the incision site and the spiral pattern is repeated. The whole procedure is repeated twice more, with fresh sponges at each step, and a sterile gauze sponge is placed over the incision. The animal is then transported to the surgical suite, positioned, and tied to the surgical table and the surgical scrub is performed.

The sterile surgical scrub should be performed wearing sterile gloves, cap, and mask to reduce the potential for contamination of both the patient and the surgical suite. The technique is the same as for the preliminary scrub (three alternating scrubs) except that timing is critical when using povidone-iodine. The contact time for iodophors should be at least 5 minutes.

In some cases, the veterinarian may request a one-step prep, which may be painted on the area and left there without performing the alternating scrub. Some veterinarians may prefer that the one-step prep be painted only on the incision site itself, after the alternating sterile surgical scrubs. Preliminary scrubbing should always be performed to remove dirt and oils that might interfere with the action of the one-step prep formulas.

Draping

The drape has a number of functions. It can absorb bodily fluids such as blood and increases the size of the sterile field. It also prevents contamination of the surgeon's hands and instruments. Draping should only be performed by the surgeon or a surgical assistant in proper surgical attire (see Preoperative Preparation of the Veterinarian and the Surgical Assistant) in order to maintain asepsis. The anesthetist or the nonsterile assistant should open the outer covering of the pack on the Mayo stand. The surgical assistant will then open the second wrap and prepare to drape the animal. In general, there should be four huck towels and a sterile drape within the pack. The four huck towels should be applied first in an overlapping rectangular pattern. They will be clipped to the patient using towel clamps which should be tucked under the towels to prevent possible contamination. Towel clamps are considered contaminated once they have penetrated the skin. The sterile drape is placed over the towels. The drape may be **fenestrated** (meaning it has a hole in it) or it may be an adhesive plastic or paper drape that requires cutting in the shape of the incision.

Maintenance of the Surgical Field

Once the pack is open and the surgical drape is in place, aseptic protocol should be in place in the surgery room. In order to prevent contamination, everyone in the surgical suite, including the anesthetist and any other personnel, should have a cap, mask, and booties. Someone may be designated to leave the surgical suite to retrieve missing instruments and other items; that individual will be less sterile than the core operating team.

Excessive movement and noise should be avoided in the surgery, and nonsterile items should be kept away from everything in the sterile field. The sterile field is a sphere that includes the portion of the animal that is draped, the front of the surgeon and the surgical assistant, the Mayo stand and pack, and anything else that has been sterilized and prepared for surgery. The surgeon and the surgical assistant should not turn their backs on the sterile field and should keep their hands between waist and shoulder height to prevent contamination.

Extra items needed during surgery should be opened by the nonsterile assistant. The exterior wrap of the pack should be opened carefully and the surgical assistant or the veterinarian can then lift the material from the opened pack. If an envelope pack of suture or a scalpel blade is needed, the nonsterile assistant should open the wrapper with both hands so the veterinarian or the surgical assistant can remove it from the wrapper with a pair of needle holders or forceps.

Preoperative Preparation of the Veterinarian and the Surgical Assistant

Anyone in close proximity to the surgical site must be properly prepped for surgery including proper attire, scrubbing of the hands and arms, gloving, and gowning. This will help to prevent contamination of the surgical site. Another value of the ritual of surgical preparation is increased awareness of asepsis and focus on the patient. The time required to prepare for the surgical procedure is often used for mental preparation by the surgeon and the team.

Proper attire includes surgical scrub pants and top, a surgical bonnet or cap, a mask, and booties. These items must be worn during scrubbing, gowning, and gloving as well as during the surgical procedure itself. Booties should be removed prior to leaving the surgical suite. Technicians and surgeons should not have acrylic nails and should keep their nails trimmed short. Nails are a great place for bacteria to hide. Acrylic nails are porous, allowing bacteria and fungi to colonize between the acrylic and the nail. The same is true for nail polish. For the purposes of the following sections on scrubbing, gowning, and gloving, the term **surgeon** will be used to describe any person in the aseptic field of the patient.

Scrubbing

The surgical hand scrub removes dirt and oils that have accumulated on the hands. Any dirt or oil can carry bacteria into the surgical site. Gloves often have tiny holes and should not be relied upon for sterility. Although their surfaces are sterile, any holes in the gloves may allow moisture to wick bacteria from the hands into the incision. Once scrubbing begins, the hands should be kept above the waist and below the shoulders and that person is considered clean and must avoid contamination. If the forearms or hands come into contact with any nonsterile item, the scrub should be repeated.

Prior to beginning the scrub, the technician should remove all jewelry, open the gown and glove packs, and don the surgical cap, mask, and booties. The gown pack should contain a towel for drying the hands and arms. If it does not, a separate towel pack should be opened.

Chlorhexidine or povidone-iodine scrub may be used for the surgical hand scrub. Most sensitivity reactions are a result of povidone-iodine scrub, but have also been reported with chlorhexidine, so any redness or irritation should be monitored.

During the scrubbing procedure, the hands should always be kept higher than the elbows. Soap and water should be allowed to drip into the scrub sink from the elbows. The first step in the scrub procedure is wetting down the hands and forearms. Water helps establish a better contact with the scrub soap and increases the effectiveness of the scrub. The hand, the wrist, the forearm, and then the elbow should be run under the faucet (in that order) slowly to ensure maximum wetting. Surgical scrub is then applied to the hands and a lather is formed. A nail brush is used to scrub the nails. The nails are then cleaned with a nail cleaner to remove any debris beneath the nail. The hands are rinsed thoroughly and more surgical scrub is applied to the hands. The scrub brush is used to scrub each quadrant of each finger, each hand, each wrist, each distal forearm, and each proximal forearm. One hand and arm should be completed before the other is begun.

The quadrants are based on the anatomy of the finger. Each surface has four quadrants: medial, lateral, dorsal, and palmar. The lateral quadrant is usually the interdigital (between the fingers) area and should receive extra attention during the scrub. On the hand to the wrist, each quadrant should get 25 scrubs, and the rest of the arms should get 10 scrubs per quadrant. The contact time with the antiseptic surgical scrub should be a minimum of 5 minutes prior to rinsing.

Rinsing should be in this order: finger, dorsal surface of hand, palmar surface, wrist, forearm, elbow. Again, hands should never be below the level of the elbow. If a nonsterile surface is contacted, the procedure should be repeated starting at the beginning. The arms should be allowed to drip dry for a few seconds, then proceed to the drying step.

Drying the hands must be performed with a sterile towel. The towel is grasped at one corner and laid over the top of the opposite hand. The grasping hand dries the covered fingers, then the hand, then the wrist, then the forearm. The towel is then grasped by the dry hand, the side that was not used to dry the other hand is draped over the wet hand, and the process is repeated. The towel is then dropped onto the table or the floor for cleaning, with care taken to avoid contaminating any sterile items that may be on the surface if the towel is dropped on a table or counter.

Gowning

The surgical gown acts as a secondary sterile barrier between the surgeon and the animal. Gloves do not extend past the wrist, so an additional barrier must be used to cover the hair and skin of the forearms. Remember, hair is always considered contaminated. Even though the arms and hands are clean and disinfected, they are not considered aseptic. Gloves and gowns come out of the package sterile and if they are properly put on, the external surfaces remain sterile. Since this is the surface that comes into contact with the animal, asepsis is maintained.

Gowns may be either muslin or disposable paper. In either case, the gown should be folded in accordion pleats with the internal surface of the gown facing the surgeon assistant. The surgeon then grasps the interior of the neck (or tie strings) and brings the gown toward him or herself, allowing it to fall open by gravity. The hands are placed into the sleeves and a nonsterile assistant ties the internal ties. If the surgeon is performing closed gloving, the hands remain inside the sleeves of the gown. The surgeon can then hand the external tie to the sterile assistant who can then complete the gowning procedure and proceed to gloving. (See **Gloving**.)

If the surgeon is performing open gloving, the hands will come through the cuffs, with care taken not to contaminate the front of the gown. The surgeon will then proceed to gloving prior to completing gowning. Closed gloving is preferred because open gloving increases the risk of gown and glove contamination.

Gloving

Open gloving allows the surgeon to visualize the hands and guide them successfully into the glove. **Closed gloving** is more challenging because the surgeon cannot see the hands, but it provides increased safety.

The procedure for open gloving is performed with the hands outside of the gown cuffs. The surgeon uses the dominant hand to grasp the interior of the glove cuff (the side that touches the surgeon's skin). The nondominant hand is inserted into the glove and the cuff is pulled down to meet the cuff of the gown without flipping the cuff of the glove. The sterile side of the nondominant hand is then inserted into the cuff of the other glove (the side that touches the patient's skin) and the dominant hand is inserted into the glove. The cuff of the dominant hand glove is inverted over the cuff of the gown. The dominant hand then is used to invert the cuff of the nondominant hand glove over the gown cuff. If this has been done correctly, the only surfaces touching the animal will be sterile.

The procedure for closed gloving is a little different. In this case, the hands remain inside the cuff of the gown and are not exposed to the exterior. The glove is picked up so that the thumb is touching the thumb of the hand to be gloved through the gown, with the fingers facing the elbow along the inner surface of the arm. The edge of the cuff is grasped by the opposite hand (still through the gown) and pulled over the hand and gown cuff. The fingers are fed into the fingers of the glove and the cuff is adjusted. The procedure is repeated for the opposite hand. If done correctly, there is no chance of contamination of the external surface of the gown or gloves. This is the preferred method of gloving.

Once the gown and gloves are in place, the surgeon is considered sterile. Hands should remain above the waist and below the shoulders. They should touch no nonsterile surfaces or items. Any contamination will necessitate repeating aseptic preparation. The surgical team should now proceed from the prep room into surgery.

Intraoperative Procedures

In the surgical suite, the patient should already be prepped, with all monitoring equipment in place by the time the surgeon and surgical assistant walk into the room. This reduces the time the patient is under anesthesia and decreases the possibility of complications.

Maintaining the sterile field (the area of the surgical drape and the front of the surgeon and the surgical assistant and any other equipment) is very important. Communication should be maintained between all people in the surgical suite. Any nonsterile persons who must come close to the sterile field should announce themselves and inform the surgeon where they are in relation to the field. This will help to prevent breaks in asepsis because of accidental bumping. The surgeon should also be informed of any new instruments or materials placed within the sterile field and their location.

Patient Monitoring

Patient monitoring includes anesthetic monitoring, monitoring patient vital signs, and monitoring the equipment. The veterinary technician may be the person assigned as the anesthetist, the surgical assistant, or the nonsterile assistant. In some cases, the veterinary tech may even be both anesthetist and nonsterile assistant.

The anesthetist is in charge of anesthetic and vital sign monitoring. Vital signs include temperature, pulse, respiration, and heart rate; equipment readings include pulse oximeter, ECG, capnometer, blood pressure, gas anesthetic and oxygen flow rates, and anesthetic monitoring of reflexes (palpebral, corneal, jaw tone, and withdrawal), fluid flow rate, and planes of anesthesia.

Vital signs should be taken every 5 minutes during an anesthetic procedure. Preprinted reference charts are available that allow the technician to plot the points on a graph. This helps to establish trends that can alert the technician and the veterinarian to potential problems during anesthesia. The plotted anesthesia chart should become part of the patient's permanent record after recovery. Although a number of machine monitors are available, with audible alarms and flashing lights that alert the operator to problems, no machine can take the place of excellent nursing care. A vigilant anesthetist may make the difference between a survivable complication and an anesthetic death. More information on anesthetic monitoring can be found in Chapter 11.

The veterinarian should be informed of any dangerous trends during anesthesia. Shock symptoms (increased CRT, increased pulse rate, increased respiratory rate, decreased blood pressure) are some warning signs. Other dangerous trends include deepening plane of anesthesia past stage III and arrhythmias. The anesthetist should be familiar with the operating manuals of the various monitoring equipment available and be able to troubleshoot problems. Most anesthetic complications are due to problems with either anesthetic or oxygen flow. Therefore, the anesthetist should also be familiar with the anesthesia machine and the air-flow pattern in order to troubleshoot issues with the system. Never rely completely on a machine; instead rely on your hands, your eyes, and your brain.

Veterinarian

The veterinarian is the surgeon, pharmaceutical prescriber, and diagnostician. The surgeon will recommend the anesthetic cocktail for the procedure and any other drugs that may be required for the case. The technician should always ask the veterinarian for this information prior to the procedure. The veterinarian will also perform the procedure. During the procedure, the veterinarian may ask for additional materials or items. It is the job of the nonsterile assistant to bring materials to the sterile field (see Maintenance of the Surgical Field on page 95). The nonsterile assistant may also be given items from the sterile field for further testing (culture and sensitivity, cytology, or histopathology). Once the veterinarian has finished the procedure, the technician staff will be responsible for patient recovery.

Function of the Surgical Assistant

The surgical assistant helps the veterinarian during the surgical procedure. This may involve handing instruments to the veterinarian, organizing the pack materials, counting gauze sponges (to make sure none are left inside the animal), retracting tissues within the sterile field, and acting as an extra set of eyes for the veterinarian. In some states, skin closure is within the scope of the technician practice act. Whatever their duties, surgical assistants should be in surgical attire (sterile gown and gloves, hair cover, and mask) and must remain sterile until released by the veterinarian.

Postoperative Procedures

Postoperative procedures are just as important as pre- and intraoperative procedures. The proper postoperative maintenance of equipment, instruments, and the surgical suite is just as important as patient recovery in the smooth function of a surgical facility.

Patient Monitoring

Many fatal surgical complications occur during recovery and can be avoided with proper monitoring. Machine monitoring should continue until **extubation**, or the removal of the endotracheal tube from the animal. The patient's vital signs—TPR (temperature, pulse, and respiration), reflexes, and capillary refill time—should continue to be monitored until the animal is sternal, a sure sign of recovery. Periodic monitoring of vital signs (every 15 to 20 minutes) should continue until the animal leaves the facility.

Monitoring equipment should be inspected at least daily for proper function. Cords should be inspected, surfaces should be disinfected, and any other maintenance (such as battery changes) should be performed prior to putting the equipment away. A checklist for equipment maintenance should be maintained in the surgical suite to ensure quality control. This saves precious time during a surgical procedure. If the equipment is not functioning, the patient may not be monitored while the technician is troubleshooting or finding other equipment. This is dangerous to the patient.

Patient Recovery

The anesthetized patient is unable to control body temperature, posture, reflexes, and other biological processes, and depends on the surgeon and technicians for all of these functions. It is the technician's responsibility to maintain the patient's body temperature by using external heat sources (circulating water blankets, forced air warmers, bubble wrap, and the like) and warmed fluids. Animals recover from anesthesia much faster if they are maintained close to normal body temperature for the species. Proper body temperature assures that normal chemical reactions can occur in the animal's tissues. Reptiles should be kept within their optimum temperature zone during surgery for the same reason.

Recovering animals should be placed in normal body posture after surgery as well. An animal in lateral recumbency (lying on its side), will not be able to fully ventilate the down side of the lungs. Sternal recumbency allows both lungs to inflate fully, which will increase the rate of gas exchange (oxygen and carbon dioxide) and facilitate exhalation of anesthetic gases such as isoflurane. Discontinuing the gas anesthetic and placing the animal on 100% oxygen will also facilitate the exchange of anesthetic gases. Care must be taken to disconnect the endotracheal tube from the anesthetic machine prior to moving the animal to prevent accidentally removing the tube or damaging the trachea.

Monitoring reflexes will help to assess when the patient is ready to be extubated. In general, the first reflex to return after anesthesia is discontinued is the blink, or palpebral, reflex. The next is the withdrawal reflex and the last one is the swallow reflex. The animal should not be extubated until the swallow reflex is present. If the animal swallows twice, it is ready. Brachycephalic animals with short, broad heads, such as pugs, should be kept intubated until they begin to chew the tube. These animals have elongated soft palates, small nares (nostrils), and small tracheas, so they are already compromised. Maintaining an endotracheal tube for longer time in these animals ensures better airway maintenance during recovery.

The animal should be closely monitored until he is on his feet and walking under his own power. Recovering animals have altered states of consciousness and may have behavioral issues that they do not have when awake. They are also ataxic (unsteady) and may injure themselves during this period.

Postoperative Instrument and Equipment Care

Surgical instruments are expensive pieces of equipment. They require care and maintenance in order to perform their function properly. Surgical instruments are generally made from stainless steel. They can range in price from $14 to $1,400 for a single instrument. Improper care or mishandling can result in broken, corroded, or misshapen instruments that must be replaced.

The entire pack should be brought to the surgical prep area and broken down as soon as possible after surgery. All gauze sponges (soiled and fresh) and instruments should be counted and checked against the pack inventory. Missing sponges or instruments may be in the animal. It is best to use gauze sponges with a radio-opaque line woven in. These sponges can be seen on a routine radiograph if they are accidentally left in the animal. Stainless steel instruments will also show up on a routine radiograph. After counting, the instruments should be opened (open the ratchet or lock box) and placed in cold water to prevent sticking of debris. Another cold water bath will help to loosen blood from muslin drapes and towels.

Cleaning

Detergent is added to warm water and the instruments should have all surfaces scrubbed with a soft brush. After the initial cleaning, the instruments should be placed in an ultrasonic cleaner to remove hidden debris, and then rinsed and dried. Instruments with hinges and lock boxes should be sprayed down with lubricant surgical milk and dried again. They are now ready for the autoclave. Instruments should be sterilized with the lock boxes in the open position for all methods except dry-heat sterilization. Dry-heat sterilization sterilizes by conduction of heat which is transmitted through the body of the instrument. All other methods sterilize by surface contact.

Prior to being packed for sterilization, fabric items such as gowns, drapes, and towels should be rinsed well, then laundered separately from other clinic materials such as bedding.

Common Surgical Procedures

Many surgical procedures are considered routine in veterinary medicine because they are performed either frequently in the practice or on an elective basis. However, no surgical procedure is without risk. Any procedure requiring general anesthesia and/or entering a body cavity poses a potential danger to the patient. It is important to minimize the risks as much as possible by providing excellent nursing care and following routines in surgery that minimize mistakes. This will enable the technician to be prepared if an emergency arises and anticipate both the veterinarian's and the patient's needs.

The most common complication during a surgical procedure is shock. Excellent patient monitoring enables the technician to anticipate potential problems with shock, which is a decrease in systemic blood pressure or cardiac output. During surgery, shock can occur secondarily to hemorrhage, pain, anesthetic overdose, oxygen deprivation, or dehydration. Treatment may be as simple as turning down the anesthetic flow rate, putting the patient on 100% oxygen, increasing patient body temperature, and providing increased fluid flow rates. Drugs can also increase cardiac output or stabilize arrhythmias due to shock.

Another possible postoperative complication is wound dehiscence (separation of the wound edges). This may occur secondary to infection, traumatic injury (usually due to self-mutilation), suture reaction, or poor surgical technique. Dehiscence can occur in the internal layers or in the skin. Internal dehiscences may occasionally be referred to as incisional herniation. Prevention of infection has already been discussed in the surgical preparation section. Prevention of traumatic injury includes keeping the patient quiet and preventing excessive activity including running, jumping, or excessive play activity during the postoperative period. Since wound healing normally requires 10 to 14 days, the patient should be kept at a decreased activity level for that time period. If external sutures have been used, the animal may go back to normal activity levels after suture removal. It is good practice to recommend a recheck after 7 to 10 days to assess the animal for postoperative complications.

Suture selection can play a role in postoperative recovery. Sutures comes in various sizes from 7-0 (smallest ophthalmic suture) to 3 (large-animal suture) and are either absorbable or nonabsorbable, natural or synthetic, inert or reactive, and monofilament or braided. **Absorbable** suture material may be left in the patient and is made to be absorbed over time. A **nonabsorbable** suture may either be left in the patient or removed after healing. Inert substances (such as stainless steel) may be left within the animal because the body will not react. Reactive materials (such as some plastics) may need to be removed to prevent the body from having a foreign-body reaction (inflammation).

The ideal suture does not exist. The ideal suture would retain its strength in tissues until the tissue is completely healed, then dissolve. It would not cause foreign-body reaction and would produce minimal inflammation. It would have enough friction to hold a surgical knot without untying but would have minimum tissue drag, and it would be flexible. Because this magic suture does not exist, veterinarians develop preferences for one or more types of suture depending on their characteristics.

Natural, absorbable, reactive, monofilament suture material is surgical gut made from the submucosa of the intestines of a sheep. It is highly reactive and is broken down by inflammation and phagocytosis (neutrophils) in the animal. Because of this inflammatory reaction, it breaks down quickly (within 1 to 3 weeks) and can lead to dehiscence. On the other hand, it forms excellent knots and handles well.

Synthetic, absorbable, inert, monofilament suture material, such as PDS™ (polydiaxinone), has decreased tissue drag (as a monofilament) and retains its shape, but requires multiple throws to maintain knot strength. It maintains its strength for 2 to 4 weeks in tissues and will actually remain in the tissues for 6 months before breaking down completely. Maxon™ (polyglyconate) has similar characteristics to PDS. Monocryl™ (polyglecaprone) is a monofilament that breaks down quickly (like gut), but does not cause the intense reaction of gut. It does not have the strength of the other synthetic monofilaments. Monocryl Plus™ is a coated monofilament that decreases the bacterial colonization. Biosyn™ (glycomer 631) is similar in use to Monocryl and breaks down quickly, but has the strength of Maxon and PDS.

Natural, nonabsorbable, reactive, braided suture material, such as silk, is made from the cocoon of the silkworm. It is strong and has excellent handling characteristics including knot holding. On the other hand, it causes severe tissue reaction and can act as a wick for bacterial contamination. It usually degenerates after 6 months in the body. Cotton and linen have similar characteristics to silk, but are rarely used in veterinary medicine.

Synthetic, nonabsorbable, inert, braided suture material, such as polyester, has good handling ability, but has increased tissue drag and knots tend to slip. It tends to wick bacteria. Polymerized caprolactam (Braunamid™ or Supramid™) is similar to polyester in characteristics, but is coated to reduce tissue drag. It will also wick bacteria.

Synthetic, nonabsorbable, inert, monofilament suture material, such as stainless steel, does not support bacterial growth and retains its strength even in the face of severe tissue reaction due to infection. On the other hand, it does not handle well and tends to kink. Nylon (polyamide) comes in both monofilament and braided forms. While it does not cause tissue reaction, it does not handle well (knots can slip). There is little chance of wicking. Prolene™ (polypropylene) is similar to nylon but maintains its strength for longer periods of time. Novafil™ (polybutester) is also similar to nylon, but has significant stretch; it is commonly used for ligament and tendon surgeries.

Synthetic, absorbable, inert, braided suture material, such as Dexon™ (polyglycolic acid), has excellent handling characteristics (knot tying and holding) and good initial strength, but it breaks down rapidly in tissues (1 to 2 weeks). It has increased tissue drag and can cause bacterial wicking if used as an external suture. Vicryl™ (polyglactin 910) is a coated suture material that has similar characteristics to Dexon. Polysorb™ (glycolside-lactide copolymer) is another suture material similar to Dexon.

Small Animals

Surgeries are more commonly performed on small animals (dogs and cats) than on large animals. Although surgical procedures ranging from open heart surgery to limb amputation are seen in veterinary practices, elective surgeries are the most frequently performed. An **elective surgery** is one that is not essential to maintaining the life or function of the animal and may be scheduled at the owner's or the veterinarian's convenience. A **nonelective surgery** is one that must be performed as quickly as possible to maintain the life or function of the animal. Elective surgeries may also be performed as nonelective procedures in certain circumstances. This will be discussed more thoroughly in the following sections.

Ovariohysterectomy

The **ovariohysterectomy** (OHE), more commonly known as spaying, is the most common elective procedure in female dogs and cats. The procedure requires complete removal of the uterus and the ovaries and is performed electively as a means of preventing pregnancy or on a nonelective basis to treat such diseases as pyometra (infected uterus), dystocia (difficult birth), ovarian cysts, or uterine or ovarian neoplasia. Dogs spayed prior to 6 months of age have a much lower incidence of mammary cancer later in life. If possible, the bitch should be in anestrus or between 4 and 6 months of age to minimize the size of the uterus and uterine blood supply.

Because this is an abdominal surgery, postoperative pain control should be considered.

Instrumentation

A full surgical pack including 4 towels, a drape, a spay hook, several hemostatic and Kelly forceps, a pair of needle holders, scalpel blade handle, tissue forceps, towel clamps, scissors (surgical, Mayo, and Metzenbaum), and multiple sterile gauze sponges should be prepared. A #10 scalpel blade, several types of suture material (of the veterinarian's preference), and additional gauze sponges in a separate pack should also be available if needed. For a nonelective spay, additional clamps, bowls, retractors, and saline flush may be needed.

Technique

The ventral midline of the animal is prepared as stated in the section on Preoperative Preparation. The incision will be along the ventral midline somewhere between the umbilicus and the pubis, so the shaved area should be from approximately 2 cm above the umbilicus to the pubis. Veterinarians differ as to the size of the incision they prefer, but the initial cut is usually 1 to 2 cm below the umbilicus and extends caudally. In cases of a nonelective spay, the incision may be much larger and extend farther cranially, requiring a larger area to be shaved and prepped. The surgical prep is performed by the nonsterile assistant.

Once the animal is prepped, towels are placed in a square around the proposed incision and a sterile drape is placed. These two steps must be performed by the sterile assistant or the veterinarian. Once the animal is draped, the veterinarian begins the procedure. The skin is incised first, then the subcutaneous fat, then the abdomen is penetrated by incising the linea alba. The linea alba is an **aponeurosis** (fascia connection) between the two sides of the abdominal musculature. The peritoneum is the internal layer of the linea alba. This is the same approach used for an exploratory **laparotomy** or any other abdominal surgery. For cranial abdominal surgeries, such as gastrotomy (stomach surgery), liver, or spleen, the incision will extend cranially to the umbilicus.

Once the abdomen has been entered, the uterine horns are located and exteriorized. The ovaries are located and a clamp is placed on the connective tissue between the ovary and the uterine horn and over the ovarian artery/vein stump. The ovarian blood vessels are then ligated (tied off with suture), and cut above the suture. The suspensory ligament between the ovary and the crus of the diaphragm may need to be separated in order to exteriorize the ovary. The other uterine horn is located and the procedure is repeated.

Once both ovarian stumps are ligated, the clamps should be removed and assessed for bleeding. Bleeding stumps should be reclamped and religated. The uterine horns are followed caudally to the uterine body, which is clamped and double ligated. The clamps are removed and the uterine stump is again assessed for bleeding.

The incision is closed beginning at the muscle layer in a simple interrupted pattern. The subcutaneous and cutaneous tissues may be closed in a va-

riety of patterns, but should be closed separately from each other. External sutures may also be used. These should be removed 10 to 14 days after surgery. In most states, it is within the technician's scope of practice to perform skin closures. The most common skin closure is the simple interrupted pattern.

Possible complications include hemorrhage of the ovarian or uterine stumps; ligation of the ureter, which can cause renal failure; and dehiscence.

Orchidectomy

Orchidectomy, more commonly known as neutering or castration, is the second most common elective surgical procedure in small animals. This is the complete removal of the testicles. Advantages to orchidectomy are numerous: prevention of pregnancy, prevention of testicular cancers, prostatic hypertrophy/prostatitis and perianal adenomas, decreased roaming behaviors, possible decreased aggression, and decreased urine odor in cats. The procedure may be performed at any time, although, in cats, castration at 6 to 7 months of age may prevent urine spraying and fighting due to testosterone. Nonelective orchidectomy may be performed in animals with testicular tumors (most of which are benign), perianal adenomas, or prostatic problems. Removal of the hormones that lead to these problems may result in complete resolution of symptoms.

Both testicles must be removed. Cryptorchid (hidden or retained testicle) animals may have the testicle in the inguinal canal or in the abdominal cavity. Such animals require an abdominal approach to remove the hidden testicle (**cryptorchidectomy**). Retained testicles have a higher incidence of testicular cancer than scrotal testicles and should be removed.

Instrumentation

The canine neuter requires a full surgical pack including a scalpel handle, thumb forceps, hemostatic forceps and Kelly forceps, a needle holder, and scissors (surgical and Mayo). Full draping (including towels, towel clamp, and drape) is generally performed. A #10 scalpel blade and absorbable suture material are generally used.

The feline neuter requires only a scalpel handle, thumb forceps, and hemostatic forceps. Although this is performed using aseptic technique, the area is rarely draped prior to the incision. A #10 scalpel blade is used. Absorbable suture may be used in some cases.

Technique in the Canine

The anesthetized dog should be placed in dorsal recumbency in a frog-legged position. Preparation for the canine neuter involves shaving the prepuce, inguinal, and prescrotal areas with a #40 clipper blade. The veterinarian may prefer not to shave the scrotum itself to prevent irritation and clipper burns that may increase self-mutilation after surgery. The prescrotal area and scrotum is then prepped as previously with alternating scrubs, toweled in with towel clamps, and draped. The veterinarian pushes the testicle into the prescrotal area and makes an incision through the prescrotal skin on the midline over the displaced testicle. The testicle is exteriorized through the incision and an incision is made through the vaginal tunic encasing the testicle. The testicle, testicular artery, vas deferens, and pampiniform plexus can then be visualized, clamped, and ligated. The testicular artery, pampiniform plexus, and vas deferens are then cut between the clamp and the testicle is removed. The stump is then examined for bleeding, and the procedure is repeated on the other side. Simple closure of the subcutaneous and skin is all that is needed. This procedure is called an open castration because the vaginal tunics are opened and the testicle and blood vessels are visualized.

Closed castration means that the vaginal tunics remain closed. In this type of castration, the covered testicle and blood vessels are exteriorized and a clamp is placed. A suture ligature is placed around the entire stalk and the entire structure is cut and examined for hemorrhage. The advantage of the closed castration is that it maintains the integrity of the inguinal canal. Incorrect ligation of the blood vessels in a closed castration may cause severe abdominal hemorrhage and should be corrected if it occurs. Closure is the same as for the open procedure.

In cases of cryptorchid testicles, an abdominal approach is needed. The abdominal approach requires a skin incision made around one side of the penis and prepuce. Once the skin has been incised, a ventral midline approach through the linea alba is made. The vas deferens and pampiniform plexus are located, clamped, and ligated and the testicle is removed. The muscle layer and skin are closed as described in the ovariohysterectomy section.

Technique in the Feline

The anesthetized cat is generally placed in either lateral recumbency or dorsal recumbency with the legs forward depending on the preference of the veterinarian. The hair is generally plucked from the scrotum by pulling the hair with the pad of the thumb and index finger until all hair has been removed. Shaving will generally cause more irritation than plucking and should be avoided. The area is aseptically prepared with alternating scrubs. The surgeon should wear surgical gloves and a gown.

An incision is made directly into the scrotum and the testicle is exteriorized. An incision is made through the vaginal tunic and the blood vessels are clamped and ligated. Another technique is to tie the entire cord in a knot, or to separate the pampiniform plexus and vas deferens and tie them together in a square knot. The last two techniques avoid possible suture reaction at the site, but may increase the chance of hemorrhage. The stumps of the blood vessels are allowed to retract within the tunic and the incisions are left to drain without suturing.

Complications of feline orchidectomy include hemorrhage, swelling, and self-mutilation. Elizabethan collars and proper preparation of the area may reduce the incidence of self-mutilation and checking stumps prior to leaving surgery will reduce the incidence of hemorrhage and swelling.

Onychectomy

Onychectomy, or declawing, is the removal of the claw and the associated third phalanx. This is an amputation. There are many different techniques for this procedure. The veterinarian will use whatever technique he or she has been trained to perform. This procedure is very painful for the cat, and owners should be made aware of this prior to having their pets undergo the procedure. In some countries, declaws are no longer allowed because of the pain involved. Many veterinarians recommend only declawing the front feet because the cat will still be able to defend itself and might be able to still climb trees if it still has rear claws.

Although the onychectomy is painful and may seem barbaric, it has its place. It will prevent destruction of furniture and can decrease injury to children, the elderly, and immunosuppressed or diabetic people. Cats that might otherwise need to be relinquished to the humane society may be kept in a home if they are declawed.

Cats have a retractable third phalanx to which the claw is attached. The musculature allows retraction of the claw into a sheath of skin rather like a switchblade when it is at rest (this actually puts the joint in extension). The extension of the claw occurs through action of the deep digital flexor tendon on the ventral side of the phalanx. The only feline that does not have retractable claws is the cheetah. Cats do not walk on the third phalanx, so removal should not affect ambulation (the ability to walk). Dogs use their third phalanx and claws to ambulate, so declaw should never be performed in canines unless medically necessary.

Instrumentation

Instrumentation for onychectomy is as varied as the techniques used. In general, a scalpel blade (either #11, #12, or #10 blade depending on preference), a blade handle, and a pair of Kelly or Carmault forceps or towel clamps are used. In some cases, a pair of guillotine nail trimmers may be used instead of the scalpel blade and forceps. Some practices use a laser to cut the tissues. Laser surgery may decrease bleeding and postoperative swelling.

Technique

The feet are prepped using alternating scrubs of chlorhexidine and alcohol. Long-haired cats should always be clipped, but some surgeons prefer leaving the feet unshaved to reduce postoperative inflammation and pruritis.

A ring block using Lidocaine with epinephrine should be placed at the carpus or tarsus. The block should begin at the lateral styloid process of the ulna/lateral malleolus, medially at the radial insertion/medial malleolus, then at the carpal or tarsal pad. All blocks should be in place a minimum of 5 minutes prior to the first incision to allow maximal efficacy of pain control. The ring block should be effective in controlling intraoperative and postoperative pain for a few hours and preventing wind-up (see Chapter 11).

A tourniquet is then placed at the elbow or the tarsus and the forceps are used to grasp the toenail or claw and extend it fully from the sheath. Incision is made on the dorsal surface of the claw proximal to the third phalanx, cutting through the lateral collateral ligaments, the extensor tendon, and the digital flexor tendon. The entire third phalanx must be removed to prevent regrowth of the claw. Care should be taken not to cut through the digital pad because that would interfere with healing.

Once the claw has been removed, the resulting hole should be checked and the skin closed with surgical glue such as Nexaband®. The procedure should be repeated on all five claws on the front feet (four claws on the rear). The foot should then be bandaged with gauze sponges and surgical tape or vet wrap and the tourniquet removed.

Postoperative pain control is a must after onchyectomy even though regional nerve blocks have been used. Opiates such as buprenorphine provide excellent analgesia. Some veterinarians use a single dose of the NSAID meloxicam prior to surgery. This will last 24 to 30 hours postoperatively for pain control. Clay and clumping litter should be avoided. Newspaper litter is safer in these cases.

Complications of onchyectomy include hemorrhage, infection, and dehiscence.

Caudectomy and Dewclaw Removal

Caudectomy, or tail dock, and dewclaw removal are often performed on purebred puppies from breeds for which the AKC recommends specific tail length and no front or rear dewclaws. Terriers, corgis, and other breeds are subject to those standards. The veterinarian and technician must be sure to consult the AKC and the owner about the desired length of the tail, especially in show animals. Incorrect tail length may disqualify the animal. These procedures are usually performed 2 to 3 days after birth without general anesthesia. Local anesthesia may be used for the caudectomy procedure.

Instrumentation

A pair of Mayo scissors and a pair of mosquito forceps along with needle holders and absorbable suture are usually all that is required for these procedures.

Technique

The puppy is held with the tail up and the ventral side facing the surgeon. The feet are restrained. The tail is prepped with alternating surgical scrubs and the veterinarian grasps the tail to reduce blood flow, counts the required number of vertebrae and cuts the tail with the Mayo scissors distal to that point. Sutures are then placed in the skin to cover the stump. Sutures are generally clipped short to prevent the dam from removing them while grooming the pup.

The puppy is then flipped on its side and each individual leg is restrained to give the veterinarian access to the dewclaws. Each dewclaw is grasped at the base (proximal to the pad) with a pair of mosquito forceps and twisted to remove the dewclaw or cut with scissors. Any remaining piece of bone from the dewclaw should also be removed to prevent regrowth. The resulting skin defect should then be sutured.

The major complication with this procedure is wound dehiscence from overgrooming by the dam. This may result in excessive scarring or even keloid formation.

Large Animals

Many large-animal procedures are performed with the animal either awake or in twilight or standing anesthesia with a local anesthetic. Putting a large animal under general anesthesia requires specialized instrumentation such as a lift table. General anesthesia has many risks for large animals, including bloat in ruminants (cattle, goats, and sheep), broken limbs in horses (during recovery and induction), myositis and myoglobinuria (in all large animals), and malignant hyperthermia in pigs.

If a large animal is to be placed under general anesthesia, an entire team and a great deal of preparation are needed to prevent injury to the animal, the veterinarian, and the rest of the team. The induction area must be free of protrusions that can injure the animal, the room should be thickly padded, and the animal's hooves should be wrapped in tape to prevent self-injury.

Horses and pigs are generally intubated prior to surgery. A 12-hour preoperative fast will help to empty stomach contents and prevent aspiration in pigs. In horses, vomiting does not occur, but a 12-hour fast will make respiration easier by emptying the stomach. In ruminants, a 24- to 30-hour fast may be needed prior to surgery to empty out the stomach. A nasogastric tube may be inserted to prevent gas bloat in these animals.

Although general anesthesia is rare in ruminants, sheep and goats are commonly used as research animals and may require general anesthesia for certain procedures. General anesthesia is far more common in equines for orthopedic injuries and colic surgeries. The techniques covered in this section will focus on procedures performed in general practice, not at equine surgical specialty centers.

Orchidectomy (Gelding or Castration)

This procedure is usually performed in the field either as a standing procedure or in lateral recumbency. This is the most common procedure in the horse. Cryptorchids can also be castrated as a standing procedure through the inguinal canal. Technicians usually participate in surgical prep, anesthesia, and animal restraint.

Instrumentation

The instrumentation required for castration is minimal. A scalpel blade handle and a #10 blade and an emasculator are often all that is needed for horse castrations. The veterinarian should have sterile surgical gloves with sleeves.

For ruminant castration, the same instruments are generally needed.

Technique

For standing castration, the horse is heavily sedated and the scrotum and inguinal cord are injected with local anesthetic. The scrotum is incised over the testicles, the testicles are pulled through the opening, and an emasculator is placed around the spermatic cord. It is important to orient the emasculator properly so that the cord is cut distal to the crush. In common parlance, it should go nut-to-nut which means that the side of the emasculator with the nut on it should be closest to the testicle. The incisions are left open to drain and the horse is put on stall rest for 24 hours, then on minimal exercise for 3 to 4 days.

If the animal is to be under general anesthesia, it should be placed in lateral recumbency with the upper leg pulled forward to expose the scrotum. The procedure is otherwise the same.

Ruminants generally are done as standing castrations. They are restrained in a squeeze chute and the scrotum and spermatic cord are injected with local anesthetic. The scrotum is incised circumferentially and the emasculator is used in the same fashion. The incision is allowed to drain.

Caslick's Procedure

Caslick's procedure is the most commonly performed procedure in female horses. Many thoroughbreds have insufficient vaginas, which means that the vulva extends too far dorsally. This can result in air and feces entering the vagina, which can lead to infection. Caslick's procedure will prevent that from occurring by decreasing the length of the vulvar slit.

Instrumentation

The instrumentation required is fairly minimal and includes a scalpel blade holder, a #10 blade, a pair of thumb forceps, and a pair of Mayo scissors.

Technique

The tail is diverted to one side and the vulva is prepped aseptically. The veterinarian wears sterile surgical gloves. The horse is sedated and local anesthetic is infiltrated into the lips of the vulva. The dorsal vulva is incised on both sides by the veterinarian and the freshened edges are sutured together to shorten the length of the slit using a continuous suture pattern.

Practice Questions

1. Which of the following means the removal of visible soil from a surface?
   a. cleaning
   b. disinfecting
   c. antisepsis
   d. sterilization

2. Which of the following will NOT result in fewer postoperative complications?
   a. use of analgesics during surgery
   b. intraoperative fluid therapy
   c. maintenance of asepsis in the surgical suite
   d. All of the above will result in fewer postoperative complications.

3. Glutaraldehyde is which of the following?
   a. a cleanser
   b. a disinfectant
   c. an antiseptic
   d. all of the above

4. Your clinic had four dogs with parvovirus come in. The disinfectant that you use says it is effective against this infection at a 1:50 dilution. Which of the following should you do?
   a. Mix the solution until it is the right color in the bucket.
   b. Make a double-strength solution because the whole clinic is infected.
   c. Mix according to label directions.
   d. Use Nolvasan® because the disinfectant smells bad.

5. You are prepping an animal for surgery. The veterinarian would like you to use povidone-iodine. Which of the following should be used as the alternating scrub?
   a. alcohol
   b. saline
   c. chlorhexidine
   d. Povidone should not be used an alternating scrub technique.

6. Which of the following is true of quaternary ammonium compounds?
   a. They are inactivated by soft water.
   b. They cannot be used on cotton.
   c. They can be used as antiseptics.
   d. They work best on gram-positive organisms that have a sugar cell wall.

7. Which of the following works by coagulation of proteins in the bacteria?
   a. steam autoclave
   b. plasma
   c. ethylene oxide
   d. irradiation

8. Which of the following works by free radical production?
   a. steam autoclave
   b. plasma
   c. ethylene oxide
   d. irradiation

9. Which of the following is true of steam sterilization?
   a. Rubber cannot be sterilized in a steam autoclave.
   b. Steam should be at 100° Celsius for 15 minutes for sterilization.
   c. The autoclave door should be opened completely after the cycle is completed to dry the pack adequately.
   d. Indicator tape is sufficient indication that the instruments in the pack are sterile.

10. How long should instruments remain in a cold sterilization bath before they are considered sterile?
   a. 5 minutes
   b. 30 minutes
   c. 3 hours
   d. 24 hours

11. Where should surgical packs be stored to ensure the longest maintenance of sterility?
   a. in the surgical suite in an open cabinet
   b. in an open cabinet outside the surgery
   c. in a closed cabinet inside the surgery
   d. in a closed cabinet outside the surgery

12. Which of the following will NOT invalidate pack sterility?
   a. putting a sterilization indicator strip inside the pack
   b. getting the pack wet
   c. overcrowding the autoclave
   d. forgetting to write the date of sterilization on the pack

13. A veterinary assistant packed the packs last week. You are in surgery with the doctor and notice that the box locks are all closed on the instruments. The pack had been sterilized in a steam autoclave.
   a. You allow the veterinarian to proceed with the surgery because the pack is fine.
   b. You ask the veterinary assistant to get you another pack from two weeks ago.
   c. You ask the veterinarian what he or she would like to do.
   d. You lecture the veterinary assistant in front of the doctor.

14. Which of the following is true of packing instruments and packs?
   a. The pack should be wrapped as tightly as possible.
   b. The pack should contain as many gauze sponges as are able to fit.
   c. The pack should be labeled with the technician's name and the date of sterilization.
   d. The instruments do not need to be counted prior to wrapping.

15. Which is NOT one of the *four rights* of surgical procedures?
   a. right animal
   b. right owner
   c. right sex
   d. right body part

16. Which of the following is important for preoperative preparation of the owner?
   a. estimate of costs
   b. consent forms
   c. education on the risks of anesthesia and surgery
   d. all of the above

17. Why should all pharmaceuticals that will be given to the animal during induction and anesthesia be drawn up prior to surgery?
   a. to minimize distraction of the technician
   b. to smooth induction
   c. to save time
   d. all of the above

18. Which of the following should NOT be recorded in the anesthetic record?
   a. time of induction
   b. response of the animal at induction
   c. time of preanesthetic administration
   d. dose and concentration of drugs

19. How often should the animal's temperature, pulse, and respiration be monitored on the anesthetic record?
 a. every minute
 b. every 5 minutes
 c. every 15 minutes
 d. only if the animal is having a problem

20. An animal under anesthesia is turning blue. There is no evidence of blockage of the tube and the anesthetic machine appears to be working fine (the oxygen is on, the tubes are not kinked, the Sodasorb® is fresh). Which of the following is likely?
 a. the cuff is overinflated
 b. the tube diameter is too wide
 c. the tube is inserted too far
 d. some other problem

21. Which of the following is NOT an identifying structure of the glottis?
 a. hyoid apparatus
 b. vocal cords
 c. epiglottis
 d. arytenoid cartilage

22. Where is the epiglottis normally found?
 a. at the base of the mouth
 b. between the arytenoid cartilages
 c. hooked over the soft palate
 d. in the esophagus

23. Which of the following animals should NOT have a cuffed endotracheal tube?
 a. a rabbit
 b. a pig
 c. a horse
 d. a parakeet

24. Which of the following is true regarding clippers?
 a. A #10 blade should be used to perform a surgical clip.
 b. Clipper burn can increase self-mutilation postoperatively.
 c. Clipper blades should be stored dry to prevent contamination.
 d. Clippers should be held at a 45-degree angle to the skin to prevent clipper burn.

25. Which surgical scrub should be performed wearing surgical gloves?
 a. preliminary scrub
 b. sterile surgical scrub
 c. neither; they can both be done wearing exam gloves
 d. both **a** and **b**

26. How should a surgical scrub be performed?
 a. spiraling out from the incision site
 b. in stripes with the first stripe being over the incision site
 c. spiraling in from the outside edges of the incision site
 d. in stripes, with the second stripe being over the incision site

27. Which of the following is an acceptable method of sterile surgical scrub?
 a. chlorhexidine alternating with povidone-iodine
 b. povidone-iodine alternating with alcohol
 c. one-step prep painted on the surgical site and removed with alcohol
 d. chlorhexidine alternating with alcohol

28. Which of the following is true of draping?
    a. huck towels are placed prior to draping
    b. huck towels are placed after draping
    c. huck towels may be used in place of the drape
    d. huck towels are completely unnecessary

29. Which of the following is NOT considered part of the sterile field?
    a. the drape
    b. the thighs of the surgeon, covered by the gown
    c. the suture material used for closure
    d. the arms of the surgical assistant

30. Which of the following is NOT considered appropriate attire for the surgeon or the surgical assistant?
    a. surgical scrubs (tucked in)
    b. a surgical bonnet
    c. a wedding ring covered by tape
    d. a mask

31. What is acceptable nail care for surgeons and surgical assistants?
    a. nails should be kept short unless they are acrylic
    b. acrylic nails are acceptable if they are scrubbed an extra 5 minutes
    c. nail polish seals the nail and prevents bacterial colonization
    d. nails should be scrubbed and picked prior to the rest of the hand

32. Which of the following is true?
    a. Once a mask has been put on, it is acceptable to touch the nose with the gloved hand.
    b. It is proper to keep the hands in the prayer position above the waist once gowning and gloving have been completed.
    c. The back of the surgeon and the surgical assistant are considered sterile once gowning and gloving are completed.
    d. Water should be allowed to drip from the hands prior to drying with a towel.

33. How many scrubs should each quadrant on the hand get?
    a. 5
    b. 10
    c. 20
    d. 25

34. How many scrubs should each quadrant on the arm get?
    a. 5
    b. 10
    c. 20
    d. 25

35. How many zones should be scrubbed?
    a. each finger 4 quadrants, the hand 4 quadrants, the wrist 4 quadrants, the distal forearm 4 quadrants, the proximal forearm 4 quadrants
    b. each finger 4 quadrants, the hand 4 quadrants, the distal forearm 4 quadrants, the proximal forearm 4 quadrants
    c. each finger 4 quadrants, the hand 2 quadrants, the distal forearm 4 quadrants, the proximal forearm 4 quadrants
    d. each finger 4 quadrants, the hand 2 quadrants, the forearm 4 quadrants

36. For maximum asepsis, how long should the hand scrub last?

  a. 1 minute

  b. 2 minutes

  c. 3 minutes

  d. 5 minutes

37. Surgeons need to wear a gown even if they are wearing gloves. Which statement does NOT apply?

  a. The hair on the forearms is considered contaminated even after sterile surgical scrub.

  b. The sterile field is considered the entire draped area, which is larger than the length of the surgical gloves.

  c. The gown acts as a secondary sterile barrier between the surgeon and the animal.

  d. The surgeon may lean against the surgical table while performing surgery.

38. Which statement about gloving in NOT correct?

  a. Open gloving has the highest possibility of contamination.

  b. Closed gloving means that the hands are outside the gown and the glove pack is closed prior to proceeding.

  c. Once the surgeon is gloved, if he or she touches a nonsterile surface, aseptic preparation should be repeated.

  d. A surgeon performing closed gloving may hand the outside tie of the gown to the assistant prior to donning gloves.

39. Which of the following is NOT important in a surgical suite?

  a. communication

  b. music

  c. monitoring

  d. awareness

40. Which of the following is NOT an anesthetic complication?

  a. shock

  b. blood loss

  c. stage IV anesthesia

  d. arrhythmias

41. Which of the following is NOT a reflex commonly monitored during anesthesia?

  a. palpebral

  b. patellar

  c. jaw tone

  d. withdrawal

42. Which of the following is NOT a job of the veterinary technician?

  a. recovering the animal

  b. administering anesthesia

  c. maintaining and operating patient monitoring and anesthesia equipment

  d. deciding which anesthetic protocol to use

43. Which of the following statements regarding extubation is correct?

  a. Animals should be extubated when they have tongue movement.

  b. Animals should be extubated when they are swallowing.

  c. Animals should be extubated when they are chewing.

  d. Appropriate time to extubate an animal may vary according to breed.

44. Which of the following is true regarding postoperative instrument care?
  a. Instruments should be soaked in hot water after use to loosen blood and fat.
  b. Instruments should immediately be placed in the ultrasonic cleaner.
  c. Instruments should be sprayed with instrument milk prior to cleaning.
  d. Instruments should be cleaned with detergent and a soft brush.

45. Which of the following is NOT a cause of wound dehiscence?
  a. use of reactive sutures
  b. failure to place external sutures
  c. self-mutilation
  d. increased activity after surgery

46. Which suture is the least likely to cause suture reaction or wicking of bacteria?
  a. silk
  b. Monocryl™
  c. stainless steel
  d. Vicryl™

47. What is an elective surgery?
  a. one that requires preoperative bloodwork
  b. one that is done at the convenience of the veterinarian and the owner
  c. one that has no inherent risks
  d. one that is medically necessary

48. Which of the following is a nonelective surgery?
  a. an ovariohysterectomy for pyometra
  b. an orchidectomy for prostatic hypertrophy
  c. a declaw for malignant melanoma of the nail bed
  d. all of the above are nonelective

49. Which of the following are NOT common general anesthesia complications in the horse?
  a. fractures
  b. hemorrhage
  c. bloat
  d. myositis/myoglobinuria

50. Which statement about castration is false?
  a. It is often performed as a standing procedure in both cattle and horses.
  b. The emasculator should have the side with the nut on the side of the spermatic cord with the testicle to prevent severe hemorrhage.
  c. Incisions are usually left open to drain postoperatively.
  d. Local anesthesia is generally placed in the scrotum only.

Answers and Explanations

1. a. Cleaning is the removal of visible soil from a surface. Disinfecting is the removal from a surface of living organisms to an acceptable level, antisepsis is the removal of organisms from a living surface to an acceptable level, and sterilization is the complete removal of all living organisms.

2. d. All of the above will result in fewer postoperative complications. Analgesics will decrease pain, intraoperative fluid therapy may prevent shock and will maintain kidney function and hydration, and maintenance of asepsis will prevent secondary bacterial contamination.

3. b. Glutaraldehyde is a disinfectant or sterilant. It will kill living tissues, so it cannot be used as an antiseptic, and it has no cleaning activity.

4. c. You should mix according to label directions. Mixing to color does not guarantee the right concentration and double strength of the solution may decrease the efficacy of the disinfectant.

5. b. Saline. Alcohol will inactivate povidone-iodine's residual antiseptic properties.

6. b. Quaternary ammonium compounds are inactivated by contact with cotton. They are inactivated by hard water and should not be used on the skin. They work best on gram-negative organisms because those organisms have a lipid wall. Quaternary ammonium compounds are detergents, so they dissolve lipids.

7. a. Heat (direct or steam) acts by causing coagulation of proteins inside the cell. Plasma causes free radical oxidation, ethylene oxide causes alkylation of DNA, and irradiation causes DNA disruption.

8. b. Plasma causes free radical oxidation. Heat (direct or steam) acts by causing coagulation of proteins inside the cell, ethylene oxide causes alkylation of DNA, and irradiation causes DNA disruption.

9. a. Rubber will break down in a steam autoclave. Steam should be at 121° Celsius for 15 minutes to cause sterilization. The autoclave door should be cracked open after the cycle is completed. Fully opening the door will cause condensation and invalidate the sterilization. Indicator strips should be included within every pack to ensure that the interior of the pack achieved the correct temperature and pressure.

10. c. Three hours is the minimum amount of time for glutaraldehyde to completely kill organisms. Lock boxes should be in the open position.

11. d. Surgical packs should be stored in a closed cabinet to increase longevity. Prevention of dust contamination is important. The reason they should be kept outside of the surgery is to reduce clutter and the possibility of contamination by dust.

12. a. Putting an indicator strip in the pack ensures sterility. Getting the pack wet will result in wicking of bacteria. Overcrowding the autoclave impairs steam circulation. Forgetting to write the date of sterilization on the pack will invalidate the sterilization because there is no way to know how old the pack is.

13. b. Hopefully, you were the one who made the packs two weeks ago. Locking the box locks prevents adequate penetration of the steam. Lecturing the assistant in front of the veterinarian would be poor communications and management practice. The correct thing to do is to get another pack, even if the veterinarian says it is all right to use the present one.

14. c. The pack should be labeled with the technician's name and the date of sterilization. All instruments and gauze sponges should be counted prior to wrapping the pack. It is not necessary to add huge numbers of gauze sponges to the surgical pack. They can also be wrapped separately. The pack should be wrapped so that the steam can penetrate the interior. This means tight enough that it will not come apart, but loose enough to allow steam to penetrate.

15. b. Right owner. Although this is important, right animal, right sex, right body part, and right procedure are far more important.

16. d. The owner should be informed of the estimated costs and the potential risks of surgery and anesthesia. Consent forms should be prepared for the surgery itself and preferably for CPR in case of complications.

17. d. All of the above. Drawing up medications prior to induction will save valuable time and smooth the induction process. It will also allow more attention to be given to the animal and to patient monitoring.

18. b. The response of the animal at induction is not important for the record. The time of administration of the induction agent and the preanesthetic are important, as are the dosage and concentration of the drug.

19. b. The animal's TPR should be monitored every 5 minutes so that trends may be established.

20. c. The tube has probably been inserted into a single bronchus. An overinflated cuff would be noticed after surgery because of the potential for subcutaneous emphysema (air under the skin) from a tracheal rupture or necrosis. Too large a tube would have been noticed at induction.

21. a. The hyoid apparatus cannot be seen within the glottis region. It is a basket that encloses the entire larynx and is connected to the tongue. It pulls the larynx forward when the tongue is extended, allowing easier intubation.

22. c. The epiglottis is normally found hooked over the soft palate. It is connected to the base of the arytenoids.

23. d. The parakeet has complete tracheal rings and has a higher incidence of tracheal pressure necrosis from cuffed tubes. All the other species have c-shaped rings and a trachealis dorsalis muscle that allows some stretch of the trachea.

24. b. Clipper burn can increase self-mutilation postoperatively. A #40 blade should be used to perform surgical clipping and the blade should be oriented as close to parallel to the skin as possible to avoid burns. Clipper blades should be stored in disinfectant/lubricating solution.

25. b. The sterile surgical scrub should be performed wearing sterile surgical gloves. The preliminary scrub may be performed wearing exam gloves.

26. a. The surgical scrub should spiral out from the incision site without recontaminating any area already scrubbed. Starting at the edges and working in would contaminate the incision area.

27. d. Chlorhexidine alternating with alcohol. Alcohol will inactivate povidone-iodine and should not be used with it. One-step prep should not be removed with anything other than a dry gauze sponge.

28. a. Huck towels should be in place prior to draping. They allow an expanded surgical field and absorb fluids from the surgical site.

29. b. The drape, the surgeon from the waist to the shoulders, and the arms are all considered part of the sterile surgical field.

30. c. Wedding rings and other jewelry should be removed prior to scrubbing. Surgical scrubs, a bonnet, and a mask should be worn by everyone in the surgical suite.

31. d. The nails should be picked and scrubbed prior to scrubbing the rest of the hand. Nail polish or acrylic nails can be a source of contamination because they allow bacteria to hide.

32. b. Keeping hands in the prayer position minimizes the chance of contamination. It is never acceptable to touch the nose or the mask with the gloved hand. The back of the surgeon is considered contaminated. Water should be allowed to drip from the elbows after the scrub. The hands should always be kept above the level of the elbows during surgical scrubbing.

33. d. Each quadrant on the hand must get a minimum of 25 scrubs.

34. b. Each quadrant on the arm should get a minimum of 10 scrubs.

35. a. Each finger, each hand, and the arm should be treated as a cylinder with four quadrants. The arm should be further subdivided into wrist, distal forearm, and proximal forearm.

36. d. Five minutes is the minimum time of scrubbing in order to achieve maximum asepsis.

37. d. The surgeon should *never* lean against the surgical table. Gowns are required to extend the sterile field of the gloves. Hair is always considered contaminated, so the forearm is a contaminated area.

38. b. The gloving procedure where the hands extend past the sleeves of the gown is called open gloving and has the highest possibility of contamination. In closed gloving, the hand is kept within a sterile field and the surgeon may hand the assistant the outside tie prior to donning the gloves. Once the surgeon is gloved, contamination requires repeating aseptic preparation.

39. b. Music is nice to listen to, but may be distracting. Communication, monitoring, and awareness are of paramount importance in the surgical suite.

40. b. Blood loss is the only surgical complication. The other three answer choices are anesthetic complications.

41. b. The patellar reflex is not commonly monitored during surgery. The palpebral and withdrawal reflex and jaw tone are commonly monitored.

42. d. The decision on anesthetic protocol is the (prescribing) veterinarian's. Recovery, anesthesia, and equipment are the technician's responsibility.

43. d. Animals should generally be extubated when they are swallowing. Brachycephalic dogs are usually extubated when they are chewing.

44. d. Instruments should be soaked in cold water, scrubbed with detergent and a soft brush, then placed in the ultrasonic cleaner, then lubricated with instrument milk.

45. b. External sutures may not be needed if the surgeon performs a subcuticular closure. Reactive sutures can increase inflammation at the incision, which can cause dehiscence; self-mutilation and increased activity can result in dehiscence or herniation.

46. c. Stainless steel is the only nonreactive monofilament on the list.

47. b. Elective surgeries are performed either at the request of the owner or at the veterinarian's and the owner's convenience. Bloodwork may or may not be required, and every surgical procedure has inherent risks.

48. d. All these surgeries are nonelective because there is a pathological condition that makes the surgery necessary.

49. c. Bloat is a complication of general anesthesia in cattle. Fractures and myositis are common in horses during recovery. Hemorrhage is a complication of any surgery in any animal.

50. d. Local anesthetic is placed in both the scrotum and the spermatic cord. The cremaster muscle is sensitive to pain. The procedure is performed in the standing position with an emasculator and the incision is generally left open to drain unless there is cryptorchidism and a large inguinal ring. In that case, herniation of abdominal contents through the inguinal ring may occur, so closure of the inguinal ring is sometimes performed to prevent this.

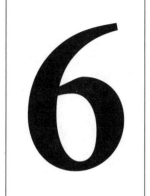

CHAPTER

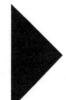

DENTISTRY

CHAPTER OVERVIEW

Being familiar with dental procedures and techniques is very important in the modern veterinary practice. Basic preventative treatment to maintain dental health and avoid problems in the future is an essential part of most veterinary practices and is a standard part of the veterinary technician's job description. What does vary from state to state is the level of responsibility for a vet tech. For example, California allows veterinary technicians to do surgical extractions, but many other states do not.

Veterinary dentistry has become increasingly important as dental techniques have improved with more research into animal health and veterinary medicine. At the same time, our pets (like ourselves) are living longer and this increasingly aging pet population means more dental challenges. In humans, dental health can add to overall patient health because infections and inflammations in the mouth can quickly spread throughout the body and affect major organs such as the heart or liver. A pet's improved dental health also increases well-being by reducing pain, often leading to increased activity and better health. Owners are often astonished how quickly improved dental health will lead to decreased halitosis (bad breath). In fact, bad breath is usually a sign of dental problems in an animal.

Key Terms

alveolus

anisognathic

apex (apical)

aradicular

arcade

biofilm

brachyodont

buccal

calculus

caries

carnassial

cavitation

cementum

coronal

crown

curette

deciduous

dentifrice

dentin

elevator

elongation

enamel

endodontics

epulis

exodontics

foreshortening

furcation

gingiva

gutta percha

hypsodont

kilovoltage

labial

lingual

malocclusion

mandibular

maxillary

mesial

milliamperage

occlusal

oronasal fistula

ostium

palatal

pellicle

periodontium

plaque

prophylaxis

pulp

radicular

retropulse

scaler

stomatitis

sulcus

tartar

Concepts and Skills

Knowledge of the following six concepts and skills is essential in veterinary dental assisting:

- dental anatomy
- instrumentation
- dental radiography
- anesthesia and analgesia
- dental techniques
- dental pathology

Dental Anatomy

Knowledge of veterinary dental anatomy is essential in veterinary dentistry. It is the study of the animal tooth structures, and the identification, naming, and locating of the various teeth in the animal's mouth. The veterinary technician plays a central role in the dental exam of each patient. Often, the veterinary professional will conduct the oral examination of the patient with the technician recording the results, but increasingly technicians are conducting these exams themselves. In fact, some states such as California allow certified dental technicians (CDTs) to do many extra tasks such as surgical extractions. A vet tech must be familiar with the dental anatomy of the patient in order to record dental diseases of the teeth, gums, bone, and surrounding tissues.

Charting, that is, recording information on a dental chart, begins with tooth numbering and naming. There are two basic recording techniques: anatomic and triadan.

The anatomic system uses the four tooth types in small animals: I = incisor, C = canine, P = premolar, M = molar. Individual teeth are named either by number or by placement (i.e., the upper right third incisor is identified as URI_3). The main problem with this system is that tooth number and placement are not consistent across species.

The triadan system was originally used in human dentistry and it can be used with consistency across species. This system identifies teeth by quadrants or arcades: the upper right quadrant teeth are numbered 100–111, the upper left quadrant is 200–211, the lower left quadrant is 300–311, and the lower right quadrant is 400–411. The teeth are numbered starting at the midline of the face, for example the first upper right incisor is 101. The numbers increase as you go back toward the tonsil.

This system also has the rule of 4 and 9—the canine is always numbered 4 (104, 204, 304, 404) and the first molar is always numbered 9 (109, 209, 309, 409). This is important because premolar numbers are variable in animals. To be consistent, the premolars are numbered backwards from 9. In the normal cat, for example, the lower teeth consist of only two premolars and one molar. The right lower row of teeth (known as the **arcade**) would be recorded in the triadan system as: 401, 402, 403, 404, 407, 408, 409. (Notice that 405 and 406 do not exist.)

Identifying and recording the locations of the teeth is the beginning of the charting process. The tooth surfaces also need to be recorded to identify dental problems. There are seven common surfaces:

apical—toward the apex (contained within the alveolus or tooth socket)

buccal—the surface of the teeth facing the cheek or the outside of the mouth

coronal—toward the crown of the tooth (occlusal surface)

interproximal (or **interdental**)—the surfaces between the teeth

labial—the surface of the canines and incisors that face the lips

lingual—the surface of the lower teeth that faces the tongue

mesial—toward the midline of the front of the dental arch

palatal—the surface of the upper arcade that faces the palate

In addition to knowing the locations, numbering systems, and surfaces of the teeth, the veterinary technician must be familiar with the various structures related to the teeth and jaw. There are 12 significant structures associated with teeth (see Figure 6.1):

alveolar bone—the bone surrounding the alveolus

apex—the entrance into the pulp cavity at the base of the **alveolus** (tooth socket)

cementoenamel junction (CEJ)—the area at the neck of the tooth where the root and crown portions come together; this should be in the same area as the gingival margin

cementum—this substance covers the root of the tooth and is softer and more rough in texture than enamel

crown—the portion of the tooth covered with enamel, the chewing (occlusal) surface

dentin—this substance makes up most of the tooth surrounding the pulp cavity and under the cementum and the enamel

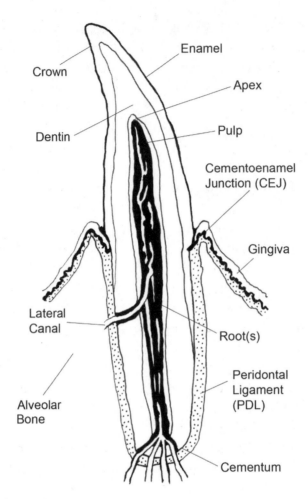

Figure 6.1 *Parts of a Tooth*

enamel—this substance covers the crown of the tooth and is the hardest substance in the body

furcation—the area in multiple-rooted teeth, such as carnassials, where the roots meet under the crown; this area is normally under the gum line

gingiva—the soft tissue covering of the interior of the mouth, which covers the alveolar bone and attaches to the periodontal ligament at the cementoenamel junction

periodontal ligament (PDL)—the attachment of the gingiva and tooth to the alveolar bone; it lines the alveolus and must be disrupted for exodontic procedures

pulp—the internal canal of the tooth containing blood vessels and nerves extending from the apex; this will decrease in size with the age of the tooth

root—the portion of the tooth covered with cementum

Canine Dental Anatomy

Since the jaws of all animals are symmetrical, only one half of the mouth is described here. The upper jaw (**maxillary arcade**) is listed first, over the lower jaw (**mandibular**) teeth. An adult dog has three incisors (I3), one canine (C1), four premolars (P4), and two molars (M2) in the upper jaw (maxillary). In the lower jaw (mandibular), it has three incisors (I3), one canine (C1), four premolars (P4), and three molars (M3). Thus, the adult dog dental formula is $I\frac{3}{3}$, $C\frac{1}{1}$, $P\frac{4}{4}$, $M\frac{2}{3} \times 2$. (See Figure 6.2.)

All the incisors, canines, and first premolars are single-rooted teeth. The second and third premolars and second molar are double-rooted teeth in the maxillary arcade. The fourth upper premolar (also called the carnassial tooth) and the first upper molar have three roots.

Carnivores in general also have deciduous (baby) teeth that will be replaced as they age with permanent (adult) teeth. In the canine, the primary incisors and canines erupt at 3 to 4 weeks of age, and the premolars at 4 to 12 weeks. There are no primary molars. The primary incisors are replaced by adult teeth at 3 to 5 months, the canines and premolars at 4 to 6 months, and the adult molars should be in by 7 months of age. Puppies have 28 deciduous teeth that fall out around 6 months of age and are replaced by a set of 42 permanent or adult teeth.

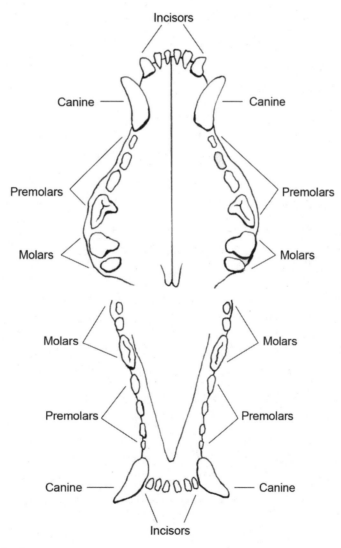

Figure 6.2 *Canine Dental Anatomy*

DECIDUOUS AND PERMANENT TEETH: DOGS		
TIME OF ERUPTION		
	DECIDUOUS TEETH	PERMANENT TEETH
Incisors	3–4 weeks	3–5 months
Canines	3–6 weeks	4–6 months
Premolars	4–12 weeks	4–6 months
Molars		3–7 months

The dental formula for deciduous teeth always uses lowercase letters. The puppy dental formula is $i\frac{3}{3}$, $c\frac{1}{1}$, $p\frac{3}{3} \times 2$.

Feline Dental Anatomy

The saying *as different as dogs and cats* certainly applies to the dental anatomy of these animals. Kittens have 26 deciduous teeth compared to puppies, which have 28. Adult cats have only 30 teeth. An adult cat has three incisors (I3), one canine (C1), three premolars (P3), and one molar (M1) in half of the maxillary arcade. It has three incisors (I3), one canine (C1), two premolars (P2), and one molar (M1). Thus, the adult feline dental formula is $I\frac{3}{3}$, $C\frac{1}{1}$, $P\frac{3}{2}$, $M\frac{1}{1} \times 2$. (See Figure 6.3.)

All the incisors, the canines, and the maxillary second premolar have one root each. The only tooth with three roots is the upper last premolar (the carnassial tooth). All other teeth have two roots.

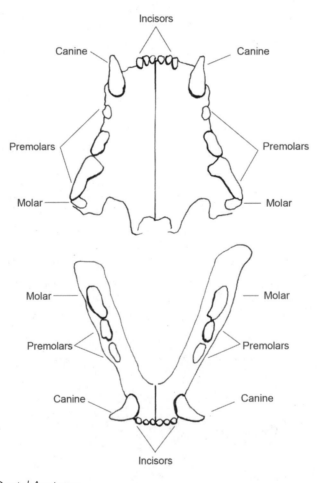

Figure 6.3 *Feline Dental Anatomy*

TABLE 6.2 DECIDUOUS AND PERMANENT TEETH: CATS		
	TIME OF ERUPTION	
	DECIDUOUS TEETH	PERMANENT TEETH
Incisors	2–3 weeks	3–4 months
Canines	3–4 weeks	4–5 months
Premolars	3–6 weeks	4–6 months
Molars		4–6 months

As with dogs, the deciduous teeth of kittens are written using lowercase letters, so the dental formula is $i\frac{3}{3}, c\frac{1}{1}, p\frac{3}{2} \times 2$.

Equine Dental Anatomy

All equine and bovine teeth are single rooted. They are also **radicular hypsodont**, which means that the apex of the permanent tooth remains open, allowing the teeth to grow continuously throughout most of the animal's life. This continued growth means that the length of the teeth is continually replaced as these herbivores wear down their teeth in aging. Older horses have closed apices, which can lead to enough tooth wear that they cannot continue to grind effectively.

Canines are usually only present in adult male horses. The first premolar may or may not be present; only 25% of horses have the first premolar. This tooth has no deciduous tooth associated with it and is called a *wolf tooth*. The wolf tooth is smaller, and located closer to the incisors. It may interfere with the bit causing pain and may be extracted to prevent this in many horses.

The upper jaw is wider than the lower jaw (**anisognathic**) and the **occlusal** surface is angled to provide increased grinding surface. Changes in this angle (10 to 15 degrees) may result in problems such as **malocclusion**. A procedure known as *dental floating* may be needed to address this problem. (For more on this see the Equine and Pocket Pet Procedures section on page 129.)

The horse has a fused mandibular symphysis, the ridge where the left and right mandibles meet. The horse also has large masseter muscles and a wider temporomandibular joint (TMJ) to enable better grinding (side-to-side motion). Horses use their lips for prehension where dogs and cats use their teeth for this. Equine teeth are covered completely with cementum, enabling the surface to be worn away when grinding. (See Figure 6.4.)

The adult equine dental formula is: $I\frac{3}{3}, C\frac{0\text{-}1}{0\text{-}1}, P\frac{3\text{-}4}{3\text{-}4}, M\frac{3}{3} \times 2$

The deciduous dental formula is: $i\frac{3}{3}, c\frac{0}{0}, p\frac{3}{3} \times 2$

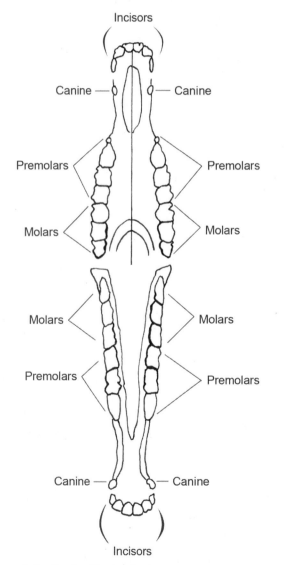

Figure 6.4 *Equine Dental Anatomy*

Bovine Dental Anatomy

Most cattle do not receive dental care. A few important anatomical features are present, however. Cattle have no upper incisors or canines. These teeth have been replaced by a rubbery dental pad over the incisive bone that forms an occlusive surface with the lower incisors. Cattle have a mandibular symphysis that is unfused.

Bovine teeth and musculature are very similar to the equine in structure and function.

The adult dental formula in the bovine is I_3^0, C_1^0, P_3^3, $M_3^3 \times 2$. (Note: lower canines may be absent.)

Lagomorph Dental Anatomy

Rabbits have a few interesting dental features. One is that they have a double set of upper incisors. The first incisor is the only tooth seen externally. However, there is another set directly behind these incisors, called the *peg teeth*, which are tiny and cannot be seen but are nevertheless important. The presence of peg teeth is unique to lagomorphs (hares, pikas, and rabbits).

Rodents and rabbits share several dental features. Rodent and rabbit incisors are chisel shaped because enamel is only found on the lingual surface. The rest of the tooth is covered in cementum, which enables wear to occur in this pattern. All lagomorphs and some rodents have **aradicular hypsodont** teeth, meaning that they grow throughout the animal's life. This is different from horses, which have radicular hypsodont teeth, where the apices close after a certain amount of time. Animals with aradicular hypsodont teeth also have a different structure of the periodontal ligament. It is typically a *plexus*, which is a grouping of blood vessels that holds the tooth in place. This allows a looser attachment to the tooth enabling the tooth to continue to erupt through the gingiva.

The cheek teeth of the rabbit are very similar to the cheek teeth of the horse in that they are chisel shaped, with the point of the chisel of the maxilla being toward the cheek (buccal). The jaw of the rabbit is anisognathic with the maxilla being slightly larger than the mandible. Rabbits have a wide TMJ and well-developed masseter muscles. (See Figure 6.5.)

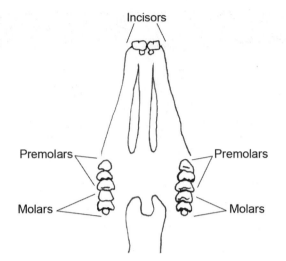

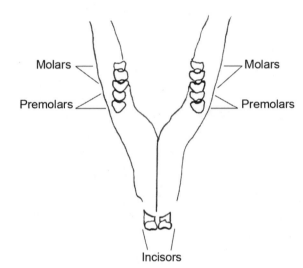

Figure 6.5 *Lagomorph Dental Anatomy*

The adult rabbit dental formula is I_1^2, C_0^0, P_2^3, $M\frac{2\text{-}3}{3}$.

Rodent Dental Anatomy

Rats and mice have aradicular hypsodont (high-crowned) incisors and **brachyodont** (low-crowned) premolars and molars.

Chinchillas and guinea pigs have aradicular hypsodont teeth throughout the mouth. They also have a structure at the back of the soft palate called the palatal ostium that makes intubation and gavage feeding very difficult. Chinchillas and guinea pigs need to have their molars checked and floated in a manner similar to horses.

The dental formula for the rat (or mouse) is: I_1^1, C_0^0, P_0^0, $M_3^3 \times 2$, and the dental formula for the chinchilla and guinea pig is: I_1^1, C_0^0, P_1^1, $M_3^3 \times 2$.

Instrumentation

It is important to use and care for dental instruments correctly in order to provide adequate dental care. Dental instruments are either manual instruments or machine-aided instruments. The instruments needed will vary depending on the procedure and technique used.

Instrumentation for Small-Animal Routine Prophylaxis

Preventative dental treatment, known as **prophylaxis** or prophy, involves tooth cleaning and polishing to prevent gum disease and cavities. There are two main ways of cleaning teeth: manually with hand scalers or using machine scalers. The latter come in two varieties, ultrasonic and sonic.

Hand Scaling

Hand scaling instruments have three parts: the shank, the handle, and the blade. The shank is connected to the handle at one end and to the blade at the other end. The blade has a tip, a face, and a cutting edge. Hand instruments should all be held in a modified pen grasp with the index finger and thumb at the join of the shank and the handle. The middle finger gives direction by resting on the shank. The ring finger and pinkie should rest on part of the animal's oral cavity in order to reduce strain on the forearm. The angle will change depending on the instrument. Scalers and curettes have a cutting surface on the blade in order to remove tartar. In general, the blade face should be kept parallel to the root or tooth surface and the curve of the instrument should be directed toward the gingiva during insertion. The angle should be increased to 60 degrees from the tooth surface and the face should be pulled coronally to dislodge tartar.

The following five instruments are used in handscaling.

curettes—these instruments have a blunt or spatulate tip; they are used for subgingival (below the gumline) scaling

explorer—this instrument has a pointy tip and looks like a shepherd's hook; used to explore the tooth surface at the gingival margin to check for rough surfaces, it may also be used to assess tooth mobility

probe—this instrument has a blunt tip and is marked with measuring bars in millimeter increments; it is used to assess the depth of subgingival pockets

scalers—these instruments have a pointy tip and one cutting blade; they are used for supragingival (above the gumline) scaling

tartar forceps—this instrument is used to remove tartar above the gumline by placing the blade against the tooth at the gingival margin and then closing the blades by pulling toward the crown

Dental instruments must always be kept sharp, because dullness results in ineffective tartar removal and possible tissue damage to the gingiva. Dull instruments can also increase muscle strain and the possibility of repetitive-motion injury for the veterinarian or veterinary technician. Instruments should be sharpened frequently using sharpening stones. To do this, the instrument should be held stationary and the stone should be moved against the face of the blade. The stone should be kept lubricated so that the fines can be removed from the blade edge as it is being sharpened. The fines are tiny pieces of metal that have been ground off the edge of the blade of dental instruments. There are two types of stone: the Arkansas stone, which should be lubricated with oil, and the Ceramic stone, which should be lubricated with water.

Machine Scaling

There are two types of machine scalers. The *ultrasonic scaler* works by piezoelectric effect and blasts the tartar and plaque from the surface of the tooth using ultrasonic vibrations at 18,000 to 30,000 cycles per second (KHz). The electromagnetic stimulation destroys bacteria and tartar by causing cavitation, which works by causing water bubbles to collapse and so create tiny shock waves. The shock waves kill the bacteria and break down the tartar. The newer models of ultrasonic scalers can be used both above and below the gumline.

The second type of machine scaler is the *sonic scaler*. It is not often used in the modern veterinary office. It operates at a much lower frequency and is less able to remove tenacious tartar.

A drill with a rounded bur may also be used to remove tartar, but there is a greater possibility of causing tooth damage.

Periodontal Instrumentation

The instrumentation for periodontal disease treatment is basically the same as for the routine dental prophylaxis. A few other instruments may also be required, such as a scalpel blade and handle, suture, tetracycline gel application, and a drill and bit for removing subgingival alveolar bone.

Endodontic Instrumentation

Endodontics is a very specialized part of dentistry dealing with the pulp of the tooth, for example, in root canals. As such, it requires very different instrumentation. Since endodontics is not within the usual scope of practice of veterinary technicians, only an overview is given here. All critical instruments used in endodontics—those that contact bone or tissue—must be sterilized in an autoclave prior to use.

> **barbed broaches**—these instruments are used to remove the necrotic pulp cavity after injecting with a dilute sodium hypochlorite solution; these come in various sizes

> **composite** or **glass ionomer**—material used to make a smooth surface and plug the cavity

> **dental drill and bits**—these instruments are used to approach the pulp cavity of the tooth by drilling through the enamel and dentin layers; bits come in various shapes

> **endodontic files**—there are two different types of endodontic files: Hedstrom and Kerr (H and K files); these are used to widen and smooth out the pulp cavity

> **endodontic sealer**—material used to fill in the space not taken up by the gutta percha points

> **gutta percha points**—a rubbery plastic filling material that is placed inside the hollowed-out pulp cavity

> **paper points**—these are used to dry out the interior of the pulp cavity prior to filling

> **plugger**—this instrument is used to tamp the filling material into the pulp cavity

> **spreader**—this instrument is used to move the gutta percha to the side walls of the pulp cavity

Some teeth may need to have a crown made after endodontic work is performed. This specialty is called *restorative dentistry*.

Exodontic Instrumentation

Exodontics is also called tooth extraction. In most states, this is not within the scope of practice of veterinary technicians, although some states, such as California, allow CDTs to extract teeth. Tooth extraction may be needed in cases of periodontal, endodontic, or orthodontic disease.

> **alveolar filling material**—this material, which may be made of bioglass or cancellous bone graft, is placed within the alveolus and the gingiva is closed over the top; new bone growth is stimulated and the alveolar bone is strengthened

drill and bits—these instruments are used to remove the alveolar bone from around the roots

elevators—these instruments are used to disrupt the periodontal ligament by inserting them between the gingiva or alveolar bone and the tooth; elevators come in various sizes depending on the tooth being extracted, and they may either be plain or winged

extraction forceps—this instrument is used to remove the tooth from the alveolus

periosteal elevators—these instruments are used to remove alveolar bone from the tooth surface

root pick—this instrument is used to extract small root tips that may be difficult to remove with elevators

scalpel and blade handle—these instruments are used to remove the gingiva from the underlying alveolar bone over the roots

suture, needle holder, and **forceps**—these are used to close the gingiva over the alveolus

Orthodontic Instrumentation

In lay terms, orthodontics is the straightening of teeth. It involves moving teeth into more normal positions by using compression and distraction forces on the alveolar bone surrounding the tooth. Models of the oral cavity must be made in order to place the appropriate dental appliances on the teeth.

brackets—anchor points placed onto the teeth that hold wire or rubber tracks placed to move the teeth into the preferred position

calcium alginate—used to take an impression of the oral cavity, this product is a powder that forms a gel when mixed with water

dental stone—powder used to make a model of the oral cavity; it forms a product similar to concrete as it dries

model—a positive impression formed by placing the dental stone into the calcium alginate mold

mold—a negative impression of the oral cavity obtained from the calcium alginate

Interceptive orthodontics may also be performed, where exodontics (extractions) are performed on specific teeth that obstruct the normal architecture of the mouth by causing interference with other teeth. The instruments would be the same as for exodontic procedures.

Equine and Pocket Pet Dental Instrumentation

The term *pocket pet* generally refers to small, nonexotic mammals kept as household pets; it includes hamsters, gerbils, and guinea pigs. Horses, rabbits, chinchillas, and guinea pigs all require similar instrumentation to get adequate dental care. This is because they all have at least some aradicular hypsodont teeth. Rats, mice, and squirrels have brachyodont teeth for molars and premolars, so they only need specialized equipment for the incisors. The technique used to care for aradicular hypsodont teeth is called floating. The technique for care of the incisors of rabbits and rodents is called tooth trimming.

diamond wheel—this attachment on a dental drill trims the incisors without fracturing them

files—these instruments have cutting surfaces that only work on the forward stroke

molar cutters—these instruments can be used to trim the points off the molars prior to use of the rasp or file

oral speculum—this instrument allows adequate visualization of the oral cavity; because most of these species have lip comissures, where the lips join together, located rostrally, or toward the nasal area, visualization can be a problem; rodents also have redundant, or extra, folds in the buccal area, which can be especially problematic in rodents with cheek pouches, so rodent and rabbit speculums have cheek retractors

rasps—these instruments have cutting surfaces that can work in both directions (on the forward and the backward strokes)

Dental Radiography

Dental radiography (x-ray technology) is important for planning how to perform dental procedures. X-rays are also used to assess the postsurgical results in endodontic and exodontic procedures. This subject is more fully discussed in Chapter 10.

Equipment

Although regular x-ray machines may be used to perform dental radiography, they are difficult to position correctly and they require the animal to leave the veterinary treatment table. Dental x-ray machines allow much more flexibility for positioning, have a set distance that is easily measured, and have lower electrical requirements. Most veterinary practices have a dental x-ray machine.

Dental film is small (film sizes range from 0 to 4) and is flexible, making it easier to insert into the mouth. This film does not have screens; this amplifies the image of x-ray light, so it is a direct image. The film is packaged in a plastic sleeve, backed by a lead sheet and paper, which must be removed when it is processed.

The dental x-ray machine may be mounted on the wall or it may be moveable on wheels. It consists of three parts: the control panel, the arm, and the tube head. The arm and the tube head may be positioned in various ways in order to conform to the view needed. The control panel generally has set **kilovoltage** (kVp) and **milliamperage** (mA) and may only allow adjustment of the time.

Kilovoltage (kVp) controls how deep the radiation will penetrate by controlling the speed of the electrons leaving the cathode and striking the anode. This controls the contrast of the resulting image. Milliamperage (mA) controls the number of light and dark photons leaving the tube head. The amount of radiation is usually multiplied by exposure time to give mAs.

The tube head has a position-indicating device that sets the distance; this is used to maintain the appropriate distance between the tube head and the dental film and ensure the best image. This device is lined with lead to reduce scatter radiation.

The timer switch must be located a minimum of 6 feet from the tube head to assure radiation safety for the technician. In addition, proper personal protective equipment (PPE) containing lead must be worn (gloves, thyroid collar, body apron). To prevent irradiation of the technician's hands, the film should never be held in the patient's mouth by hand. The dosimetry badge, which measures exposure to radiation, must be worn outside of the apron near the thyroid.

The developing process is similar to the process for regular radiographic plates. Some practices have digital x-ray film that contains phosphor crystals. These crystals give off an energy signal that is interpreted by the computer and converted to digital images. This not only saves developing costs, but decreases the need for silver recovery systems and file storage.

Radiographic Techniques

Several techniques are used to take radiographs of the oral cavity. The particular approach used depends on the tooth to be assessed. The three main radiographic techniques are parallel, bisecting angle, and extraoral.

Parallel Technique

The parallel technique is used only for the mandibular cheek teeth (premolars and molars) in small animals. There is enough soft tissue in the intermandibular space to allow a true lateral view of the tooth roots. The film is placed intraorally between the tongue and the tooth (parallel to the tooth) and the beam is directed at a 90-degree angle to the film. The other teeth all have bony interference that does not allow this view.

Bisecting Angle Technique

The bisecting angle technique is used for non-mandibular teeth in small animals. The film is placed as close to parallel to the tooth axis as possible and an imaginary line is drawn bisecting the angle made by the tooth axis and the film. The beam is directed at a 90-degree angle to that imaginary line. The problem with this technique is that the image may end up distorted. If the root appears longer than normal, the distortion is called **elongation**. If it is shorter than normal, the distortion is called **foreshortening**. This can confuse the image and make it difficult to assess apical abnormalities. Carnassial teeth and molars can be very difficult to image correctly because of the overlapping multiple roots crowded together. Several views of multiple-rooted teeth may be necessary to assess all roots and the crown.

Extraoral Technique

The extraoral technique may be necessary in order to assess one or more roots of multiple-rooted teeth in carnivores. It is usually needed for assessing cheek teeth in equines, rodents, and lagomorphs. This technique may use either a screen type cassette or dental film. The x-ray beam may be intraoral (in which case it is a bisecting-angle type technique), or it may be the same view as a lateral skull in the case of the horse, the rodent, and the rabbit.

Anesthesia and Analgesia

Anesthesia and analgesia (pain control) are extremely important in veterinary dentistry. Although these topics are covered in detail in Chapter 11, we include a short review here in the interests of completeness. The oral cavity and the muscles of mastication are innervated by the trigeminal nerve (cranial nerve V). Each individual tooth is supplied by nerves (known as innervation), and the alveolar bone is also highly innervated. The oral cavity, joints, and muscles of mastication contains almost 60% of the proprioceptors for dogs (which is the only animal that has been so measured), so there is high sensitivity in the oral cavity and associated structures. Proper anesthesia and analgesia are necessary before, during, and after the procedure to ensure proper healing after dental procedures.

General Anesthesia

General anesthesia is required for every veterinary dental procedure. All these procedures require intra-oral manipulation and, unlike human patients, animals cannot be convinced to cooperate. This increases the danger to the vet tech or other individual performing the procedure. Endotracheal tube placement is extremely important to prevent possible aspiration. Endotracheal tubes should be cuffed.

Local Anesthesia

True local anesthesia occurs when the gingiva around a particular tooth is infiltrated with a local anesthetic such as bupivicaine. It is extremely important to check the maximum dosage of the particular local anesthetic. With local anesthesia, the potential for toxicity is higher because high doses of anesthetic are needed, especially if more than one tooth needs to be anesthetized. All local anesthesia should be performed a minimum of 5 minutes prior to the dental procedure to ensure adequate anesthesia of the area.

Regional Anesthesia

Regional anesthesia occurs by performing specific nerve blocks that anesthetize a region of the oral cavity. All nerve blocks are unilateral. As with local anesthesia, this should be performed a minimum of 5 minutes prior to the dental procedure to ensure adequate anesthesia of the area.

  infra-alveolar block—performed by injecting the anesthetic at the medial side of the angle of the mandible; it anesthetizes the entire mandible on that side

infraorbital block—performed by injecting the anesthetic into the infraorbital foramen located in the maxilla above the carnassial tooth (upper fourth premolar); it anesthetizes the entire maxillary arcade on that side

mental block—performed by injecting the anesthetic into the mental foramen located in the mandible under the canine tooth; it anesthetizes the mandible cranial to the lower first premolar on that side

Dental Techniques

Any dental procedure begins with the physical exam; this exam should precede any anesthesia event. Additional in-depth examination of the head and neck should also be performed. This should include examining the muscles of mastication, an ophthalmic exam (including retropulsion of the globes to assess for retro-orbital masses), an assessment of facial symmetry, range of motion of the TMJ, breath odor, nasal discharge, and extraoral pain. These are all indicators used to assess overall dental health. A good cranial nerve exam is also very important because 9 of the 12 cranial nerves can be affected by or cause oral disease including:

CN I—olfactory
CN II—optic
CN III—oculomotor
CN IV—trochlear
CN V—trigeminal
CN VI—abducens
CN VII—facial
CN IX—glossopharyngeal
CN XII—hypoglossal

The function of the olfactory nerve may be affected by chronic sinusitis due to chronic dental disease. The optic, abducens, and trochlear nerves can be affected by retrobulbar masses from the oral cavity as well as abscesses of the posterior root of the carnassial tooth. The trigeminal nerve is the innervation for the oral cavity, so any dental disease will affect this nerve. The facial and oculomotor nerve may be affected by a cervical injury, Horner's syndrome, or Bell's palsy causing a lip and face droop, decreased salivation, decreased lacrimation, and a miotic pupil. The glossophyaryngeal nerve and hypoglossal nerves can both cause tongue movement abnormalities and decreased sensation. The glossopharyngeal nerve is also responsible for the sense of taste.

Once the animal is anesthetized and intubated (a tube is placed into the trachea to protect the airway), a more thorough oral exam may be performed. The buccal cavities and the interior of the lips should be assessed, the tongue should be lifted, the pharynx, the tonsils, and the hard and soft palates evaluated. All areas should be assessed for firmness and the presence of masses, ulcerations, and other lesions. After all of the soft tissues have been evaluated, the teeth may be assessed. Occlusion should be evaluated, tooth number and condition and gingival surfaces should be assessed. All deviations from normal should be recorded in the permanent record. Photographs may be helpful in following lesions over time.

Each tooth should be assessed separately, beginning with the middle incisor and working out from the midline. The probe should be used first. This is inserted gently between the gingiva and the tooth and the depth of the periodontal sulcus is measured in mm increments, using the mm markings on the probe. This should be done at a minimum of 6 different sites around the tooth circumference. Any sulcus greater than 3 mm in the dog or 1 mm in the cat should be recorded.

The explorer should be used next. This is also inserted into the gingival sulcus and run along the subgingival tooth surface. Any vibrations received from the tip should be recorded and reassessed after the dental prophylaxis or prophy (tooth cleaning) has been completed. The explorer may also be used to assess any superficial lesions of the supragingival tooth surface. The explorer should not catch on enamel. If it meets a surface not covered with enamel, it will vibrate or stick, and these lesions should also be recorded.

Any lesions should receive dental radiography to assess both condition of the alveolar bone (including tooth attachment) and the pulp cavity. Failure to radiograph may result in the overall failure of the dental procedures. Any endodontic treatment requires both pre- and postoperative radiography.

Procedure for Dental Prophylaxis

After the dental exam is completed, the dental prophylaxis (commonly known as teeth cleaning) begins. The first step is to remove the supragingival plaque and tartar. **Plaque** is the matrix of calcium-impregnated protein and aerobic gram-positive oral flora normally found in the mouth after eating. Over time, this matrix becomes more impregnated with calcium and the aerobic gram-positive flora gets replaced with gram-negative anaerobic flora (*Porphyromonas gulae*). This matrix then produces a more acid medium that affects the health of the gingiva.

Large pieces of tartar and calculus are removed with tartar forceps. Care should be taken not to damage the gingiva with the forceps.

Remaining supragingival tartar is removed with the scaler. Scalers may be either *universal* (able to be used on any tooth crown) or *area specific* (meant to be used only on specific teeth that have a sharper curvature). Care must be used with the universal type, or sickle scaler, because it has two cutting surfaces rather than one and can cause gingival trauma. The scaler is used between 45 and 90 degrees of the tooth surface and is pulled coronally to dislodge plaque and tartar.

Once the supragingival tartar is removed, the subgingival tartar needs to be removed using curettes. Curettes have a rounded tip and a rounded base of the curvature to prevent gingival trauma. They may be used for supragingival scaling but are generally used for subgingival scaling and root planing. They are inserted at 0 degrees to the tooth surface, then rotated to 45 to 90 degrees and pulled coronally to smooth subgingival cementum and remove the bacteria that can become lodged in the cementum. The most commonly used curettes are called Gracey curettes. Each type of Gracey is double ended (right and left) and has individual curvatures depending on the tooth it was designed for.

If machine scaling is used, it may be performed on both supra- and subgingival surfaces. The sonic scaler will not be reviewed here because most practices use the ultrasonic scaler. This tool converts electrical energy to mechanical/vibrational energy in the range of 18 to 50 kHz. Water is also used to cool the tooth surface and the tip of the instrument. Cavitation causes disruption of the bacteria and tartar and also requires water. Appropriate PPE (gloves and shields or masks covering the eyes, nose, and mouth) is essential because bacteria are aerosolized along with tartar. The animal must be intubated with an inflated cuff in place to reduce the possibility of inhalation of the same material. Tips should be replaced annually and the stacks should be checked frequently. If the stack is bent, or splayed, so that the sheets do not make contact with each other, they should be replaced. To prevent damage to the enamel and the tip of the scaler, the tip should not be placed at a 90-degree angle to the tooth. The tip should have a shallow angle to the tooth surface. It should be moved constantly and should not remain in contact with an individual tooth for more than 30 seconds, to prevent excessive heating of the pulp cavity. In addition, use a low RPM setting to avoid excessive heating up of the teeth.

After the curette or machine scaler has been used, the subgingival surface is again assessed with the explorer and the tooth surfaces are rinsed to remove tartar. The next step is polishing. Polishing should always be performed after every prophy, whether using manual or power scaling. Polishing smoothes out any microscopic imperfections in the tooth surface. There are many options for dental polish (**dentifrice**), most containing pumice. The rubber cup should be filled with the pumice paste and the prophy unit should be placed on low speed. Even at low speed, the procedure will cause heat buildup in the tooth pulp, so the prophy head should only be in contact with the tooth for one to three seconds to prevent damage. The cup should not contact the gingiva if possible.

The oral cavity should then be flushed out with either plain water, saline solution, or a diluted chlorhexidine rinse to remove debris. The oral cavity should again be assessed and any foreign material removed to prevent it from entering the lungs (known as aspiration) on recovery.

Periodontal Treatment

Periodontal treatment deals with the tissue and bone that surround teeth, and it is an extension of the dental prophy. In cases of deep periodontal pockets, additional treatment may be needed, including periodontal flap formation and root planing. Root planing involves removal of the infected cementum by curettage. Periodontal flap formation may include removal of the infected portion of the gingiva over the exposed root in order to facilitate more appropriate dental hygiene.

Doxycycline may be injected into the subgingival tissue to kill off anaerobic bacteria. Alternatively, an osteoconductive material such as Consil® (Bioglass®) or cancellous bone allograft may be used to stimulate new alveolar bone formation. This procedure will be covered further in the section on Dental Pathology, although it is beyond the scope of practice for veterinary technicians in most states. Familiarity with the materials required is important for procedure preparation.

Endodontic Treatment

Endodontic treatment, also called root canal, may be used to extend the life of a tooth after an injury. Endodontics is the replacement of pulp material with a bioinert filler in order to maintain dental architecture and decrease attrition. This procedure is beyond the scope of practice for veterinary technicians, but it is becoming more common for veterinarians in general practice to perform it. Vet techs must be familiar with endodontic procedures and be prepared to assist the veterinarian with them.

An important first step in endodontics is the radiograph. Dental radiography can help to assess whether there is other pathology besides the pulp disease that may affect the success of the procedure. A fracture of the root, severe curvature of the root tip, severe periodontal disease, or dentigerous cysts may all affect the ability to clean and fill the pulp cavity properly. A complete dental prophy is usually necessary prior to proceeding. Regional anesthesia and general anesthesia are a must for endodontic therapy.

The next step is to drill an access hole into the pulp cavity. For single-rooted teeth, only one access is needed. For multiple-rooted teeth, an access point is needed for each root. A round burr is used on a high-speed drill. It is very important to use water irrigation to decrease heat production by the drill bit. Although the pulp cavity is being removed, the surrounding alveolar bone and periapical nerves might be affected and become necrotic.

Once access has been obtained, the pulp cavity is flushed with a dilute sodium hypochlorite. This will decrease bleeding and kill microorganisms found in the pulp cavity. A barbed broach is then inserted into the cavity, rotated, and removed. Several different sizes of the instrument may be needed to completely clean out the cavity. The canal is flushed again to remove any remaining debris.

K or H files are then inserted, rotated, and pulled in increasing size until the canal is widened enough to fill. Remaining material is flushed out using dilute sodium hypochlorite solution, and paper points are inserted to dry the resulting canal.

The dry canal is then filled with gutta percha and a dentinal filler, using as much gutta percha as needed to fill the canal by using pluggers and spreaders.

The defect created by the dental drill is then filled with either composite or glass ionomer. In addition, a metal crown may be placed to provide additional support and prevent repeat fracture of the tooth.

Exodontic Treatment

Despite all the advances in veterinary dentistry, there are still times when teeth must be extracted. This is know as exodontics. Some states allow veterinary technicians to perform extractions. Check your individual practice act. In general, extractions should not be attempted without sufficient postgraduate training. This training may be obtained at most large veterinary meetings from AVDS (American Veterinary Dental Society) and AVDT (Academy of Veterinary Dental Technicians) members around the country. Problems that can arise from improper technique or preparation include jaw fracture, tooth root fracture and retention, bruising, gingival trauma, retrobulbar abscess or direct damage to the eye or sinuses, oronasal fistulas, and a host of other problems.

Extractions may be necessary in cases of severe tooth fracture where endodontics are unfeasible, severe (grade III to IV) periodontal disease, severe gingival disease (feline lymphocytic/plasmacytic gingivitis), or some types of malocclusions. The need for extraction will be determined by the veterinarian and will be assessed by tooth mobility, severity of the lesion, and owner preference for treatment. Prior to extractions, the owner should be informed of the probable number of extractions to be performed and given a cost estimate. A full dental exam with radiographs and a dental prophylaxis should be performed. Radiographs are important in order to determine the quality of the alveolar bone and the morphology of the tooth root. If there is a change in the number of extractions, or their difficulty, the owner should be told before proceeding.

Adequate regional anesthesia should be in place prior to beginning extractions. A minimum of 5 minutes after the injection of anesthetic should be allowed prior to beginning the extraction, in order to prevent ramp-up of the pain response and decrease the need for postoperative pain control. Radiographs may be taken after the injection to decrease the time under anesthesia. All instruments should be adequately sharpened and sterilized in an autoclave prior to use.

Single-rooted teeth can usually be extracted using what is called a *closed* technique. This means that the periodontal ligament is separated from the tooth using either a scalpel, a dental luxator, or an elevator. The appropriate size dental elevator is then inserted and gentle pressure is used to insert the instrument between the tooth and the alveolar bone. Slight rotation of the instrument helps to fatigue the periodontal ligament, the pressure is then let off, the elevator is advanced and rotated and held again. Progressively larger elevators can be used. Patience is needed to ensure that there is no alveolar bone or tooth root fracture. Generally the routine is *insert, rotate, hold rotation 10 seconds, release rotation, advance, repeat.* The procedure may be done around the circumference of the tooth to loosen the entire tooth from the periodontal ligament. The loosened tooth may be easily removed with either extraction forceps or even the fingers. The gingival defect should be closed with 3-0 to 5-0 monofilament absorbable suture material.

The *open,* or *surgical,* technique should be used for all multiple-rooted teeth and may be helpful for larger single-rooted teeth such as the canine. A gingival flap is created that raises the gingiva from the alveolar bone on the buccal side of the tooth using either a scalpel blade or a periosteal elevator. A round burr is then used to remove alveolar bone from the lateral side of the tooth root. With multiple-rooted teeth, the tooth is sectioned and the individual roots will be removed as single-rooted teeth. Elevators are then used in the same method as in the closed technique to remove the roots. The flap is sutured for closure. Osteoconductive material may be used under the flap to stimulate new alveolar bone growth.

Aftercare following extractions is very important. Animals should not receive hard food or chew toys for 14 days after the operation to avoid impaction of debris into alveolar sockets and possible jaw fracture from weakened alveolar bone. Proper dental hygiene including tooth brushing with enzymatic dentrifices, oral rinses (containing chlorhexidine or zinc sulfate), foods containing hexametaphosphate, or dental-cleaning diets may help to increase time between dental procedures. Current wisdom is that every other day tooth brushing is sufficient to prevent tartar and plaque buildup.

Orthodontic Procedures

If a malocclusion is seen and an orthodontic procedure is recommended, a model of the oral cavity should be made in order to track the progress of tooth movement and make any necessary appliances. Generally, a three-step procedure is recommended:

Step 1: The dental prophy will provide a smooth surface of the teeth so that the calcium alginate will not stick.

Step 2: The calcium alginate impression is made by placing the calcium alginate powder in a rubber bowl and mixing it with water according to directions on the label. The resulting gel is placed in the dental impression tray, with care taken to eliminate all air bubbles. The tray is placed over the animal's teeth, with care taken to keep lips and hair away from the tray. The tray is held in place for 5 minutes or until the gel sets to the consistency of rubber. The tray is then carefully removed from the mouth in the direction of the long axis of the teeth in one smooth motion. Going too slow will result in fracture of the impression. The impression is then inspected, rinsed with water, and dried thoroughly.

Step 3: The dental stone model is made by placing the dental stone powder in a bowl and mixing it with water according to label directions. It is then placed on a vibrator in order to get rid of air bubbles that might be trapped in the mixture. The calcium alginate impression is then placed on the vibrator and small amounts of stone are added to it in order to fill the negative impression. If this procedure is performed too quickly, air bubbles will be formed, which will cause artifacts in the model. Once the model has been filled, it should be allowed to sit on the vibrator to set for 10 minutes. It can then be removed from the vibrator and allowed to sit for one additional hour, and then removed from the calcium alginate impression.

The remainder of the orthodontic procedure is outside the scope of practice of a veterinary technician.

Equine and Pocket Pet Dental Procedures

The nature of aradicular hypsodont teeth sets up equines and pocket pets for a host of problems. Many of the dental problems seen in the horse, the rabbit, the chinchilla, and the guinea pig occur either because of a congenital or acquired malocclusion or because of incorrect food intake. Animals fed mostly hay diets tend to have fewer dental problems than animals maintained on food pellets.

The incisors of rodents and lagomorphs continue to grow after birth. If a congenital abnormality prevents the upper and lower incisors from meeting properly, or if a tooth trimming was performed incorrectly, one or more of the four incisors will grow in the wrong direction. Because the upper incisors are curved, continued growth will eventually lead to penetration of the hard palate by the upper incisors. The lower incisors could grow through the upper lip. These animals should be assessed frequently and have tooth trimming performed as needed. Tooth trims should be performed under sedation using a diamond wheel bit or dental floats (rasps and files). The teeth should be trimmed to maintain the chisel shape at a 45-degree angle. If malocclusion is severe and tooth trimming needs to be done too frequently, the incisors may be removed. It is important to remove both the incisor and the peg tooth in rabbits to prevent regrowth.

The technique for rodent or lagomorph incisor removal is different from other small-animal exodontics. The incisor is loosened from the spongy periodontal ligament with a luxator using the standard technique. These teeth are very fragile and will fracture easily. Extraction forceps are used to remove the tooth from the alveolus (following the curvature of the tooth to prevent fracture). The empty socket should then be cleaned taking special care to avoid leaving the apical tooth bed filled with osteoconductive material, and closed with absorbable sutures. If the apical tooth bed is not removed, the tooth may regrow in 4 to 6 months or cause a sterile abscess.

Equine incisors generally will not overgrow like those of rodents. They may have a wry mouth (abnormal bite alignment toward one side), but this is usually correctable by floating both the incisors and the cheek teeth using rasps and files. Recall that rasps work on both the pull and push stroke, while files work only on the pull stroke. In horses, it is common to use power equipment similar to Dremel® tools to copy or form a natural oral architecture.

Cheek teeth of horses, rabbits, chinchillas, and guinea pigs may also need to be floated. Most other rodents have brachyodont premolars and molars, so do not need this procedure. Dental examinations should occur annually at a minimum. If there are malocclusions, examinations should be more frequent.

Exodontics in horses, rabbits, chinchillas, and guinea pigs is difficult because of the aradicular nature of the teeth. Periodontal disease is very common in guinea pigs and horses, and cheek tooth abscesses are common in all species. The procedure for extraction is very similar to that for small animals although visualization is difficult. Buccotomy (cutting through the cheek to access the alveolar bone) or repelling (coming up through the alveolar bone from the ventral surface of the mandible and pushing the tooth up

into the oral cavity) may be necessary. Buccotomy should be avoided if possible because of the presence of cheek pouches in most of these species.

Dental Pathology

A number of dental pathologies are important in veterinary medicine. In human medicine, dental **caries** (cavities) are significant, but other dental pathologies are of greater importance in veterinary clinics. Treatment for these diseases is similar in the human and veterinary fields.

Significant Dental Diseases in Small Animals

There are seven leading dental diseases in small animals. These are periodontal disease, tooth fractures, feline odontoclastic resorptive lesions (FORLs), lymphocytic plasmacytic gingivitis/stomatitis (LPG/S), epulis, oral malignancies, and malocclusions. We will examine each in turn.

Periodontal Disease

The primary oral pathology seen in dogs, cats, and ferrets is periodontal disease. This is caused by inflammation and destruction of the periodontal ligament attachment between the gingiva and the tooth. It is the primary cause of tooth loss in most of our domestic animals. Associated disease from the presence of bacteria in periodontitis can cause a host of problems such as lung, kidney, and liver disease and may be associated with bacterial endocarditis and endocardiosis.

Periodontal disease begins with the formation of plaque, which is made up of glycoproteins in the saliva (the **pellicle**) mixed with bacteria that begin to colonize. The bacterial colonization takes 6 to 8 hours. The dead and dying bacteria at the tooth surface absorb calcium and form **tartar** or **calculus**. The normal bacteria living in the plaque are gram-positive aerobes. As the tartar gets thicker, less oxygen is available to the bacteria and the colonies change from gram-positive aerobes to gram-negative anaerobes, including spirochetes. This change in bacteria along with direct gingival irritation by the tartar sets up inflammation of the gingiva. Inflammatory mediators cause tissue damage and eventual recession of the gums.

The grading scale for periodontal disease is set up to differentiate the degree of gingival inflammation and the recession of the gingiva from the tooth surface.

> **Grade I** (early gingivitis)—gum is mildly red and irritated at the gum margin and there may be sponginess of the gingival **sulcus**; this usually occurs within the first week after plaque accumulation and is reversible with dental prophylaxis
>
> **Grade II** (advanced gingivitis)—subgingival plaque is formed, supragingival tartar may be present, and gingiva may become irregular; there may be up to 25% of loss of the gingival attachment to the tooth; usually reversible with dental prophylaxis
>
> **Grade III** (early periodontal disease)—subgingival tartar and plaque are present, root exposure has begun, 25 to 50% of the gingival attachment may be lost; may be reversible with root planing and gingival curettage and/or periodontal surgery with placement of osteoconductive material; injection of doxycycline gel may be required
>
> **Grade IV** (severe periodontal disease)—there is usually mobility, >50% loss of attachment of the gingiva, and possible pus; usually irreversible and may require extraction

Periodontal disease may result in such severe bone loss that the alveolar bone becomes spongy and can either fracture the jaw (usually the mandible) or form a hole into the maxillary cavity (an **oronasal fistula**).

The most important thing to remember with periodontal disease is the follow-up appointment. Once periodontal disease has occurred, the animal must be followed closely and dental prophylaxis appointments should be set up two to four times a year depending on the severity of disease and the owner's willingness to establish good home care. Disrupting the formation of plaque within the first 24 hours is the most important aspect of home care for these patients.

Tooth Fractures

Tooth fractures are very common in dogs because they tend to chew on inappropriate items such as hard toys, wood, or rocks. The most common site for tooth fractures is the carnassial tooth (upper fourth premolar) or the mandibular first molar. Dogs used for protection training or bite work may also fracture canine teeth. Cats tend to fracture the canines as well.

Fractures of the carnassial tooth are usually slab fractures, in which the buccal surface is sheared off parallel to the axis of the tooth. Many of these fractures expose the pulp cavity of the tooth, allowing bacteria to colonize the pulp cavity. Because the pulp cavity is narrow, the infection can exit through the apex of the tooth and may cause swelling or a draining tract (fistula) seen in the infraorbital area. This is called a carnassial tooth root abscess.

Canine teeth are usually sheared off perpendicular to the tooth axis (transverse fracture). This may cause nasal discharge on the same side as the fracture.

Tooth fractures must be treated with either endodontics or exodontics. Abscessed teeth may be inappropriate candidates for endodontics because of the presence of apical infection. Fresh fractures in puppy and kitten teeth may be treated with vital pulpotomy which leaves the pulp in place and caps it with composite or glass ionomer. This is important in order to maintain normal architecture in the mouth and prevent orthodontic issues in the future. These teeth will be replaced with the adult teeth and be shed normally.

Feline Odontoclastic Resorptive Lesions

Feline odontoclastic resorptive lesions (FORLs) occur in 70% of cats and, despite the name, in 20% of dogs. The lesions are found at the cervical line, also called the neck of the tooth or the cementoenamel junction. This pathology is often seen on radiographs before it is visible clinically. Once it begins to develop, the overlying gingiva becomes hyperplastic and covers the lesion with granulation tissue.

Oriental breeds of cat, such as Siamese or Burmese, are predisposed to FORLs. There is evidence that they may be caused by a defect in vitamin D metabolism.

The dental explorer can identify these lesions better than the naked eye. Restorations may be performed but they tend to have very high failure rates. Often the root reabsorbs faster than the crown. If the tooth root is poorly differentiated from the underlying alveolar bone on radiographs, the crown should be removed and the alveolar bone smoothed with a round bur. The overlying gingiva should then be closed over the defect. If tooth root absorption is not present, the tooth should be extracted.

Lymphocytic Plasmacytic Gingivitis/Stomatitis

Lymphocytic plasmacytic gingivitis/stomatitis (LPG/S) is common in cats and may occur in dogs. If the lesions are confined to the gingiva, it is called gingivitis. If it is found throughout the oral cavity, it is called **stomatitis**. In cats, the most common cause is an immune mediated disease, although anything causing inflammation may cause the pathology (viral, uremia, allergy, and so on). The clinical signs can include halitosis, drooling (ptyalism), anorexia, and bloody saliva. In cats, it appears to be an inflammatory response to plaque (sometimes in the presence of calicivirus or herpesvirus). Generally, dental prophy is not helpful and some cats may need full-mouth extractions to control the lesions (80% of cats with full-mouth extractions exhibit a reduction or absence of lesions). Cyclosporine and corticosteroids may be helpful in reducing inflammation and pain.

Epulis

An **epulis** is an overgrowth of the gingival tissues that is very common in brachycephalic breeds. Epulis has now been split into two categories: the local and relatively benign peripheral odontogenic fibroma, which does not invade surrounding bone and does not recur; and the acanthomatous ameloblastoma, which is invasive and requires wide (1-cm) margins and radiation. Mandibulectomy or maxillectomy may be preferable treatments to radiation because there may be malignancies that occur at or near the site of radiation therapy.

Oral Malignancies

Oral malignancies are generally highly invasive and metastatic. Surgical excision is difficult because of the need to maintain appropriate dental architecture, enabling the animal to eat and drink. Owners may be affected by the appearance of the animal after the operation, which can have an impact on the human-animal bond.

Malignant Melanoma

Malignant melanoma is the most common oral cancer found in dogs and the second most common found in cats. These tumors are highly metastatic and invasive and may be pigmented or unpigmented (amelanotic melanomas). Treatment is generally by a combination of surgery and a new vaccine, known as Oncophage®, that has been shown to increase survival times. Melanoma spreads very quickly to the body and is highly vascular, making treatment and surgery difficult.

Squamous Cell Carcinoma

Squamous cell carcinoma (SCC) is the most common oral cancer found in cats and the second most common found in dogs. This tumor is highly invasive and moderately metastatic. Treatment is by radical surgery with radiation. These tumors appear flat and ulcerated.

Fibrosarcoma   Fibrosarcoma is the third most common tumor in both dogs and cats. The tumors are flat, smooth, and usually not ulcerated. Treatment is the same as for squamous cell carcinoma.

Malocclusion

Misaligned teeth, or malocclusions, are extremely common in veterinary medicine because of changes in fashion and breed standard. Malocclusion is most common in dogs, but also occurs in cats, horses, and rabbits. Brachycephalic animals have the highest incidence of malocclusion, but it may occur in any animal. Causes can include chronic trauma during tooth bud development, failure of deciduous teeth to shed, and congenital abnormalities. The normal occlusion is called a *scissor bite*. Scissor bite means that the maxillary incisors are slightly **rostral** to the mandibular incisors, the mandibular canine is forward of the maxillary canine, and the premolars and molars meet in a zigzag fashion.

Malocclusion is any deviation from this normal pattern. Three classes of malocclusions are listed in most literature.

> **Class I**—Both jaws are normal length but one or more teeth are in an abnormal position. Base narrow canines occur when the deciduous canines do not shed normally and the adult canines come in medially. Interference with the upper canines or even the palate can lead to oronasal fistulas. Another example is a crowded second incisor that is displaced rostrally and interferes with the upper incisors. This is called a *crossbite*. A *lance tooth* is a canine tooth that projects rostrally.
>
> **Class II**—The maxilla is longer than the mandible. This may be due to an excessively long maxilla (maxillary prognathism) or an excessively short mandible (mandibular brachygnathism). It used to be called *overshot jaw* or *parrot mouth*.

> **Class III**—The maxilla is shorter than the mandible. This may be due to an excessively short maxilla (maxillary brachygnathism) or an excessively long mandible (mandibular prognathism). This is considered normal in many brachycephalic breeds.

Practice Questions

1. What would be the appropriate care for a tooth fracture with exposed pulp that occurred two weeks ago?
   a. antibiotics and sealing the tooth defect with glass ionomer
   b. subgingival curettage and placement of an osteoconductive material in the alveolar bone
   c. nothing; this will heal on its own
   d. remove the pulp, fill with gutta percha, seal with glass ionomer

2. How do the nerves and blood vessels enter the tooth?
   a. at the apical delta
   b. at the cementoenamel junction
   c. at the periodontal ligament
   d. at the alveolus

3. The majority of the tooth is made of what?
   a. enamel
   b. cementum
   c. dentin
   d. pulp

4. What should be used to anesthetize 406?
   a. a mental block on left
   b. an infra-alveolar block on the right
   c. an infraorbital block on the right
   d. a local infiltration of the PDL around the lower left first premolar

5. What is the hardest substance in the body?
   a. enamel
   b. bone
   c. cementum
   d. lens epithelium

6. What instrument is used during endodontic therapy?
   a. periosteal elevators
   b. rasps
   c. curettes
   d. barbed broaches

7. Which statement regarding dental radiography is *incorrect*?
   a. Dental radiographs are essential both pre- and postoperatively in endodontics.
   b. Dental radiography usually uses nonscreen film.
   c. Dental radiography requires the same PPE as routine radiography.
   d. One lateral view is all that is generally needed for adequate dental radiography.

8. Which of the following animals do not have brachyodont teeth?
   a. rats
   b. dogs
   c. ferrets
   d. horses

9. What is the most common dental pathology seen in the dog?
   a. malignant melanoma
   b. epulis
   c. periodontal disease
   d. tooth fractures

10. What oral pathologies are most commonly associated with calicivirus?
    a. FORL
    b. lymphocytic plasmacytic stomatitis
    c. squamous cell carcinoma
    d. periodontal disease

11. Which of the following statements is *incorrect* regarding rabbit dentistry?
    a. rabbits get periodontal disease
    b. rabbits have aradicular hypsodont teeth
    c. rabbits have two sets of lower incisors
    d. rabbits have cheek tooth problems similar to chinchillas

12. What instrument should only be used supragingivally?
    a. hand scaler
    b. hand curette
    c. ultrasonic scaler
    d. elevator

13. A puppy comes into the clinic with a fairly normal bite except that the lower middle incisor is in front of the upper middle incisor. What is this called?
    a. scissor bite
    b. Class I occlusion
    c. spear or lance tooth
    d. brachygnathism

14. What is the correct order for dental prophylaxis?
    a. probe, explore, scale, radiograph, polish
    b. probe, explore, scale, polish, radiograph
    c. radiograph, probe, explore, scale, polish
    d. radiograph, scale, probe, explore, polish

15. What is the correct order of procedures for endodontic treatment?
   a. drill, barbed broach, file, gutta percha, composite
   b. drill, file, barbed broach, gutta percha, composite
   c. drill, barbed broach, gutta percha, file, composite
   d. drill, composite, barbed broach, file, gutta percha

16. What is a possible cause of FORLs?
   a. herpes virus
   b. feline leukemia virus
   c. anaerobic bacteria
   d. vitamin D problems

17. When is epulis commonly seen?
   a. in cats
   b. in animals with resorptive lesions
   c. in brachycephalic canines
   d. in animals with periodontal disease

18. What is the anaerobic bacterium found in many dogs with severe periodontal disease?
   a. *Pseudomonas*
   b. *Porphyromonas*
   c. *Leptospirosis*
   d. *Staphylococcus*

19. When is doxycycline gel used?
   a. endodontics
   b. exodontics
   c. periodontal treatment
   d. routine prophylaxis

20. Which of the following statements is correct?
   a. Radiographs of the upper premolars should be taken using the parallel technique.
   b. Radiographs of the lower canines should be taken using the parallel technique.
   c. A radiograph to diagnose a draining tract in the infraorbital area should be taken using the bisecting angle technique.
   d. Radiographs of rabbit cheek teeth are best taken using the bisecting angle technique.

21. Cyclosporine and corticosteroids are often used to decrease the pain associated with what condition?
   a. FORL
   b. epulis
   c. tooth fractures
   d. lymphocytic plasmacytic stomatitis

22. Which of the following statements is true?
   a. Canine teeth are susceptible to slab fractures.
   b. Carnassial teeth rarely fracture.
   c. Tooth root fracture can be diagnosed without a radiograph.
   d. Fractures can be treated with endodontic therapy.

23. Which of the following species has a palatal ostium?
   a. chinchilla
   b. mouse
   c. hamster
   d. rabbit

24. Which of the following species has no upper incisors?
   a. horse
   b. cow
   c. hamster
   d. ferret

25. Which of the following statements is true of rodent and rabbit incisors?
   a. They only have enamel on the labial surface.
   b. They are brachyodont.
   c. The upper incisors will penetrate the bottom lip if they overgrow.
   d. They should be trimmed with nail trimmers.

26. Which of the following statements is true of cattle?
   a. They only have lower canines.
   b. They have brachyodont teeth.
   c. They have well-developed temporalis muscles.
   d. They have a narrow temporomandibular joint.

27. A neurologic exam is a central part of the dental assessment. Which cranial nerve is NOT important to the dental exam?
   a. the olfactory nerve
   b. the trochlear nerve
   c. the vagus nerve
   d. the hypoglossal nerve

28. During a dental exam you notice that the left side of a dog's face is drooping. Which cranial nerve is probably affected?
   a. the trigeminal nerve
   b. the facial nerve
   c. the glossopharyngeal nerve
   d. the hypoglossal nerve

29. A dog is unable to swallow and the tongue is pulled to the right side. Which cranial nerve might be affected?
   a. the oculomotor nerve
   b. the trigeminal nerve
   c. the glossopharyngeal nerve
   d. the vagus nerve

30. During a dental exam you notice that the right side of the cat's head seems to be depressed. You attempt to do an oral exam and notice that the mouth does not seem to open as far as it should. There is no history of head trauma. Which muscle is affected?
   a. the temporal
   b. the pterygoid
   c. the masseter
   d. the digastricus

31. An owner complains that the cat has had halitosis (bad breath) for several weeks. You perform an oral exam and notice a 1-cm plaque-like lesion with what appears to be some ulcerations and no pigment. Which of the following is the *least* likely?
   a. fibrosarcoma
   b. squamous cell carcinoma
   c. lymphocytic plasmacytic stomatitis
   d. epulis

32. Which statement about machine scaling is *false*?
   a. Machine scaling can be performed both supra- and subgingivally.
   b. Ultrasonic frequencies are in the range of 18 to 50 kHz.
   c. The tip of the scaler should be at a 90-degree angle to the tooth surface.
   d. The tip must be kept in constant motion to prevent etching the enamel.

33. What type of interference can base narrow canine teeth cause?
   a. The mandibular canine will be caudal to the maxillary canine tooth.
   b. The mandibular canine will interfere with the lateral incisor of the maxilla.
   c. The mandibular canine will penetrate the palate.
   d. The mandibular canine will interfere with the maxillary canine tooth, resulting in fracture.

34. Which of the following statements is true about retained deciduous canine teeth?
   a. They should be removed at 3 months of age to prevent orthodontic abnormalities.
   b. They have fragile roots that can fracture if removed incorrectly. These roots can cause orthodontic problems.
   c. They can prevent the first premolars from breaking through.
   d. They can lead to lance teeth.

35. Which of the following statements is true about periodontal disease?
   a. Formation of the pellicle occurs within one hour of eating a meal.
   b. Gingivitis occurs when the aerobic, gram-positive bacteria changes to gram-negative, anaerobic bacteria.
   c. Feeding a sodium hexametaphosphate-containing food is all that is needed to prevent periodontal disease.
   d. Once-a-week tooth brushing is adequate to prevent the formation of dental calculus.

36. What are supernumary teeth?
   a. the same as retained deciduous teeth
   b. extra adult teeth
   c. teeth with extra exposed crown
   d. teeth with extra roots

37. Endodontic procedures require the canals be flushed with what?
   a. dilute sodium hypochlorite solution
   b. dilute glutaraldehyde solution
   c. normal saline solution
   d. distilled water

38. What is the purpose of the water spray from the scaler?
   a. to cool the tooth surface and the tip
   b. to remove debris by flushing
   c. to provide a medium for cavitation to occur
   d. all of the above

39. What is calcium alginate used for?
   a. making a positive dental model
   b. an endodontic sealer
   c. making an impression
   d. periodontal treatment

40. What is the term for radiation that is reflected from the patient?
   a. scatter radiation
   b. primary beam
   c. ionizing radiation
   d. background radiation

41. In the triadan system, what is the correct numbering for the upper right second premolar in the cat?
   a. 105
   b. 106
   c. 205
   d. 206

42. What is the anatomical designation for 410?
   a. lower left first molar
   b. lower left second molar
   c. lower right first molar
   d. lower right second molar

43. When is a dental bur used?
  a. endodontics
  b. periodontal surgery
  c. exodontics (surgical)
  d. all of the above

44. How many roots does the carnassial tooth have in carnivores?
  a. one
  b. two
  c. three
  d. four

45. Why should oral radiographs be taken for dentistry?
  a. to assess roots
  b. to assess periodontal attachment
  c. to assess the success of endodontics
  d. all of the above

46. Which of the following statements is true about polishing after dental prophylaxis?
  a. A smooth surface is more resistant to bacterial attachment.
  b. Polishing makes the teeth noticeably whiter.
  c. Polishing removes additional plaque.
  d. Polishing kills more bacteria.

47. Which of the following statements about dosimetry badges is true?
  a. They protect from radiation absorption.
  b. They should be worn on the scrub pocket.
  c. They measure the amount of radiation exposure.
  d. They are only necessary when taking full-body films.

48. Which dental specialty deals with diseases of the supporting structures of the tooth?
  a. orthodontics
  b. periodontics
  c. exodontics
  d. endodontics

49. Which dental specialty deals with diseases of the tooth itself?
  a. orthodontics
  b. periodontics
  c. exodontics
  d. endodontics

50. Which dental specialty deals with abnormal orientation of teeth?
  a. orthodontics
  b. periodontics
  c. exodontics
  d. endodontics

Answers and Explanations

1. d. The fracture is two weeks old so it will need endodontic treatment because of bacterial contamination. If it were a fresh tooth fracture with pulp exposure, vital pulpotomy would be appropriate. Teeth do not heal on their own, and subgingival curettage only treats the external surface of the tooth.

2. a. The apical delta is where the blood vessels and nerves enter the tooth. It is the only connection of the pulp cavity to the alveolar bone.

3. c. The majority of the tooth is made up of dentin. Cementum and enamel are only coverings over the tooth. The alveolus is the socket into which the tooth is inserted.

4. b. Infra-alveolar block will anesthetize the entire right mandibular arcade. 406 is the right mandibular second premolar.

5. a. Enamel is harder than any other substance in the body.

6. d. Barbed broaches are used to remove the diseased pulp from the pulp cavity during endodontics. Periosteal elevators, curettes, and rasps are used to treat the external surface of the tooth.

7. d. Multiple views are needed for adequate dental radiography. All other statements are true.

8. d. Horses have only hypsodont teeth. Rats have both hypsodont and brachyodont teeth and dogs and ferrets have only brachyodont teeth.

9. c. Periodontal disease is the most common dental disease in the dog. Malignant melanoma is the most common oral tumor seen in the dog.

10. b. Lymphocytic plasmacytic gingivitis/stomatitis is common in cats with viral diseases such as calicivirus and herpesviruses. FORL lesions may be associated with vitamin D metabolism problems. Squamous cell carcinoma is the most common oral tumor in the cat. Periodontal disease is common in all species but does not depend on viruses.

11. c. Rabbits have two sets of upper incisors. All other statements are true.

12. a. The hand scaler should only be used supragingivally because of the pointy tip and, in the case of the universal scaler, the double blade edge.

13. b. Class I occlusion. Scissor bite is the normal orientation with the maxillary incisors all slightly rostral to the mandibular incisors. Brachygnathism means a short jaw, which affects all teeth. Lance teeth are canine tooth abnormalities.

14. c. Radiograph prior to beginning the prophy, which includes scale, probe, explore, and polish.

15. a. The pulp should be removed prior to filing. So, first would come the drill, then the barbed broach, the file, gutta percha, and then the composite.

16. d. Vitamin D metabolism problems may be associated with FORLs in cats. Diet is being looked into as a causal factor. Viruses are associated with lymphocytic plasmacytic gingivitis/stomatitis. Anaerobic bacteria are associated with periodontal disease.

17. c. Epulis is very common in brachycephalic dogs such as boxers and bulldogs. It may predispose animals to periodontal disease because of increased entrapment of food and hair between the gingiva and the tooth, but this is not a cause of epulis.

18. b. *Porphyromonas gulae* has been implicated as a periodontal pathogen in dogs. The other bacteria listed are either aerobic or microaerophilic.

19. c. Doxycycline gel is used to treat deep periodontal pockets and kill off bacteria in the cementum and superficial alveolar bone.

20. c. Draining tracts in the infraorbital area are usually associated with carnassial tooth root abscesses. Maxillary cheek teeth are best radiographed using the bisecting angle technique. The only teeth that should be radiographed using the parallel technique are the lower cheek teeth (molars and premolars).

21. d. Lymphocytic plasmacytic gingivitis is an inflammatory disease that may respond to immune suppressants such as corticosteroids and cyclosporine. These would be contraindicated in any infectious process and are unnecessary in epulis or FORLs.

22. d. Tooth fractures should be treated with either endodontic therapy or exodontics. Canine teeth are more susceptible to transverse fractures. Carnassial teeth are more prone to slab fractures. All fractured teeth should be radiographed to assess alveolar bone and apical abscesses.

23. a. Chinchillas have a palatal ostium that may make intubation difficult.

24. b. The cow has no upper incisors or canine teeth. The upper incisors are replaced by an incisive pad of tissue.

25. a. The incisors of rodents and rabbits have enamel only on the labial surface. The rest of the tooth is covered in cementum. This allows wear of the posterior surface of the teeth and the formation of a chisel shape. Overgrowth of the incisors usually causes penetration of the upper palate because the teeth grow in a curve. Rabbit and rodent teeth should only be trimmed using a saw because they are brittle and tend to fracture if clipped with nail trimmers.

26. a. Cattle only have lower canine teeth. When present, they are usually only found in males. They only have hypsodont teeth, a wide TMJ, and well-developed masseter muscles for lateral grinding.

27. c. The vagus nerve (CN X) is not important to the oral cavity. The olfactory nerve (CN I) is found in the sinus cavity and may be affected by severe dental disease. The abducens and trochlear nerves (CN IV) may be affected by retrobulbar abscesses, which are common in carnassial tooth root abscesses. The hypoglossal nerve (CN XII) affects the function of the tongue.

28. b. The facial nerve (CN VII) controls the facial muscles. The trigeminal nerve (CN V) is more involved with the muscles of mastication, the glossopharyngeal nerve (CN IX) controls swallowing and taste, and the hypoglossal nerve (CN XII) controls tongue movement.

29. c. The glossopharyngeal nerve (CN IX) controls the ability to swallow and works with CN XII (hypoglossal) to control tongue movement. The oculomotor nerve (CN III) controls pupillary light responses, the trigeminal nerve (CN V) controls the muscles of mastication, and the vagus nerve (CN X) controls the autonomic responses.

30. a. The temporal muscle covers the parietal bone and controls the ability to open and close the mouth. The masseter muscle allows side to side movement of the jaw, the pterygoid is found within the mouth, and the digastricus is found between the sides of the mandible.

31. d. Epulis is rare in the cat. All the other choices could fit the symptoms.

32. c. The tip of the scaler should never be oriented at 90 degrees because of the jackhammer effect. This can cause damage to both the tooth and the tip of the instrument. All the other answers are true.

33. c. Base narrow means that the lower canines are closer together than the maxillary canines. This is usually caused by retained mandibular deciduous canines. The mandibular canines can either interfere with the palatal surface of the upper canines causing attrition, or they can actually penetrate the hard palate.

34. b. When permanent canine teeth do not erupt and force out the deciduous teeth, the two sets of teeth appear alongside one another. This condition is known as retained deciduous canine teeth and these have fragile roots that fracture easily. These deciduous teeth should be removed at 4 to 5 months of age.

35. b. Gingivitis occurs when the bacterial flora change and begin releasing inflammatory mediators. Tooth brushing should be performed a minimum of every other day. All the other answers are false.

36. b. Supernumary teeth are extra adult teeth.

37. a. Pulp cavities should be flushed with a dilute sodium hypochlorite solution. Distilled water and saline will not disinfect and glutaraldehyde will damage the surrounding tissues (it is a chemical sterilant; see Chapter 5).

38. d. All of the above. Water is required to flush away debris such as plaque and tartar. The ultrasound frequencies cause cavitation of the water molecules, which blast apart debris. Water also removes heat from the tip of the scaler and the tooth and rinses the surface after plaque destruction.

39. c. The teeth are placed into the calcium alginate gel in order to make a negative impression from which the model (dental stone) is made. Ceramic or glass ionomer is used to seal the tooth during endodontic treatment.

40. a. Scatter radiation is that which is reflected from either the patient or the surface that the patient is on. The primary beam is the direct radiation from the tube. Ionizing radiation is either x-rays or gamma rays that can cause changes in somatic cells. Background radiation is normal radiation from the sun or the surrounding room that people are exposed to on a regular basis.

41. b. Triadan numbering 205 and 206 refer to the upper left quadrant, not the upper right. The right maxillary arcade is the 100 series of teeth, but cats do not have a tooth 105. Count backwards from 109, which is the first molar, and 106 is the upper right second premolar.

42. d. The lower right arcade is the 400 series. The first molar is 409, so the second molar is 410.

43. d. All of the above. The dental bur (drill) is used to approach the pulp cavity in endodontics, to approach the roots in surgical exodontics, and to remove diseased cementum and alveolar bone in periodontics.

44. c. The carnassial tooth has three roots.

45. d. All the above. Oral radiographs can assess alveolar bone attachment, root fractures, apical abscesses, and the quality of endodontic filling.

46. a. Polishing smoothes out the microscopic defects caused by the scaling procedure. The plaque bacteria have more difficulty attaching to a smooth surface. Note: This is the principle behind the use of wax dental sealants.

47. c. Dosimetry badges are monitoring devices only. They should be worn outside the lead apron and collar as close to the thyroid area as possible.

48. b. Periodontics is the dental specialty that deals with the supporting tissues of the tooth (gingiva, periodontal ligament, and alveolar bone).

49. d. Endodontics is the dental specialty that deals with the tooth itself. Exodontics does not treat the disease, it removes it. Orthodontics deals with mouth architecture, and periodontics deals with the supporting structures.

50. a. Orthodontics deals with orientation and occlusion within the oral cavity.

7 ▶ LABORATORY PROCEDURES PART 1

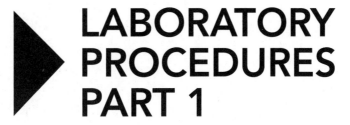

CHAPTER OVERVIEW

Laboratory procedures are a significant part of the veterinary practice. This is such a significant topic and so central to any veterinary practice that we were forced to divide it into two chapters. This chapter discusses hematology, coagulation and bone marrow testing, cytology/histology, clinical chemistry, and immunology/serology. The next chapter covers the second half of lab work, parasitology, urinalysis, and microbiology.

The ability to perform and interpret laboratory information is necessary to diagnosis and treatment of animals because they are unable to tell the veterinarian what their symptoms are and evaluate how they "feel." The ability to bring together and evaluate information obtained from laboratory tests is important to communication between the doctor, the technician, and the client.

Knowledge of subjects such as blood science, testing, clinical chemistry, and immunology are central to a modern veterinary practice. Hematology is the study of blood and blood-related diseases, and testing the blood is one of the most common ways of discovering the health of an animal. These tests are generally fairly simple to perform and inexpensive, which is why hematologic testing is one of the keystones of any veterinary practice.

Key Terms

acidosis

agglutination

alkalosis

anticoagulant

azotemia

chemotaxis

ejaculate

hematochezia

hematologic indices

hematopoiesis

hemoglobin

hemolysis

icterus index

leukogram

lipemia

malabsorption

malassimilation

maldigestion

marginating pool

mean corpuscular hemoglobin (MCH)

mean corpuscular hemoglobin concentration (MCHC)

mean corpuscular volume (MCV)

melena

negative feedback

pellet

phlebotomy

plasma

polychromatophil

polydipsia

polyuria

reticulocyte

serology

serum

supernatant

turbidity

uremia

Vacutainer®

venipuncture

viscosity

Concepts and Skills

This chapter will include questions that focus on the first part of laboratory procedures, covering six primary concepts:

- hematology
- coagulation testing
- bone marrow testing
- cytology and histopathy
- clinical chemistry
- immunology and serology

Hematology

Hematology can provide the veterinary practice with valuable information about the animal's ability to carry oxygen, organ function, and immunologic status. Calculations based on hematologic values allow us to classify anemias and the animal's ability to respond to invaders. The ability to perform and interpret the CBC (complete blood count), hematologic indices, and leukogram are integral to the operation of a veterinary practice.

Hematologic Testing

Proper interpretation of blood work requires good phlebotomy (blood drawing), knowledge of appropriate blood tubes and appropriate storage techniques, and the ability to make a diagnostic blood smear. Failure in any of these areas can lead to artifacts that can interfere with proper interpretation of results and can invalidate any results obtained.

Phlebotomy: Drawing a Good Blood Sample

Phlebotomy is the art (and science) of getting blood from a vein, usually for the purposes of diagnostic blood testing. Drawing an adequate blood sample begins with knowledge of the appropriate quantity of blood to be obtained. Blood can be drawn from an animal up to $\frac{1}{4}$ of the total blood volume. Blood tubes are labeled with the quantity of blood needed to fill the tube. They are maintained in a vacuum so that the appropriate amount of blood will be added to the tube when a **Vacutainer®** system is used. This is especially important in tubes containing an **anticoagulant**. Inappropriate quantities of blood added to anticoagulant tubes can result in artifacts on the blood smear and in dilution for packed cell volume (PCV) and total protein (TP) measurements. Drawing blood with a needle and syringe is common in practice, but may cause problems with **hemolysis** (red blood cell rupture and release of hemoglobin), which will interfere with many chemistry results. In general, it is best to take too much blood than too little.

Blood Tubes

Blood tubes have tops that designate the additive (or lack of an additive) and the purpose of the tube. Most tubes are used to separate the liquid from the cellular components of the blood. The resultant liquid is either plasma or serum, depending on whether it is allowed to clot prior to centrifugation. If it is allowed to clot, it is called **serum** and does not contain the clotting proteins. The total protein (TP) of serum will be slightly lower because of this. **Plasma** still contains fibrinogen.

BLOOD TUBES			
COLOR OF TUBE	ADDITIVE	USES	SPECIAL TECHNIQUES
Red top	none	serum tests (chemistry); should NOT be used for blood glucose determination (will decrease blood glucose)	blood must be in tube for a minimum of 60 minutes prior to centrifugation to assure clot formation
Tiger top (red and black)	clot activator and agar gel	serum tests (chemistry); should NOT be used for blood glucose determination (will decrease blood glucose)	blood must be in tube for a minimum of 30 minutes prior to centrifugation to assure clot formation
Tiger top (yellow and gray)	thrombin clot activator (causes very rapid clot formation) and agar gel	serum tests (chemistry); may be used as preliminary screening for blood glucose	blood must be in tube for a minimum of 5 minutes prior to centrifugation to assure clot formation
Green top	heparin anticoagulant	plasma tests CBC in reptiles the tube should be inverted several times to ensure adequate mixing	if used for chemistry, centrifuge immediately after mixing and remove the plasma with a pipette to a red top tube; label as *heparinized plasma*
Blue top	sodium citrate	coagulation studies (PT, aPTT) the tube should be inverted several times to ensure adequate mixing	if used for coagulation studies, centrifuge immediately after mixing and remove the plasma with a pipette to a red top tube; label as *citrated plasma*
Lavender top	EDTA anticoagulant (ethylene diamine tetra acetic acid)	CBC in mammals the tube should be inverted several times to ensure adequate mixing	EDTA binds calcium, which is needed for the coagulation cascade

(continued)

COLOR OF TUBE	ADDITIVE	USES	SPECIAL TECHNIQUES
BLOOD TUBES (continued)			
Gray top with label Gray top with label	sodium fluoride calcium oxalate	blood glucose determination blood glucose determination	sodium fluoride should be used for blood glucose determination because it stabilizes the glucose in the plasma
Gray top without label	diatomaceous earth	activated clotting time (ACT)	

Technique

Performing phlebotomy properly without causing artifact is one of the most important skills for a veterinary technician in practice (or research). The primary sites for venipuncture are:

Cat and dog: jugular vein, cephalic vein, lateral saphenous, common saphenous/femoral vein (cats only)

Horse: jugular vein, facial vein, tail vein

Cow: jugular vein, tail vein

The most important part of **venipuncture** is atraumatic technique. This requires the ability to visualize the vein and a basic knowledge of anatomy. Visualization can be improved by clipping the area and wetting it with isopropyl alcohol, which will cause blood vessel dilation. The needle should follow the path and direction of the vein. The vein should be held off between the venipuncture site and the heart to increase the back pressure of blood in the vein and allow it to stick out. You should not try to fish for the vein because this will cause tissue damage with the release of tissue thromboplastin, which will cause platelet activation and clotting in the syringe and the blood tube. As stated, Vacutainer® systems should be used if possible. If coagulation studies must be performed, a Vacutainer is essential. If Vacutainers are not available, care must be taken not to collapse the vein by using excessive back pressure when pulling back on the syringe. Collapsing the vein will also cause tissue damage and increase platelet activation.

Use of appropriate needle and syringe size is also important when performing phlebotomy. All materials needed for venipuncture should be collected *prior* to beginning the process. The needle should be the maximum size that can comfortably fit into the vein without causing damage to the vessel wall. Use of a very small needle will cause hemolysis by increasing turbulence inside the needle and disrupting the red blood cell membranes. **Hemoglobin** in the plasma is also possible from certain diseases (blood parasites and autoimmune hemolytic anemia, for example), so iatrogenic hemolysis (hemolysis caused by bad technique) may cause a misdiagnosis of another problem.

Blood Storage

In general, blood should be processed as quickly as possible after being drawn and centrifuged. Many chemistry values (such as ammonia and glucose, for example) will be invalidated by prolonged time between blood draw and processing and blood cell morphology will also be affected. Platelets will aggregate and lyse after 6 hours of storage. Ideally, whole blood should be kept refrigerated and processed within 6 hours. Plasma should be frozen if not processed within 6 hours. Serum should be kept refrigerated and processed within 8 hours.

Artifacts

As stated, hemolysis and platelet activation are the most common artifacts seen from improper blood handling. **Lipemia** (increased fat and cholesterol in the plasma) may also interfere with machine blood counts and several chemistry tests. Lipemia may be caused by metabolic diseases (hypothyroidism, hyperadrenocorticism, diabetes), be an inherited problem (congenital hypertriglyceridemia), or be caused by eating prior to blood draw. For this reason, animals should be fasted for 10 to 12 hours prior to drawing blood for analysis. Postprandial lipemia usually occurs within 2 to 3 hours of a meal.

Making a Good Blood Smear

With the advent of better machine blood cell counters, many veterinarians and veterinary technicians have lost the art of making and reading a good blood smear. This technique is extremely important. Without hand evaluation of blood smears, many pathologies will be missed including parasitism, hematopoetic cancers (leukemias), certain toxicities (lead, zinc, maple leaf, acetaminophen) and other cellular inclusion diseases (*Ehrlichia*, anaplasma, hemobartonella, distemper). In general, a blood smear should be performed if any abnormality on the machine CBC is seen or if the animal is ill.

A good blood smear has three parts: the body, the monolayer, and the feathered edge. No matter which technique is used, the smear should look like a flame, with the base being made of the body and the feathered edge as the flickering outer portion of the flame. The sides of the smear should not make contact with either edge, and the monolayer should be of adequate size to analyze for the white blood cell differential.

The key to making a good smear is the size of the drop. It should be small enough that the contact with the spreading slide does not bring the blood to the slide edges, but big enough that the smear is adequate size. The slide for the sample should be clean and free of scratches and the spreading slide should have a smooth edge for making contact with the blood drop.

The drop of blood is placed on the sample slide approximately one-fifth of the length of the slide away from the edge. The edge of the spreader slide is placed on the sample slide at a 45-degree angle and is backed into the blood drop and smoothly pushed across the length of the slide. The blood will be drawn along with the spreader slide to make the characteristic flame shape. The body is the portion of the smear closest to the original drop. This section is the thickest area and cannot be evaluated because the cells are piled on top of one another, making individual morphology (cell shape and staining characteristics) difficult. The monolayer is the diagnostic area. This region is thinner and contains cells in a single layer (red, white, and platelets) that can be evaluated for cellular morphology. The feathered edge is where the heaviest items are seen, including clumps of platelets, parasites (trypanosomes and microfilaria), and destroyed red blood cells. This area should not be used to evaluate white blood cell morphology, but should be used for platelet estimation in cases of artifactual platelet clumping.

Once the smear is made it should be stained with a Romanowsky type stain (an alcohol-based stain) such as Diff-Quick. Diff-Quick has three parts: the fixative (methyl alcohol), the eosin stain (which stains the proteins of the cell red), and the basophilic stain (methylene blue stain) which stains the nucleic acids of the cell blue. Artifacts can result from staining. These include the following:

water artifact—a refractile artifact (highly reflective bubbles in the cytoplasm of cells) resulting from water contamination of the alcohol fixative; may be mistaken for parasitic infection

stain precipitate—a purple aggregate of small crystals that may be mistaken for platelet clumping; usually found in a different focal plane on the microscope than the cells

Both of these artifacts can be prevented by appropriate maintenance of the Diff-Quick stain by changing out the alcohol and stains and cleaning the staining jars regularly. Staining solutions and alcohol fix should not be topped off with fresh solution because this will increase artifacts.

Red Blood Cell Indices

Evaluation of anemias and polycythemias is within the scope of practice of veterinary technicians. Such an evaluation will result in a *laboratory diagnosis*. The method for making laboratory diagnosis of anemias is to perform **hematologic index** calculations. Laboratory diagnosis is the responsibility of the technician while medical diagnosis is the responsibility of the veterinarian.

Hematocrit

The hematocrit (HCT) is arguably the most important piece of laboratory information obtained from the patient. A total of ten items of interest may be obtained from the HCT: the icterus index (II), packed cell volume (PCV), buffy coat (BC), total protein (TP), and occasionally microfilaria can be seen by direct examination. Estimated red blood cell count (RBC), estimated hemoglobin (HB), mean cell hemoglobin concentration (MCHC), mean corpuscular hemoglobin (MCH), and mean cell volume (MCV) can be obtained by calculations based on the HCT.

The HCT is performed by collecting blood into a microhematocrit tube approximately two-thirds full, sealing one end with clay, and placing the tube into a balanced high-speed microhematocrit centrifuge. The tube is spun for 3 to 5 minutes on high speed. This separates the various blood components (serum, white blood cells and platelets, and red blood cells).

Icterus Index

The **icterus index** (II) is the color of the serum. Normal serum is clear to straw colored (in herbivores, it may appear yellow to orange because of the amount of beta carotene or vitamin A in the diet). Other colors may indicate disease or iatrogenic problems with blood handling. The serum color is evaluated by placing the tube in front of a white piece of paper and assessing the color.

ICTERUS INDEX		
COLOR OF SERUM/PLASMA	**PIGMENT**	**CAUSE**
Red	hemoglobin	intravascular hemolysis from autoimmune disease (autoimmune hemolytic anemia) or red blood cell parasites that cause red blood cell lysis
	myoglobin	muscle breakdown (myositis)
Yellow	bilirubin	cholestatic disease (gall bladder or bile stasis)
		extravascular hemolysis* from red blood cell parasites that increase splenic RBC breakdown, toxicity reactions, red blood cell fragmentation diseases (hemangiosarcoma, iron deficiency anemias)
	carotenoids	yellow serum may be normal in herbivores with high levels of carotene or vitamin A in the diet
White	fat/lipemia	hypothyroidism, hyperadrenocorticism, diabetes, postprandial
Pink/opaque	hemolysis and lipemia	
Bright orange	hemolysis and icterus	

*Extravascular hemolysis is red blood cell destruction that happens in the tissues (usually spleen and liver). Destruction of red blood cells by the macrophages in these tissues causes hemoglobin to be broken down into its components: heme, iron, and globulin. The heme is then further broken down into bilirubin in the liver, where it is released into the serum.

Packed Cell Volume

The packed cell volume (PCV) tells us the percentage of red blood cells per milliliter of whole blood. It is an estimate of anemia but should not be evaluated without also checking the total protein (TP). The PCV is read by placing the hematocrit tube against a Read-o-crit scale. The top of the clay and the top of the serum column are lined up with the bottom and top lines of the scale and the interface between the buffy coat and the red blood cell column is located. That line corresponds to the PCV.

The reason the PCV should not be evaluated by itself is that it depends on the hydration of the animal. If an animal is dehydrated, there will be less water and thus less serum in the whole blood. The total protein will be elevated because the protein will be more concentrated. The PCV will, therefore, appear increased. If the PCV is elevated in the face of a high total protein, that is not a real value. If it is elevated and the TP is low or normal, that is a real value and pathology should be suspected.

Buffy Coat

The buffy coat (BC) is a rough estimate of the white blood cell count. It is made up of white blood cells and platelets and should be the smallest component of the HCT. It should be 1 to 2% of the column and should be measured when the PCV is measured. If microfilaria are present due to heartworm disease or *Dipetalonema*, they can be visualized at the BC serum interface by examining the tube at low power under the microscope. Buffy coat smears may be made, which will allow visualization of white blood cell parasites such as *Ehrlichia*. The technique is the same as for a normal blood smear except that the sample will consist of the buffy coat material only.

Total Protein

The total protein (TP) concentration must be evaluated along with the PCV, as described. Most of the proteins in the blood are made in the liver.

The highest concentration of protein in the blood is albumin. Albumin is the protein that con-

trols osmotic pressure (maintenance of blood volume inside the blood vessels). In general, a drop in TP means a drop in albumin concentration. The most common cause of decreased albumin concentration is liver disease.

The second highest concentration of proteins in the blood is fibrinogen. Fibrinogen may cause an increase in TP in animals with inflammation (especially cattle).

The rest of the TP is made up of the globulins, including the immunoglobulins.

Estimates

Two estimates can be obtained from the PCV: the red blood cell estimate and the hemoglobin estimate. The red blood cell estimate may be vastly different from the actual count and should not replace it. The hemoglobin estimate may have to be used in animals with severe lipemia or hemolysis because both of these artifacts will interfere with machine calculations of hemoglobin concentrations.

$$\text{RBC est} = \frac{\text{PCV}}{6} \times 10^6/\mu l$$
$$\text{HB est} = \frac{\text{PCV}}{3} \text{ g/dl (grams per deciliter)}$$

Mean Cell Hemoglobin Concentration and Mean Corpuscular Hemoglobin

Mean corpuscular hemoglobin concentration (MCHC) and **mean corpuscular hemoglobin** (MCH) are the two calculations that will estimate the amount of hemoglobin present in the blood. Although the MCHC is more accurate, the MCH is still used in practice. These calculations are important because, along with the MCV, they will help us to give a laboratory diagnosis of an anemia. Young red blood cells contain less hemoglobin than adult red blood cells. This means that they will not be able to carry as much oxygen as adult cells. On cellular morphology, they will appear blue-tinged by the stain because they still contain ribosomes for hemoglobin manufacture. These cells are called **polychromatophils** because they vary in color from the adult RBCs. A regenerative anemia will have a decreased MCH and MCHC because there will be more polychromatophils present resulting in a decreased hemoglobin concentration. This is called a hypochromic anemia (low-color anemia). The hyperchromic (too much hemoglobin) state is not possible. The calculations for MCH and MCHC are:

$$MCH = \frac{HB \times 10}{RBC} \text{ pg (picograms are one-trillionth of a gram)}$$

$$MCHC = \frac{HB \times 100}{PCV} \text{ g/dl (grams per deciliter)}$$

Mean Corpuscular Volume

The **mean corpuscular volume** (MCV) estimates the average size of the red blood cell. This is important for similar reasons to the MCH and MCHC. Young red blood cells are larger than adult red blood cells so, if a regenerative anemia is present, the MCV will be increased. This is called macrocytosis. If we have very old red blood cells or the cells are being damaged (fragmentation hemolysis), we may have a low MCV. This is called microcytosis.

To review, if we have a low PCV with a low MCHC and a high MCV, we would call that a hypochromic, macrocytic anemia, which would generally indicate a regenerative anemia. If, on the other hand, we have a low PCV with a normal MCHC and a high MCV, we would call that a normochromic, macrocytic anemia, which would probably indicate something like an iron deficiency anemia (inadequate production of hemoglobin because there are low iron stores).

Although machines can calculate these values, the machine will not be able to read the hemoglobin concentrations in cases of hemolysis and lipemia. The ability to calculate HB estimates, the MCHC, and the MCV may help the veterinarian diagnose a case. The MCHC and MCV results should always be checked against a reticulocyte count (see Reticulocyte Counts).

Hematologic Inclusions and Abnormalities

Blood cell morphology (shape and staining characteristics) can be very important to the diagnosis of various diseases including viral, bacterial, and parasitic disease. Toxicities can affect cellular morphology as well.

Red Blood Cell Inclusions

The function of the red blood cell is oxygen distribution. Oxygen is carried on the hemoglobin molecule, which consists of proteins (heme and globin) bound to ionic iron. The reason for blood's red color is oxidation of the iron ion. It literally rusts the iron, making it red.

Normal blood cells in most mammals are anuclear (having no nucleus), round, and biconcave (indented on both sides). Camellid (alpaca, camels, vicuna, llama) blood is elliptical in shape. Erythrocytes stain red/orange with Diff-Quick stain in the adult form. As stated, young red blood cells are called polychromatophils and stain various shades of blue with Diff-Quick. Polychromatophils are generally larger than adult red blood cells and are generally not biconcave. Very young circulating red blood, *metarubricytes*, cells may still have a nucleus. They usually have a dark blue cytoplasm and a dark, condensed nucleus. The nucleus is expelled from the cell when it becomes a polychromatophil. Incomplete expulsion results in Howell-Jolly bodies, which are nuclear remnants in adult red blood cells.

Reptile, avian, and fish red blood cells are elliptical and nucleated. The nuclei are dense and oval and the cytoplasm is pink. The polychromatophils have more open nuclei and bluish cytoplasms. Metarubricytes and other young red blood cells look similar to those of mammals.

Viral Inclusions

Distemper virus results in intracytoplasmic inclusions in all blood cells and epithelial cells. The inclusions generally stain pink and are round and varied in size.

Bacterial Inclusions

Hemobartonella/Mycoplasma organisms are atypical bacteria that lack cell walls.

Anaplasma marginale is the most prevalent tick-borne disease in livestock. It is a rickettsial bacterium and an obligate intracellular parasitic bacterium. The bacterium produces toxins that eventually destroy the blood cells (extravascular hemolysis).

BACTERIAL INCLUSIONS				
GENUS/SPECIES	VECTOR	SYMPTOMS	DIAGNOSIS	TREATMENT
Mycoplasma felis	fleas	severe anemia; common with feline leukemia	bacterial aggregates in rings or clumps on or around RBC	tetracyclines
Mycoplasma canis or mycoplasma haemocanis	ticks (may be zoonotic)	severe anemia; usually only pathogenic in splenectomized dogs	chains of organisms on RBC	
Anaplasma marginale	ticks	anemia, extravascular hemolysis, jaundice, bilirubinuria	single or multiple organisms on the margins of RBC on blood smear	

Parasitic Inclusions

Most of the parasitic inclusions, or hemosporidians, infect red blood cells exclusively. Leukocytozoon also infects white blood cells. They have varying pathogenicity depending on the species and most are fairly host specific. Their clinical signs and treatments will be discussed in the Parasitology section in Chapter 8. Appearance on examination of the blood smear is laid out in the following table.

THE HEMOSPORIDIANS				
GENUS/SPECIES	DEFINITIVE HOST	VECTOR	SYMPTOMS	DIAGNOSIS
Plasmodium spp. (malaria)	birds and reptiles	mosquitoes	intravascular hemolysis, anemia	organism occupies red blood cell, displacing the nucleus
Haemoproteus spp.	birds and reptiles	any blood-sucking insect	nonpathogenic	organism occupies red blood cell cytoplasm, but does not displace the nucleus
Leukocytozoon	birds	simulium flies	intravascular hemolysis, anemia, and death	organism occupies all types of blood cells, displaces the nucleus, and distorts the shape of the cells.
Cytauxoon	bobcat (cats)	dermacentor ticks (probably)	nonpathogenic in bobcat in domestic cat, intravascular hemolysis and death	signet-ring shaped organism within the red blood cell
Babesia spp.	see Chapter 8	ticks	extravascular hemolysis, anemia, jaundice, hemoglobinuria	paired trophozoites in cytoplasm of the red blood cell

Toxic Inclusions

Various toxins can cause inclusions in red blood cells. These may be confused with some of the bacterial and parasitic inclusions and must be differentiated.

TOXIC INCLUSIONS				
INCLUSION	**TOXICITY**	**APPEARANCE WITH DIFF-QUICK**	**APPEARANCE WITH NEW METHYLENE BLUE**	**CAUSE OF INCLUSION**
Basophilic stippling	lead, arsenic	peppering of blue granules throughout the red blood cell	looks like a reticulocyte	aggregations of ribosomes in cytoplasm strongly regenerative anemia
Heinz bodies	acetaminophen (cats) zinc (all species) maple leaf (horses) onion and garlic (dogs)	lavender projections from the margins of the red blood cell; may see keratocytes (helmet cells) from splenic macrophage activity	dark blue projections from the margins of the red blood cell	oxidized hemoglobin (methemoglobin)

White Blood Cell Inclusions

The function of the white blood cells is in immunity. Some white blood cells directly phagocytize invaders (monocytes and macrophages), others have granules that help to digest foreign invaders (neutrophils, eosinophils, basophils), and still others manufacture proteins and mediators that destroy invaders (lymphocytes). White blood cells are divided into two groups: granulocytes and agranulocytes, depending on the presence or absence of granules in the cytoplasm. The granulocytes include neutrophils, eosinophils, and basophils. The agranulocytes include lymphocytes and monocytes.

The granulocytes have condensed, pinched-off nuclei in the adult form (segmented). In the younger forms, the nucleus is smooth and shaped like a tube or band. In very young forms, the nucleus is round and indented (metamyelocyte). All three forms contain granules.

Neutrophils are the cells involved in acute inflammatory processes. The granules of neutrophils are neutral to stain (do not stain with Diff-Quick), so the cytoplasm is clear. Neutrophils are the most numerous white blood cell in all species except cattle. Numbers increase in any inflammatory or infectious process (neutrophilias) because neutrophils respond to cell mediators from tissue damage and bacterial cell wall products. Decreases in neutrophils are called neutropenias. Neutrophils are very short lived in the blood stream (8 hours).

Birds and reptiles do not have neutrophils; their equivalent is the heterophil. Heterophils have round nuclei and a mixture of red/eosinophilic and clear granules. The function is the same as that of neutrophils.

Eosinophils are involved with allergic and parasitic diseases. The granules of eosinophils stain with eosin (they are red in Diff-Quick-stained samples). The granules may be large and round (horses), rod shaped (cats), or small and round (dogs and cattle). Eosinophil granules contain substances that directly destroy parasites and others that counteract the effects of basophils, such as histaminase. Eosinophils are usually equal in numbers to monocytes on differential cell counts. They tend to last for 8 to 14 hours in the blood stream. Elevations are called eosinophilias; decreases are called eosinopenias.

The granules in eosinophils from birds and reptiles can vary in color from red to lavender or blue (common in snakes, cockatoos, and owls). The function of these cells is the same as for mammalian eosinophils.

Basophils are also involved in allergic and parasitic diseases. Both eosinophils and basophils respond to IgE, the immunoglobulin associated with allergic disease. The granules of basophils stain with the basophilic stain (they are purple on Diff-Quick-stained samples). The granules are generally small and round and may fill the entire cytoplasm, making it difficult to see the nucleus. In cats, the granules are very small and appear as lightly dusted purple or just a diffuse purple/lavender color to the cytoplasm. Basophils contain several vasoactive amines such as histamine and heparin, which are involved in anaphylactic reactions. They also contain eosinophil chemotactic factor, which calls eosinophils to the site of degranulation (eosinophils counteract some of the damaging effects of basophil degranulation). Basophils are the least numerous of all the white blood cells. Basophil elevation (basophilia) is commonly seen in heartworm disease.

The agranulocytes are both the largest and the smallest white blood cells. Agranulocytes look the same in birds and reptiles as in mammals. They do not contain granules. They are very long lived in the circulation. Lymphocytes may remain in the tissues and circulation for years. Monocytes can go into tissues and back into the circulation (granulocytes are trapped in the tissues and cannot go back into the circulation). Most lymphocytes are found in the lymph nodes. Most monocytes convert to macrophages, which are embedded in the tissues (Kuppfer cells in the liver, Langerhans cells in the skin, etc.). Granulocytes are only seen in the tissues in inflammatory responses.

Monocytes are very large cells (about five red blood cells can fit inside a monocyte). The blast (young) forms look very similar to the mature cells. Monocytes have a bluish grey cytoplasm and a pink-purple nucleus with open chromatin (light can come through the nucleus) that varies in shape. The cytoplasm often has vacuoles and looks foamy. The nuclear-to-cytoplasmic ratio (how much cytoplasm vs. how much nucleus) is usually 1:1 (the nucleus has the same area as the cytoplasm). Monocytes are involved in chronic inflammatory processes and in processing antigens for presentation to lymphocytes. They will be increased in viral infections and chronic inflammatory disease (such as fungal infections or granulomas). Monocytes' main purpose is phagocytosis. Monocytes are often seen with red blood cells, bacteria, or other organisms in their vacuoles. An increase is called monocytosis; a decrease is called monocytopenia.

Lymphocytes are usually very small cells that are almost the same size as a red blood cell in their inactive form. The cytoplasm is light (active form) or dark blue (inactive form) and the nucleus may be either condensed (inactive form) or contain open chromatin (active form). There may be a perinuclear halo (lighter area in the cytoplasm around the nucleus) that corresponds to the Golgi apparatus that is actively making proteins (either immunoglobulins or complement) in active cells during an immune response. Lymphocytes are the second-highest number of white blood cells in the circulation in all but cattle, where they are the most numerous.

Lymphocytes are grouped into B cells and T cells depending on where the cells are labeled. B cells are labeled in the bone marrow in mammals and in the bursa of Fabricius in birds. T cells are labeled in the thymus gland. B cells are responsible for humoral immunity (making immunoglobulins) and T cells are responsible for cell-mediated immunity (making complement and causing direct death of organisms and cancer cells). Most of the circulating lymphocytes are T cells. In FIV (feline immunodeficiency virus), SIV (simian immunodeficiency virus), and HIV (human immunodeficiency virus), the T cells are depressed in number. This leaves patients open to viral infection and cancers.

The trigger for lymphocyte and monocyte increases is any antigenic stimulation. An antigen is any protein or glycoprotein that is perceived as foreign to the body. The monocyte phagocytizes the invader and presents a modified portion of the invader on its surface. This is then handed off to a B lymphocyte, which makes a specific antibody to that particular protein and clones itself so that more can be made. A T lymphocyte would make a receptor on its surface that binds to the protein so the T lymphocyte can release substances to destroy it (complement). Each B and T lymphocyte is specific to a particular protein.

WHITE BLOOD CELL PARASITIC INCLUSIONS				
GENUS/SPECIES (DEFINITIVE HOST)	VECTOR	SYMPTOMS	DIAGNOSIS	TREATMENT
Neorickettsia risticii/ Ehrlichia risticii (horse)	tick	Potomac horse fever; severe leukopenias, diarrhea, fever, abortion, laminitis	morula (purple staining inclusions) in neutrophils and monocytes; perform buffy coat smears	tetracycline derivatives; vaccine available
Ehrlichia canis (dog)	*Rhipicephalus sanguineus* (brown dog tick)	tropical pancytopenia (decrease in neutrophils, monocytes, platelets, and RBC)	ELISA tests	tetracyclines
Ehrlichia lewinii (dog)	*Amblyomma americanum* (Lone Star tick)	decrease in neutrophils, monocytes, platelets, and RBC; arthritis	ELISA tests	tetracyclines
Anaplasma phagocytophilum/ Ehrlichia equi (horse, ruminants, and man)	unknown (definitive host is actually the white-footed mouse)	decreased neutrophils	ELISA tests	tetracyclines
Leishmania (humans and dogs)	*Lutzomyia* (sand fly)	granuloma formation in the skin and visceral tissues (liver and spleen)	skin or visceral biopsy; organisms are in the macrophages and neutrophils	no effective treatment is available; vaccine is available in Mexico

Platelet Inclusions

Mammalian platelets are cell fragments that are made from cell budding of the megakaryocyte in the bone marrow. They are basically packages of coagulation mediators, calcium, and inflammatory mediators. Platelets appear as small granular purple bodies between cells in the monolayer of stained slides.

Birds, reptiles, and fish have thrombocytes, which are cells that have the same functions as platelets. Thrombocytes have dark, condensed nuclei and refractile-appearing cytoplasm on Diff-Quick stain.

Platelets (and thrombocytes) function in primary hemostasis, which is the formation of the unstable clot. The unstable clot forms and degrades within 2 to 3 minutes of blood vessel injury. Platelets are drawn to the site of a blood vessel injury by mediators produced by the blood vessel lining (vascular endothelium). Once there, they bind to the subendothelial collagen by a bridge of von Willebrand factor (vWF) and factor VIII. Binding stimulates the platelets to aggregate (come together) and adhere (become sticky). They also produce platelet chemotactic factor, which calls more platelets to the area. They initiate the secondary clotting cascade which eventually forms the stable fibrin clot.

Defects of primary clot formation can occur with too few platelets (thrombocytopenia) or decreased platelet function (von Willebrand disease, collagen deficits, uremia, etc.). Platelet counts generally must be less than 80,000/µl in order to cause clotting deficits. More information on secondary coagulation and coagulation testing can be found in the section on Coagulation Testing.

Anaplasma platys (formerly *Ehrlichia platys*) is a rickettsial organism that specifically invades platelets, causing infectious canine cyclic thrombocytopenia (ICCT). The morula can be seen in the platelet cytoplasm as a uniform purple inclusion. *A. platys* causes profound thrombocytopenia leading to bleeding disorders and fevers in dogs (epistaxis, echhymosis, petechiae, etc.). It is carried by the brown dog tick (*Rhipicephalus sanguineus*). It may be difficult to diagnose on blood smear because of the similarity in color to the platelet. ELISA, IFA, and polymerase chain reaction (PCR) testing are available and accurate for diagnosis.

Noncellular Hematologic Parasites

Some of the parasites seen on blood smears are extracellular. These are usually fairly large organisms and are usually seen on the feathered edge of the blood smear.

Hemoflagellates

Hemoflagellates are trypanosomes. Trypanosomes are protozoal organisms with a flagellum and an undulating membrane. They are generally transmitted by reduviid bugs or flies. They live between the blood cells, but the amastigote stage lives in the tissues and causes damage. *Trypanosoma cruzi* causes Chagas disease, and the amastigote stage infests muscle tissue (including cardiac muscle) and can cause cardiomyopathy. Buffy coat smears should be made if trypanosomes are suspected.

Filarial Nematodes

Filarial nematode testing can be broken down into microfilarial testing (visualization of the microfilarial stage in the blood) or serology/ELISA (testing for the presence of adult worms or the antibodies to adult worms in the blood). Testing for all but the presence of antibodies requires presence of adult worms in the heart and pulmonary vessels and will not show prepatent infections. Since heartworms migrate for a prolonged period of time in the larval form (4 to 6 months), significant damage can occur in animals prone to respiratory difficulty from heartworm migration. In cats, a combination of antibody and antigen testing may be required to obtain a diagnosis because of the low worm burden (usually only 3 to 5 adult heartworms are present in cats) and lack of microfilaria in the systemic circulation (see the Immunology/Serology section for more on ELISA testing).

Direct Microfilaria Testing. Heartworm microfilaria are usually present at high numbers in the systemic circulation in the late morning. They are at lower numbers at the time of mosquito feeding (dusk and dawn) because they are generally in the capillaries of the skin at that time. Microfilarial testing can be performed either as a direct test or as a concentration test. Direct testing is usually performed on a very small sample size and gives a high percentage of false negatives. Examples of direct tests are checking the hematocrit tube at the buffy coat/plasma interface and examining the prepared and stained blood smear at the feathered edge. Another method is examination of a drop of fresh blood that is coverslipped and examined under the microscope using the 10× objective. Because of the small sample size examined and inconsistencies of movement in microfilaria, false negatives and misdiagnosis of heartworm disease in animals infected with *Dipetalonema* is common.

Concentration Microfilaria Testing. A better method of diagnosis of microfilaria is a concentration method. The most commonly used concentration method in practice is the Difil test. In this test a filter is placed in a special chamber. One cc of blood is mixed thoroughly with 9 cc of lysing solution and the mixture is then forced through the filter and rinsed. The filter is placed on a drop of heartworm stain and examined under a coverslip on 10× objective. The best method for microfilaria testing is the Modified Knott's technique. One cc of blood is mixed with 9 cc of 2% formalin (which relaxes the microfilaria) and centrifuged on low speed for 5 minutes. The **supernatant** (liquid portion of tube contents) is poured off and the pellet is resuspended and stained with methylene blue. A drop of the resuspended pellet is placed on a glass slide, coverslipped, and examined.

CONCENTRATION MICROFILARIA TESTING		
GENUS/SPECIES	CHARACTERISTICS ON DIRECT TEST	CHARACTERISTICS ON MODIFIED KNOTT'S
Dipetalonema reconditum	move linearly	blunt heads, curved tail
Dirofilaria immitis (canine heartworm disease)	wiggle in place	pointy heads and straight tail

Reticulocyte Counts

Reticulocyte counts should be performed in any case of anemia to confirm regeneration of red blood cells (the ability of the bone marrow to make new red blood cells in response to a crisis). **Reticulocytes** are simply polychromatophils that have been stained with new methylene blue stain (NMB). NMB stains nucleic acids. Since polychromatophils are still producing hemoglobin, the ribosomes (which contain RNA) are still present. The ribosomes stain blue with NMB. Red blood cells containing these blue granules on NMB stain are called reticulocytes. They can be either punctate (one or two granules in the cell) or aggregate (multiple granules in the cell, usually in a clump). Punctate reticulocytes are closer to the adult stage of the red blood cell. Aggregate reticulocytes are younger and newly released from the bone marrow.

Bird and reptile reticulocytes have the ribosome granules in a ring around the red blood cell nucleus.

The presence of reticulocytes indicates a regenerative anemia and can confirm an elevated MCV and low MCHC. Horses will not release reticulocytes into the systemic circulation, so retics in a horse would be extremely abnormal. Evaluation of anemias in horses should be by serial PCV measurements to assess response. Increasing PCVs indicate regeneration.

Cats release punctate retics into the systemic circulation without anemia. Presence of aggregate reticulocytes is significant and indicates a regenerative anemia; therefore, only aggregate reticulocytes should be counted in cats.

In all animals other than cats and horses (including birds and reptiles), punctate and aggregate reticulocytes should both be counted. Any animal exhibiting anemia should have a reticulocyte count performed. Reticulocyte staining is performed by adding equal amounts of NMB to whole blood in a 1:1 ratio. This should be mixed thoroughly and allowed to incubate for a minimum of 10 minutes. A blood smear should then be made from the mixture and allowed to dry before examining under oil immersion (100× objective). One thousand red blood cells are then examined and the number of reticulocytes are recorded. The observed reticulocyte count percentage is then performed:

Observed reticulocyte % =
(# of reticulocytes/1000 red blood cells)
× 0.1 (units in %)

To get the absolute reticulocyte count, the observed reticulocyte percentage is multiplied by the animal's red blood cell count:

Absolute reticulocyte count =
observed reticulocyte count × red blood cell count (units in #/μl)

The corrected reticulocyte % corrects for the degree of anemia and gives a more true indicator of the regenerative nature of the anemia:

Corrected reticulocyte % =
(observed reticulocyte % × PCV of the patient)/mean PCV of the species
(units in %)

A mild regenerative anemia generally has a corrected reticulocyte of 1 to 8%, a moderately regenerative anemia generally has a corrected reticulocyte of 9 to 15%, and a marked response is >15%.

White Blood Cell Counts

The relative number of the various white blood cells on a blood smear can give a rough idea of the type of process occurring in the body. As stated, neutrophilia indicates an inflammatory response, eosinophilia and basophilia indicate an allergic or parasitic disease, monocytosis and lymphocytosis indicate antigenic stimulation. The ability to perform and analyze white blood cell counts and differentials is key to helping the veterinarian establish a diagnosis and is an integral part of veterinary technology.

Technique

Most white blood cell counts are performed on machines that have been specifically calibrated for animals. Manual cell counts must still be performed on avian and reptile blood because the red blood cells are nucleated and impedence counters measure nuclei when performing white blood cell counts. Because the Unopette® system is no longer being made, the technique for manual counts will not be discussed. It is also important to note that, in some species (cats), platelets may be misidentified as red blood cells by the impedence counters, especially in cases of megaplatelets (exceptionally large platelets). Nucleated red blood cells are also counted as white blood cells in mammalian blood. These are all reasons that a blood smear should be performed when possible.

Calculations

The three primary types of white blood cell counts are differential count, absolute differential, and corrected white blood cell count and differential.

Differential Count

When performing a white blood cell evaluation, the slide should be examined on 40× (high dry) to evaluate cell numbers and at 100× for specific white blood cell morphology. A total of 100 white blood cells should be counted and the numbers of segmented neutrophils, band neutrophils, eosinophils, basophils, monocytes, and lymphocytes should be counted. Once 100 cells have been counted, you will have a percentage of cells out of 100 cells that are each of the individual cell types.

Absolute Differential

Cell type percentage is not useful when trying to interpret disease processes. Correct evaluation of white blood cell counts requires absolute values, which are the actual numbers of cell types per microliter of blood. This calculation must be performed on each individual cell type. Adding all of the absolute values together should equal the total white blood cell count. The calculation is as follows:

Absolute differential = % of cell type × white blood cell count (units # cells/μl)

Corrected White Blood Cell Count and Differential

If more than five nucleated red blood cells are seen among 100 white blood cells, you must correct for their presence. As stated, nucleated red blood cells (metarubricytes) are recognized by cell counters as white blood cells. Correction for their presence will change the differential and may make the difference between a leukocytosis and a leukopenia. The calculation is as follows:

Corrected white blood cell count = (observed white blood cell count × 100) ÷ (% nucleated red blood cells + 100)

Once the corrected white blood cell count is performed, the absolute differential should be performed using that white blood cell count instead of the original white blood cell count.

Leukograms

Now that the differential is calculated, it should be checked against the normal range for the species. The absolute differential should be recorded in the record along with an assessment (leukocytosis/leukopenia, neutrophilia/neutropenia, eosinophilia/eosinopenia, basophilia, monocytosis/monocytopenia, lymphocytosis/lymphopenia) and any morphologic abnormalities of the red or white blood cells should also be recorded. There are specific signs associated with elevations of the white blood cells that are called **leukograms**. There are three basic leukograms: inflammatory, stress, and physiologic and they are each caused by different mechanisms. All three basic types show neutrophilias. Specific leukograms can point the veterinarian in a certain direction and aid diagnosis.

LEUKOGRAMS				
TYPE OF LEUKOGRAM	NEUTROPHILS	SHIFT?	OTHER CELLS	CAUSE
Inflammatory	increased	yes; left (more bands or blast neutrophils)	monocytosis; lymphocytes and eosinophils normal	inflammatory mediators (bacterial cell wall products, prostaglandins)
Stress	mature neutrophilia	no; neutrophils are hypersegmented (older)	lymphopenia, eosinopenia	corticosteroids (either endogenous or exogenous)[1]
Physiologic	neutrophilia	no	lymphocytosis, eosinophilia, monocytosis	epinephrine from acute stress, excitement, or exercise; short lived (minutes to hours); spleen contracts and blood cells are released from the marginating pool[2]
Reverse stress	neutropenia	no	lymphocytosis, eosinophilia	hypoadrenocorticism (decreased glucocorticoid production)[3]

[1]Glucocorticoids prevent the neutrophils from leaving the circulation so they become older in the vasculature. Older neutrophils are not as effective at killing things, so the animal is less able to fight off infection or mount an adequate inflammatory response. Glucocorticoids also cause lymphocytes to lyse (explode) or become trapped in the tissues and decrease the activity of eosinophils and basophils which can also decrease the immunity of the animal. Animals with high levels of glucocorticoids are more prone to bacterial, viral, and fungal infections and are less likely to respond to allergens because of this.

[2]The marginating pool is the group of white blood cells that are attached to the blood vessel wall waiting to be called into the tissues.

[3]Because of the low levels of glucocorticoids, the neutrophils remain in the marginating pool and are released into the tissues early. Eosinophils are increased because glucocorticoids normally decrease their activity.

Coagulation Testing

As described in the platelet section, coagulation is a complex process. If one or more of the steps cannot be performed, the whole process breaks down. Coagulation consists of three parts: vasoconstriction, primary hemostasis, and secondary hemostasis.

Vasoconstriction occurs immediately on disruption of the blood vessel wall. It mostly occurs in arteries and arterioles because of the amount of smooth muscle present in the vessel wall. This is stimulated by epinephrine release from the nervous tissue surrounding the vessel and also by release of two chemicals from the platelets: thromboxane and serotonin. Serotonin is a neurotransmitter similar to dopamine and stimulates vasoconstriction as well as

increasing pain at the site of injury (to prevent further damage to the area). Thromboxane is a prostaglandin that stimulates vasoconstriction and activates platelets. Note: aspirin inactivates thromboxane and causes increased bleeding.

Secondary hemostasis is a series of enzymatic reactions that causes the formation of the stable fibrin clot. This involves a series of 12 factors, calcium, vitamin K, and fibrinogen. All of the clotting factors (except for a small part of factor VIII) are made in the liver. Vitamin K is needed for the production of factors II, VII, IX, and X in the liver. Vitamin K is a fat-soluble vitamin that is stored in the liver. Severe liver disease will cause decreases in the clotting factors and prolonged bleeding in animals. The same symptoms may be caused by anticoagulant rodenticide poisoning. Warfarin, Coumadin®, coumarin, and brodifacoum all act by blocking vitamin K activity. Symptoms of vitamin K toxicity do not occur for days to weeks after ingestion of the rodenticide because the clotting factors last for a long time in the body.

The 12 clotting factors make one final product called thrombin. Thrombin causes the conversion of fibrinogen to fibrin. The fibrin is then acted on by factor XIII which causes cross-linkage of the fibrin strands to make a mesh which is the stable fibrin clot. This closes the defect and prevents blood loss. Heparin acts as an anticoagulant by causing increased thrombin destruction.

Once the clot is formed, it must be broken down so that blood flow can be restored. This occurs by the activation of plasmin, which breaks the fibrin clot into pieces that can then be recycled in the liver. The pieces of fibrin are called fibrin split products. Fibrin split products can decrease clotting by blocking thrombin activity.

Coagulation testing is a detective story. Some factors such as vWF (von Willebrand disease), factor XII (hemophilia A), factor IX (hemophilia B), and factor VIII (may be included in von Willebrand disease) may be checked for by genetic or protein testing directly. In an emergency situation in clinical practice, waiting 3 to 5 days for a result from the laboratory may mean death for the patient. Luckily, many laboratory tests are available to help us diagnose disease.

Platelet Counts and Estimates

Platelet counts can either be performed by a machine or manually. Hemacytometer platelet counts are generally unavailable at present and will not be discussed here. If platelet counts are suspect from the machine, a manual estimate may be performed on the monolayer. If 8 to 10 platelets are seen per oil immersion (100×) field, that is considered adequate. If decreased platelets are seen, the feathered edge of the slide should be examined for platelet clumps.

Buccal Mucosal Bleeding Times

Buccal mucosal bleeding time (BMBT) is an indicator of primary hemostasis (platelet function and presence of vWF). The procedure involves an awake animal. The lip is pulled back and a simplate (a standardized double lancet) is used to make two small lacerations in the mucosal membrane. A piece of filter paper is used to blot the blood from the lacerations every 10 seconds. Do not touch the wound with the filter paper as this will disrupt the clot. The normal time for clot formation is 1 to 3 minutes for dogs and cats. Increased BMBT indicates thrombocytopenia or platelet dysfunction. This can also be used as a screening test for von Willebrand disease. Aspirin therapy will cause increased BMBT.

Activated Clotting Time

The activated clotting time (ACT) is an indicator of secondary hemostasis (specifically the intrinsic and common pathways). It evaluates the ability of the blood to clot in the presence of a clot activator (diatomaceous earth). The procedure involves getting a venipuncture (see Hematologic Testing) and drawing the blood into a grey-top tube containing diatomaceous earth. The tube should be warmed to body temperature prior to drawing blood and maintained at body temperature throughout the test. Once the blood and the diatomaceous earth are thoroughly mixed, timing begins. The tube should be placed in a warm water bath or hot block and checked after 30 seconds by tilting the tube. After the initial check, the tube should be checked every 5 seconds until the blood becomes a gel. Timing stops at this point. In normal cats, the ACT should be <65 seconds. In dogs, between 60 and 90 seconds. Anything affecting factor XII or thrombin formation (heparin, vitamin K deficiency, liver failure, hemophilia A) will prolong the test.

Activated Partial Thromboplastin Time

The activated partial thromboplastin time (APTT or aPTT) also tests the intrinsic and common pathways of secondary hemostasis but is more accurate than the ACT. Blood should be drawn atraumatically into a blue-top (citrated) tube and centrifuged at low speed to separate the plasma. The plasma is drawn off and placed in a plain red-top tube and labeled *citrated plasma*. The plasma should be frozen and run within 4 to 6 hours. The APTT is usually sent out to a reference laboratory. The plasma is incubated with a platelet substitute that causes activation of Factor XII. Calcium is then added and fibrin formation is measured. Normal is usually between 14 to 20 seconds, depending on the laboratory. Prolonged times are abnormal. The pathologies are the same as for the ACT.

Prothrombin Time

The prothrombin time (PT) tests the extrinsic and common pathways of secondary hemostasis. Citrated plasma is again used and is added to a thromboplastin-calcium mixture and the time to formation of fibrin is again measured. The reason that this measures the extrinsic portion of the cascade is that no part of the platelet is needed to begin the cascade. The citrated plasma should be assessed within 2 hours of collection and frozen. The normal PT is 7 to 10 seconds. Prolonged PT may be a result of liver disease, vitamin K deficiency, or factor VII deficiency.

Thromboplastin Time

The thromboplastin time (TT) tests for decreased fibrinogen and is a reference laboratory test. It tests the conversion of fibrinogen to fibrin by the conversion of thromboplastin to thrombin.

Fibrin Split Products

In disseminated intravascular coagulation (DIC), there is excessive clot formation throughout the body in the small blood vessels. This occurs because of tissue damage from some other mechanism initiating the extrinsic clotting cascade (heat stroke, trauma, shock, etc.). All of the clotting factors and cofactors are used up because of the microclots, and

fibrinolysis begins so that blood flow can be reestablished. Fibrinolysis begins with the activation of plasmin. Plasmin breaks down the fibrin and causes release of fibrin split products (FSPs) that normally would be broken down and recycled in the liver. In DIC, the levels of FSPs overwhelm the system and result in bleeding because FSPs inhibit the action of thrombin.

Fibrin split products can be tested at the reference laboratory on a latex agglutination test. The blood is collected in a special latex agglutination tube. The serum is added to latex particles coated with special antibodies that bind to the FSPs. The resulting antigen antibody complex is then examined to evaluate the severity of the disease.

Bone Marrow Testing

Bone marrow testing is an underutilized technique in veterinary practice. Bone marrow evaluation can provide answers for many unexplained changes in CBC values and staging of cancers. Indications for performing bone marrow aspirates are thrombocytopenias, neutropenia without sepsis, pancytopenia (both red and white blood cell decreases), leukemias (cancer of young blood cells), polycythemia (red blood cell increases without elevated total protein). and suspicion of metastatic cancers (cancers from non–blood cell origin) such as lymphoma, melanoma, or mast cell tumors.

A CBC and reticulocyte count should be performed at the same time as bone marrow studies for comparison. This allows a full picture of the blood composition to be formed and provides better diagnostic value.

Evaluation of bone marrow consists of assessing the myeloid:erythroid (M:E) ratio (the number of white blood cell precursors divided by the number of red blood cell precursors), the number of bone spicules, the fat-to-cellular ratio (space taken up by fat cells divided by the space taken up by cells), the iron stores, the number of megakaryocytes (platelet precursors), and the differential (number of various stages of myeloid and erythroid precursors).

The M:E ratio should be roughly one (there should be one white blood cell precursor to each red blood cell precursor). The myeloid series is considered to be only the granulocyte series (young neutrophils, eosinophils, and basophils) and does not include lymphocytes and monocytes. The myeloid series has blue-gray, light cytoplasm and open chromatin in the nucleus until they become segmented. The erythrocytic series has dark blue cytoplasm and the more mature (rubricyte and metarubricytes) cells have very dark, condensed chromatin.

Bone spicules appear as dark blue areas in the bone marrow that have a large number of cells around them. Fat appears as empty spaces in the bone marrow that do not have cells or stain. There should be a one-to-one ratio of cells to fat. Iron stores appear as very dark, blue-black or brown areas. Iron is stored as hemosiderin in the macrophages of the bone marrow. Lack of iron will prevent erythropoiesis.

Megakaryocytes appear as large purple to blue cells containing multiple nuclei. They are the largest cell in the bone marrow. Young megakaryocytes have fewer nuclei and are more basophilic (more blue in color) than mature megakaryocytes. There should be 3 to 5 megakaryocytes per bone spicule.

Greater than 90% of the erythrocytic precursors should be approaching maturity (rubricytes and metarubricytes). Greater than 75% of the myeloid precursors should be approaching maturity (myelocytes, metamyelocytes, and bands).

Sites for bone marrow aspiration and biopsy include the proximal humerus (best for most small animals), the wing or crest of the ilium, and the proximal femur in small animals. In cattle, the dorsal ends of T10-12 are used. In horses, the sternum is the best site (usually performed at euthanasia). Because the bone is highly innervated by pain fibers, sedation is recommended (required in cats) and adequate local anesthesia is mandatory.

Bone Marrow Aspiration

There are several types of bone marrow aspiration needles. The Rosenthal needle is the most commonly used in practice. It is a beveled, 16–18 ga needle with a solid stylet. Care must be taken to make sure the stylet is seated correctly to prevent cortical bone getting stuck in the opening.

The Illinois sternal-iliac needle may also be used. This needle has a depth gauge to prevent the needle from going too deep into the bone.

Bone marrow aspiration must be performed aseptically. The area must be clipped and prepped as for a surgical procedure and sterile gloves should be worn. Local anesthesia should be injected along the entire route of the aspiration needle down to the bone, 5 minutes before the procedure begins. The skin over the site of insertion is incised with a #11 or #15 scalpel blade and the needle is used to penetrate the subcutaneous tissue and muscle to the level of the bone. The needle is then rotated in a clockwise-counterclockwise rotation until the cortex is penetrated. The stylet is removed, a 12–20 cc syringe is placed on the hub of the needle, and negative pressure is applied to the plunger. A flash of material should be seen in the hub. More than a flash indicates blood contamination and may invalidate the sample. Negative pressure is released and the needle is removed from the animal. The syringe is removed from the needle, filled with air, and reattached to the needle. The material is expressed onto a slide or into a lavender-top tube and a squash prep is made immediately. Bone marrow coagulates extremely quickly on exposure to air. Squash preps are made by placing a drop one-quarter the length of the slide from the end, covering with another slide at a 90-degree angle, and drawing the slide to the opposite end of the drop slide. This provides a cytology sample.

Bone Marrow Biopsy

Bone marrow aspiration may not give an adequate sample because it is only sampling a small number of cells. Bone marrow biopsy allows a core sample to be obtained that is suitable for both cytology and histology.

The sites used for obtaining a core biopsy are the same as for an aspirate. The needle used is called a Jamshidi needle. The bevel of the needle is curved inward slightly to prevent the core from being pulled out of the needle when it is withdrawn. It has a stylet similar to the Rosenthal needle. The technique is the same as for an aspirate until the needle penetrates the cortical bone. On penetration of the bone marrow cavity, the stylet is removed and the needle is advanced 1 to 2 cm further into the bone marrow and rotated clockwise and counterclockwise. This is called *stirring* the sample. The needle is then withdrawn by twisting in one direction. The needle is then inverted and the stylet is inserted into the needle end, pushing the core onto a slide. Half of the sample should be placed into fixative for histology and half made into a squash prep.

Cell Maturation Series

All blood cells derive from the pluripotential stem cell (PPSC). This cell is a mesenchymal cell that has not differentiated or matured. It can form any of the blood cell precursors.

The cell maturation series of the erythrocytic cell line is as follows:

PPSC > rubriblast > prorubricyte > rubricyte > metarubricyte > polychromatophil > red blood cell

The erythrocytic series are all varying shades of blue. They start out large and shrink with each change in cell type. The rubriblast and prorubricyte have very dark blue cytoplasms and open chromatin and prominent nucleoli (areas within the nucleus where the genes are located). These cells can still divide. The rubricyte has no nucleoli and the nucleus is becoming condensed. There is a slight pinkinsh tinge to the cytoplasm. The metarubricyte has a very condensed, pyknotic nucleus and a definite pinkish color. The polychromatophil has no nucleus.

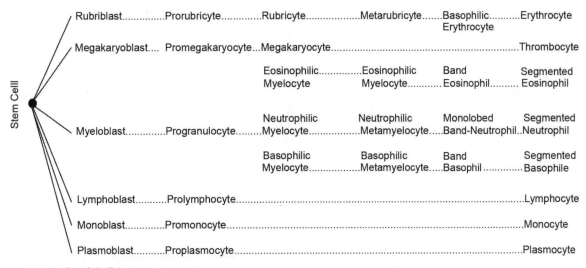

Figure 7.1 *Blood Cell Maturation*

The myeloid series is the same for neutrophils, eosinophils, and basophils. The only difference is the granules that each cell contains. Granules are seen in even very young cells (promyelocyte) making identification of the cell line possible even in young cells. The cell maturation series of the myeloid cells is as follows:

> PPSC > myeloblast > promyelocyte
> > myelocyte > metamyelocyte > band
> > segmented

The myeloid series are all lighter in both the cytoplasm and the chromatin than the erythrocytic series. The myeloblast and promyelocyte are both actively dividing larger cells with prominent nucleoli in the nucleus. The myeloblast, promyelocyte, and myelocyte all have round nuclei. The metamyelocyte has an indented nucleus (like a kidney bean). The band has a tube-shaped nucleus and the segmented granulocyte has pinches in the nucleus (generally 4 to 5).

Lymphoblasts may also be seen in the bone marrow. These lymphocyte precursors are larger than mature lymphocytes and have very open chromatin (they are a lighter pink than mature lymphocyte nuclei) and prominent nucleoli.

Cytology and Histopathology

Cytology can provide quick answers and is relatively noninvasive. Most techniques may be performed in an awake patient, while histopathology requires anesthesia and a longer turnaround time for results because of the requirements of adequate tissue preparation. Cytologic samples may be read in the veterinary clinic while the client waits in the exam room. The disadvantages of cytology are the small sample size and the difficulty of analysis if the technician is not familiar with the normal appearance of a specific tissue.

Histological analysis gives a much larger sample size that can be processed for various testing procedures including fluorescent antibody testing and special staining. The normal architecture of the various layers of tissue are preserved. Pathologists trained in tissue analysis read histologic samples and analyze the samples for the practice so there are fewer mistakes.

Cytological Techniques

The ability to perform cytology in practice can improve patient care, increase the bottom line of the clinic, and help to initiate treatment of patients sooner. Proper staining of samples is very important to cytological techniques. Improper staining or stain artifacts can invalidate results. There are three basic types of cytologic stains: Romanowsky stains, nucleic acid stains, and Papanicolaou stains.

Cells seen on cytology may be divided into three categories: epithelial, mesenchymal, and round cells. Being able to differentiate cells into these categories can aid in establishing a laboratory diagnosis of neoplasia. It is also important to divide a sample into inflammatory or noninflammatory categories.

CYTOLOGIC STAINS

STAIN	STAINING CHARACTERISTICS	SPECIAL NEEDS	TYPES
Romanowsky	alcohol based so stain penetrates cell membranes well; excellent cytoplasmic detail	increased nuclear detail can be obtained by longer staining times	Diff-Quick, Wright's Giemsa (Diff-Quick stain is in most veterinary practices)
Nucleic acid stains	water based, excellent nuclear and ribosome detail (stains nucleic acids well)	longer staining times are required to enable cell membrane penetration	NMB
Papanicolaou stains	excellent cytoplasmic and nuclear staining	complicated and expensive; require wet preps, so the cytology sample must be fixed prior to drying the slide	trichrome, Cytocolor®

THREE CATEGORIES OF CELLS

CELL TYPE	CHARACTERISTICS	LOCATION
Epithelial	cytoplasm should be larger than the nucleus, nucleus is round; have a basement membrane	linings of tissues (external and internal linings of viscera and blood vessels, skin) and glandular tissues
Squamous Simple Stratified	flat cells one cell layer thick several layers thick, go from round cells at the basement membrane to progressively flatter toward the surface	skin and lining of organs and blood vessels blood vessel lining, lining of organs skin, oral cavity, nasal cavity, vaginal mucosa
Cuboidal Simple Stratified	cells are square with nucleus and cytoplasm generally equal volume	bronchioles and bronchi are simple cuboidal; glands may be either simple or stratified cuboidal
Columnar Simple	cells have large amounts of cytoplasm and may have cilia; nuclei are displaced toward the basement membrane	internal mucosa of gastrointestinal tract from the esophagus to the rectum
Pseudostratified	cells have large amounts of cytoplasm and cilia, but the nuclei can be in various levels from the basement membrane, making them appear stratified	trachea and upper bronchi
Transitional	cells vary in appearance from cuboidal to squamous depending on need	bladder wall (areas with high stretch requirements)
Mesenchymal	spindle shaped with a central oval nucleus; equal N:C ratio.	all connective tissues
Fat	cytoplasm contains large lipid droplet, will usually dissolve on normal tissue preparation	surrounds all viscera, subcutaneous tissues, etc.
Muscle	cytoplasm usually contains striations or dense bodies	muscle tissue, surrounding blood vessels, gastrointestinal organs, and most viscera

(continued)

THREE CATEGORIES OF CELLS *(continued)*		
CELL TYPE	**CHARACTERISTICS**	**LOCATION**
Connective tissue	typical spindle-shaped cells; may have collagen associated with it	all connective tissues
Blood vessels	same as connective tissue	all tissues
Round	**round nuclei, large nucleus, smaller cytoplasm, may contain granules**	**all tissues**
Lymphocytes	round nucleus, cytoplasm stains dark blue on Diff-Quick, may have perinuclear halo	all tissues
Mast cells	round nucleus, cytoplasm contains red/purple granules containing histamine and heparin	all tissues
Melanocytes	round nucleus, cytoplasm contains black granules containing melanin	skin

Tumors of the epithelial cells are called *-omas* (e.g., epithelioma) if they are benign, carcinomas if they are malignant. A glandular benign tumor is called an adenoma; a cancer is called an adenocarcinoma. One of the hallmark signs of adenocarcinoma is acinar formation, which is a group of epithelial cells with a duct in the middle.

Benign tumors of mesenchymal cells are also called *-omas* (e.g., fibroma, hemangioma). Malignant tumors are called *-sarcomas* (e.g., fibrosarcoma, hemangiosarcoma).

Inflammatory samples have neutrophils and possibly macrophages present in the sample. Septic samples are inflammatory specimens with bacteria present. Eosinophilic infiltrates can mean allergic inflammation, autoimmune disease, or parasitic infestation. In the cat, lymphocytic infiltrates can indicate antigenic stimulation or allergic or autoimmune stimulation.

Noninflammatory samples would be tumors/ neoplasms or dysplasias (abnormal architecture or placement of cell types in the sample). Tumors usually have rapidly dividing cells. The nucleus is usually bigger than the cytoplasm (increased nuclear-to-cytoplasmic ratio), there may be nucleoli, and there may be mitotic figures present (spindle formation in the nucleus) in cells that should not be dividing. In dysplasias, the cells usually appear normal for the tissue type, but are arranged in a different pattern.

Fine Needle Aspiration

Fine needle aspirations are very quick and easy ways to obtain cells from solid or fluid-filled lesions. The area to be aspirated should be prepped with alcohol and a 22–20 ga needle on a 6–12 cc syringe should be inserted into the mass. Negative pressure should be applied. The plunger should then be released, the needle should be backed out slightly (not out of the lesion completely), and redirected. The procedure should be repeated two to three times. Negative pressure should be released and the needle should be removed from the lesion. The syringe is removed from the needle, filled with air, and reattached to the needle. Air is forced through the needle and the sample is expressed onto the slide. A squash prep is made (see Bone Marrow Aspiration) and air-dried. Air-drying will partially fix the sample onto the slide. The sample is then stained, air-dried, and examined under the microscope.

Impression Smear

Impression smears can be made either from wet ulcers or from cut surfaces of solid masses. The surface of the lesion or mass is blotted with a piece of gauze and the slide is touched to the surface. The slide is then air-dried, stained, and examined under the microscope. Wet ulcers may have secondary contamination by bacteria, so results may be suspect.

Scrapings

Scrapings can be performed on dry ulcers or areas of scaly skin. A #10 blade is drawn across the lesion at a 90 degree angle. Saline may be used ito prevent cutting the tissue if the slide will be stained. Oil should be used if the objective is to check for ectoparasites.

Swabs

Swabs may also be used on wet ulcers, on mucous membranes, or in fistulous tracts. Secondary contamination of lesions is common, so bacterial presence on these samples should be suspect. A sterile cotton swab is moistened with sterile saline and drawn across the lesion or inserted into the fistulous tract. The swab is then rolled over the surface of a slide, air-dried, and stained.

Fluid Testing

The accumulation of transcellular fluids in body cavities is abnormal. Samples of the fluid can aid in diagnosis of disease process and may be therapeutic in cases of abdominal and pleural effusions to increase patient comfort and decrease respiratory distress.

Techniques

Proper preparation of the patient and technique is an important part of the job of the veterinary technician.

Although abdominal and thoracic aspirates and tracheal washes are within the veterinary technician's scope of practice, chest tube placement is not. It is important to check your practice act because rules in various states are very different.

Abdominal Aspiration. Abdominal aspiration, or abdominocentesis, should be performed in cases of unexplained ascites (fluid accumulation in the abdomen), abdominal trauma, and puncture wounds. It is important to take fluid samples from all four quadrants (right cranial, left cranial, right caudal, left caudal) to ensure proper sampling. The area should be clipped and prepped and sterility should be maintained throughout the procedure. An over-the-needle catheter should be used if possible to help prevent bowel penetration. The sample is drawn with a 6 cc syringe and placed into a lavender-top and a red-top tube for further analysis. The sample should be tested for total protein, creatinine, BUN, and bilirubin as well as cytology. If septic inflammation is seen, the red-top tube should be submitted for bacterial or fungal culture. Cases of ureteral or bladder rupture will have elevated creatinine and urea (BUN) in the fluid. Gall bladder rupture will cause increased bilirubin. Cells that are only found in the peritoneal and pleural spaces are called mesothelial cells. Mesothelial cells are large, epithelial type cells that may be multinucleated. Mesothelial cells have brushed borders that look fuzzy on cytology. The cytoplasm is moderately basophilic. Mesothelial cells are often confused with cancer cells because they may be multinucleated or mitotic (dividing).

Thoracic Fluid Aspiration (Thoracentesis or Thoracocentesis). There is always a small amount of pleural fluid in the chest. This allows proper expansion of the lung lobes and maintenance of negative pressure in the chest. Overproduction or abnormal fluids in the pleural space cause restrictive lung disease by interfering with negative pressure. The lungs are not able to expand because the pressure in the pleural space is the same as the pressure in the alveoli. Aspiration of pleural fluid in these cases is therapeutic (makes the animal feel better) as well as diagnostic. Hemothorax (blood), pyothorax (pus), chylothorax (chyle), and hydrothorax (serum) can all be causes for thoracocentesis. Pleural fluid aspiration should be bilateral in animals with a complete mediastinum and bilateral disease. Some animals may have incomplete mediastinums and may only require thoracocentesis on one side to achieve results on both sides of the chest. The technique is similar to abdominocentesis. The patient is aseptically prepped and sterile gloves are worn. A bleb of local anesthetic is placed under the skin and a sterile over-the-needle catheter is prepared. A stopcock is attached to the syringe and an extension set is attached. The over-the-needle catheter is advanced perpendicular to the thoracic wall, withdrawn slightly, and advanced further at a 45-degree angle until a pop is felt. The pop indicates penetration of the parietal pleura. The needle is withdrawn from the catheter and the extension set, three-way stopcock, and syringe are attached. Fluid is then drawn off. Care should be taken to avoid introducing air into the pleural space as this will also cause restrictive lung disease. Cytology, triglyceride, glucose, and lactose levels and culture and sensitivities should be performed on pleural fluid. Elevations in lymphocytes and triglycerides indicate thoracic duct leakage.

Tracheal Wash or **Lavage.** Tracheal washes are performed in animals with coughs, increased lung sounds, suspicious thoracic radiographs, and anything else that causes disease of the lower respiratory tract (trachea, bronchi, bronchioles, alveoli). They will not be diagnostic for restrictive lung diseases or upper respiratory tract pathology. There are two types of tracheal washes: the percutaneous or transtracheal approach, and the endotracheal approach. The transtracheal approach yields more accurate evaluations because the animal will still have a cough reflex, so material from the lower airways will have a higher possibility of being collected. In the endotracheal approach, the animals are anesthetized, so the cough reflex is suppressed. This is the approach usually used with cats. In the percutaneous technique, the area over the larynx is clipped and scrubbed. The animal is awake for the procedure. Local anesthetic is infiltrated subcutaneously at the site of the needle insertion. The animal is restrained either sitting or standing with the neck extended. A jugular catheter is then inserted into the cricothyroid ligament (the junction between the cricoid and thyroid cartilages is palpable). The catheter is advanced through the needle to the level just above the tracheal bifurcation (this distance should be premeasured). One to two ml of sterile saline per 10 pounds of animal is injected into the trachea. When the animal coughs, the material is aspirated. The sample should be placed in a lavender-top tube for cytology and a red-top tube for culture and sensitivity. The cytology sample should be centrifuged and the pellet suspended and prepared as a squash prep. The endotracheal technique requires anesthesia and endotracheal tube placement. The endotracheal tube must be sterile and small enough to allow easy passage into the trachea. Care should be taken to avoid contamination of the tube by touching the oral and pharyngeal surfaces. The cuff should be inflated and the animal placed in lateral recumbency. A jugular catheter is advanced down the endotracheal tube until it is outside of the tube, the stylet is removed, and 1 to 2 ml sterile saline per 10 pounds of body weight is placed into the trachea. Negative pressure is applied to the syringe to aspirate some of the material. If the animal is at a very low plane of anesthesia, coughing may be caused by rolling the patient from side to side. Normal cells seen on tracheal washes include ciliated columnar cells (long, rectangular cells with the nucleus more toward one end of the rectangle and hairs at the other end) and goblet cells (columnar cells filled with a purple substance called mucin) from the trachea and cuboidal cells (square cells) from the bronchi. Occasional mast cells, monocytes, and neutrophils may also be seen, but they should be fewer than 1 cell/HPF.

Fluid Types

Fluids may be obtained from arthrocentesis, cerebrospinal taps, or body cavities. Fluids give a lot of information, especially in reference to the information obtained from a chemistry panel and CBC on the blood. The technique for obtaining fluids from body cavities has been described in the previous section.

Joint fluid evaluation is important in differentiating various joint diseases. Joints should be evaluated in cases of fever of unknown origin. Any joint aspiration should be performed with a sterile prep and gloves to prevent introduction of pathogens into the joint fluid. The carpus, tarsus, and stifle are the usual joints aspirated. Joint fluid should be relatively thick and slick (this is called **viscosity**) and have a high protein content. Viscosity can be assessed by how long a string of joint fluid can be from the tip of the needle to a slide. Two to three cm is normal. Joint fluid should be colorless and clear. Inflammatory processes will increase cloudiness (**turbidity**) and protein concentration and decrease viscosity. On cytology, joint fluid should be mostly mononuclear cells. Normal cell counts are less than 500 cells/µl. Noninflammatory or degenerative processes such as osteoarthritis cause cellularity to be 500 to 5,000 cell/µl. Increases in neutrophils over 10,000 cells/µl indicate inflammatory or septic (bacterial) processes in the joint. Increases in eosinophils usually indicate autoimmune disease.

Cerebrospinal fluid collection is usually performed by the veterinarian, but is within the technician's scope of practice in most states. The animal must be anesthetized when this technique is performed and all instruments as well as the technician and the veterinarian must be maintained in strict asepsis. Trauma to the spinal cord and brain herniation may occur when performing this procedure.

Evaluation of cerebrospinal fluid should include color, clarity, total protein, culture and sensitivity, and cytology. The fluid should be clear and colorless with a very low cellularity (less than 9 cells/µl) with mostly mononuclear cells (lymphocytes). Increased protein levels indicate pathology. Increases in neutrophils usually indicate bacterial or viral infections. Increases in lymphocytes indicate viral or degenerative diseases. Increases in eosinophils indicate parasitic or fungal diseases.

Fluids obtained from body cavities (the peritoneal and thoracic cavities) are called effusions. Effusions come in three basic types: the transudate, the modified transudate, and the exudate. Differentiation of effusions is by the protein concentration and cellularity. The fluids do not always fit well into the assigned categories, so there may be some overlap in evaluation.

FLUID TYPES				
FLUID TYPE	SPECIFIC GRAVITY/TP	COLOR	CELLS	CAUSE
Transudate	<1.018 TP 2.5 g/dl	clear to straw colored	low cell count	protein loss/hypoalbuminemia (protein-losing nephropathy, protein-losing enteropathy, liver disease, early congestive heart failure)
Modified transudate	1.018–1.025 TP 2.5–3.0 g/dl	white, amber, red, may be turbid (cloudy)	<5,000 cells/mm^3	heart disease, foreign body response, lung lobe torsions, neoplastic diseases
Exudate	>1.025 TP >3 g/dl	amber to red, turbid	5–50,000 cells/mm^3 (neutrophils)	
Hemorrhagic exudate	TP >5.5 g/dl	red, turbid (will not clot in a red-top tube)	differential should be similar to a CBC	hemorrhage
Noninflammatory exudate	same as exudate	same as exudate	mesothelial cells or cancer cells are primary cell type	neoplasia
Septic inflammatory exudate	same	same	neutrophils, organisms (bacterial, fungal)	infection
Nonseptic inflammatory exudate	same	same	neutrophils, no organisms are seen	FIP (feline infectious peritonitis), lung lobe torsions
Chylous effusions	1.007–1.040 TP 2.5–7.0 g/dl	pink, straw colored, white depending on fat content	<10,000 cells/mm^3 neutrophils, small lymphocytes, mesothelial cells	thoracic duct rupture

Histopathology

Histopathology samples are generally larger than cytologic specimens and the normal tissue architecture is maintained. Tissue samples are obtained by surgical excision of part or all of a mass. This is called biopsy. Biopsies are performed on suspicious growths (neoplasias), abnormal areas (dysplasias), and abnormal tissue locations or sizes (anaplasias and hyperplasias). Asepsis must be maintained when obtaining biopsies, and normal tissue should be included in the sample so comparisons may be made. Pathology reports should include the location of the lesion on a body map, and the size, shape, color, and texture as well as a history of the animal.

Histopathology is usually performed by veterinary pathologists and should be sent to reputable laboratories. Generally, biopsies are placed in buffered formalin for preparation. If electron microscopy is needed for viruses or other reasons, glutaraldehyde should be used as a fixative. Some studies require frozen samples or other preparation, so careful reading of laboratory requirements is important.

Clinical Chemistry

Clinical chemistries are usually run on animals as part of preanesthetic testing, as part of a diagnostic profile for disease, and to determine the effectiveness of therapy on a system. Samples may be either whole blood, serum, or plasma depending on the test. If plasma is required, heparin is the anticoagulant of choice because it does not interfere with mineral concentrations (especially calcium). EDTA, calcium oxalate, and sodium citrate form insoluble complexes with calcium that will affect levels. They will also bind to potassium in some cases. Always use the correct tube for analysis. Sodium fluoride (gray-top tube) is the anticoagulant of choice for blood glucose determination because it acts as a glucose preservative, but it should not be used for other tests.

Most chemistries can use serum for analysis and this is the preferred method if the test can use either serum or plasma. Serum must be spun as soon as possible after clot formation (30 to 120 minutes) to make sure the blood cells have minimal exposure to the serum. This will prevent further changes of values because of blood cell metabolism and degradation of proteins.

Sample volume is also important. Enough blood to run three assays will account for the possibility of technician, instrument, or reagent error. The possibility of dilution studies or add-on testing also exists, so having extra volume available is a good idea. Always fill the tube to a minimum of 75% full to ensure proper dilution with the anticoagulants and proper tube performance in clot activator tubes. Remember: the PCV is the percentage of red blood cells per milliliter of fluid, so if you draw up 10 cc of blood in a patient with a PCV of 45%, 4.5 milliliters will be cells and 5.5 milliliters will be serum or plasma.

Proper phlebotomy is as important to serum chemistries as it is to coagulation studies. Hemolysis (red blood cell lysis) and lipemia (triglycerides in the plasma/serum) will interfere with many tests by causing interference with spectrophotometric (requires the transmission of light through a sample) and colorimetric (determines the color of a sample or chemical reaction) analyses.

Proper history taking is also very important to evaluation. Young animals will have increased serum calcium, phosphorus, and alkaline phosphatase levels because of increased bone growth. Corticosteroid therapy (prednisone) will increase alkaline phosphatase and liver enzymes. Phenobarbital (seizure medication) will also increase liver enzymes. Dehydration will increase the total protein, potassium, sodium, and chloride. Low dietary protein can cause decreased total protein, low albumin, and low blood urea nitrogen (breakdown product of protein metabolism). Fluid therapy may either dilute electrolytes or increase concentrations if they are oversupplemented. Antibiotics can cause changes in some

CHEMICAL TESTS BY ORGAN

ORGAN	TESTS	SPECIAL NOTES	BLOOD TUBE
Liver			
Hepatocellular enzymes	ALT	alanine aminotransferase	RTT
	AST	aspartate aminotransferase	RTT
	SDH	sorbitol dehydrogenase	RTT
	GDH	glutamate dehydrogenase	RTT
Cholestatic enzymes	GGT	gamma glutamyltransferase	RTT
	ALP	alkaline phosphatase	RTT
Liver function tests	TP	total protein	LTT
	albumin	albumin	RTT
	PT	prothrombin time	BTT
	APTT	activated partial thromboplastin time	BTT
	bilirubin	bilirubin	RTT
	ammonia	ammonia	GTT
	BSA	serum bile acids	RTT
Secondary tests	glucose	blood glucose	sodium fluoride tube
	calcium	indirect test of albumin concentration	RTT
	cholesterol		RTT
	triglycerides		RTT
Kidney	BUN	blood urea nitrogen	RTT
	Cr	creatinine	RTT
Kidney function tests	s.g.	specific gravity (including vasopressin and water deprivation tests)	urine
Secondary tests	electrolytes	sodium, potassium, magnesium, calcium, phosphorus, and bicarbonate/total CO_2	RTT
Pancreas			
Endocrine	BG	blood glucose	sodium fluoride tube
	fructosamine	glucose bound to albumin	RTT
	glycosylated hemoglobin	glucose bound to hemoglobin	EDTA plasma
Exocrine	amylase		RTT
	lipase		RTT
	PLI	pancreatic lipase immunoreactivity	RTT, ELISA
	TLI	trypsin-like immunoreactivity	RTT
Secondary tests	calcium		RTT
	phosphorus		RTT
GI system			
Upper GI	folate	vitamin B_9	RTT
Lower GI	cobalamin	vitamin B_{12}	RTT
Function tests	fecal analysis	microscopic exam, Lugol's iodine, Sudan III or IV, gelatin digestion, etc.	feces
	fat absorption		RTT

chemistries. In general, blood should be drawn *prior* to the initiation of therapy and then be used to monitor the animal's response.

Clinical chemistries can give a glimpse into the workings of the organ systems that may be affected by disease. Some chemistries test the organ's ability to manufacture products. These are called function tests. Others test cellular integrity, or leakiness, of the cells. These are enzyme tests. Enzyme tests generally test for tissue damage, while function tests test the effective biomass of an organ (how much of the organ is able to do the job).

Most tests may be grouped together into organ systems and this is how clinical chemistries should be approached in practice. When evaluating chemistry panels, organ-related tests should be evaluated together. This avoids confusion and enables the technician to make sense of the values and decide whether or not a particular test value may have been affected by problems in another organ system. Since many of the enzymes can be produced by more than one system, this is important to the evaluation of a chemistry profile.

In this section, the tests will be discussed as they relate to systems. Ancillary tests that relate to the function or health of the specific system will also be discussed.

Liver

The liver is one of the most important organs in the body. All of the blood from the intestines comes through the liver prior to returning to the heart. The liver processes all the nutrients, detoxifies the blood, and filters bacteria. Processing of nutrients includes lipid packaging and distribution to the rest of the body, manufacturing proteins from amino acids (coagulation proteins, albumin, globulins), formation of glycogen from glucose, and conversion of maltose and fructose to glucose. It is also the primary storage site for iron, copper, and fat soluble vitamins. Detoxi-

fication includes excretion and elimination of ammonia in the form of urea (ammonia is a breakdown product of protein metabolism) and detoxification of drugs and toxins produced by intestinal bacteria. The liver also synthesizes bilirubin from the metabolism of hemoglobin from red blood cell destruction and bile acids, which aid fat metabolism.

Different pathologies will affect different enzymes and function tests depending on the type of disease.

Liver Enzymes

Some liver enzymes will be elevated when any changes occur in the liver leading to cellular damage and cell death. Cellular damage makes hepatocytes leaky. Enzyme assays check whether leakage is occurring. This is usually not quantitative (is not an assessment of how many cells are damaged). Liver enzymes will be increased with infectious, inflammatory, neoplastic, toxic, degenerative, and traumatic changes. The main enzymes associated with hepatocyte damage are ALT (alanine aminotransferase), and AST (aspartate aminotransferase).

ALT is used as a screening test for hepatocellular disease. Most of the enzyme comes from the liver hepatocytes, but some is also manufactured in the muscles, kidneys, and pancreas. In dogs, cats, and primates it is a very good indicator of liver disease. In ruminants, ALT is not a good indicator; SDH (sorbitol dehydrogenase) is better. This test should be performed on serum. Lipemia and hemolysis will cause false elevations in this enzyme. The serum should not be frozen.

AST is not liver specific and should only be evaluated if comparisons to muscle enzyme values are made—CPK (creatinine phosphokinase) levels. If muscle enzymes are elevated along with elevations of AST, then the increase in AST is probably from muscle damage, not liver damage. Hemolysis and lipemia will cause elevations in this enzyme as well.

SDH is hepatocyte specific and is the most useful liver enzyme test in large animals. It is very unstable, so serum tests must be performed within 12 hours.

GDH (glutamate dehydrogenase) is another hepatocyte specific liver enzyme test in ruminants. It is also used in birds.

Other liver enzymes will be elevated due to cholestasis (bile flow problems). Biliary obstruction can be either extrahepatic (outside of the liver) or intrahepatic (within the liver). Causes of elevations may be inflammation, infection, neoplasia, cholelithiasis (gallstones), or drugs. The cholestatic enzymes are GGT (gamma glutamyltranspeptidase), and ALP (alkaline phosphatase).

GGT is considered a liver-specific enzyme and is the most sensitive indicator of cholestasis in most species. It is only manufactured in the liver. Care must be taken to separate the red blood cells as quickly as possible because they may decrease the enzyme levels in the serum.

ALP is another sensitive indicator of cholestasis. Production of ALP is increased when there is increased pressure within the biliary system (bile backup), inflammation of the bile ducts (pancreatitis and diabetes), or the presence of drugs such as corticosteroids and phenobarbital. It is not as sensitive an indicator in cats as it is in dogs because it remains in the system for a very short time in cats (i.e., has a short half-life). The major source of ALP is the liver, although bone, the intestinal mucosa, and the kidneys also produce the enzyme. This enzyme assay is not affected by hemolysis.

Liver Function Tests

Liver function tests assess the functional integrity of the liver (ability to synthesize products). They also test the hepatic portal system (blood flow from the intestines to the liver). Tests that are considered primary hepatic (liver) function tests include total protein and albumin (both are measures of the ability of the liver to manufacture proteins), clotting factors, bilirubin (measures the ability of the liver to break down hemoglobin), ammonia (elevations of ammonia will indicate a decreased ability of the liver to convert ammonia to urea), and bile acids tests.

The total protein has been discussed in the Hemocrit section, and the clotting factors in the Coagulation Testing section. Albumin and other protein level evaluation will be discussed further in the GI Function Tests section. In general, it is important to remember that the liver is the manufacturing center and processing center for proteins. If the liver is nonfunctional, all proteins except the immunoglobulins will be decreased (immunoglobulins are made in the lymphocytes).

Albumin is exclusively manufactured by the liver. Its function is to prevent plasma loss from the capillaries by exerting oncotic pressure. Loss of albumin will result in edema. Decreased albumin will also cause decreased calcium levels because most of the calcium in the serum is bound to albumin. Most of the total protein is albumin. Albumin testing should be performed on serum.

Severe liver disease will cause coagulation defects because of the lack of clotting factors and vitamin K storage. The PT and APTT can be used to assess secondary coagulation (clotting factors). These tests should be run on citrated plasma.

Bilirubin is the breakdown product of the heme portion of hemoglobin. The liver normally clears hemoglobin from the blood by conversion to unconjugated/indirect bilirubin. Unconjugated bilirubin is then converted to conjugated/direct bilirubin which is found in the serum. Unconjugated bilirubin levels increase with excessive red blood cell destruction (prehepatic disease). Conjugated bilirubin levels increase with both hepatocellular damage and cholestasis. The serum chemistry usually gives the total bilirubin and the conjugated bilirubin levels. The unconjugated levels can be determined by subtracting the direct bilirubin from the total bilirubin. Bilirubin will be affected by hemolysis, lipemia, and light exposure. Light will decrease the unconjugated bilirubin level by 50% per hour. Hemolysis will decrease bilirubin concentrations with some assays. Bilirubin levels will not be affected by problems with the hepatic portal circulation.

Ammonia is the breakdown product of protein metabolism. Ammonia is very toxic to most of the tissues in the body, especially the central nervous system. The liver normally metabolizes the ammonia into urea. Abnormal processing of ammonia can be due to loss of portal circulation (portosystemic shunt disease) or loss of liver tissue (cirrhosis). Increased levels of ammonia will cause seizures and coma, usually in relation to feeding times. The animal eats protein, breaks it down, and the levels of ammonia rise and the animal will become comatose or have a seizure. Once the ammonia is cleared, the animal's mental status may improve. This test must be run on heparinized plasma (green-top tube) within 1 to 3 hours of phlebotomy because it is very unstable.

Serum bile acids (SBA) are synthesized in the liver from cholesterol. Most bile acids that are excreted by the liver are reabsorbed into the portal circulation and recycled, so there is a constant level maintained in the blood stream. SBA are normally stored in the gallbladder and eating a meal causes the release of bile acids into the intestines. Bile acids function in fat absorption and metabolism. Generally SBA are measured in serum samples after a 12-hour fast (preprandial). The animal is then fed and the test is repeated in 2 hours (postprandial). If pre- and postprandial levels are elevated, there is a problem with hepatic function.

Other tests that can help with evaluation of liver function are blood glucose, cholesterol levels, and triglycerides. Liver failure is often associated with mild to moderate hypoglycemia (low blood sugar) because of the inability of the liver to manufacture or break down glycogen. Cholesterol and triglycerides also rely on the liver and the bile acids for transport.

Cholesterol and triglycerides may be elevated in cholestasis.

Kidneys

The kidneys function in water and electrolyte conservation and elimination, acid base balance, elimination of urea and creatinine, conservation of glucose and protein, maintenance of blood pressure, activation of vitamin D, and red blood cell production (erythropoetin production). Renal failure indicates that the kidneys are no longer able to maintain these functions. In order to call kidney disease renal failure, over 75% of the kidney must be nonfunctional. **Uremia (azotemia)** occurs in renal failure and is the clinical syndrome associated with the loss of function.

Since the kidney's ability to concentrate urine is controlled by the pituitary and adrenal glands, these function tests will be covered in the appropriate section on hormone testing. Azotemia, or elevation of waste products in the blood, and function tests should always be evaluated along with the urinalysis because the urinalysis is often more sensitive to renal disease than the chemistries. In fact, azotemia will not increase to diagnostic levels until the kidney is >75% damaged.

Kidney Enzymes

BUN (blood urea nitrogen) and Cr (creatinine) are both products of protein metabolism. They are both excreted as waste products by the kidney. High concentrations will occur in animals with renal disease.

Creatinine is derived from muscle breakdown. It is filtered and excreted by the kidney and is maintained at fairly constant blood levels. The advantage of Cr over BUN is that it is not affected by dietary protein. Creatinine is also more specific for kidney function than BUN. Neither Cr or BUN is affected by hemolysis.

The BUN, as stated in the previous liver section, is the endpoint of protein breakdown. Increases of the GFR (glomerular filtration rate, the amount of urine produced by the glomerulus) will reduce the BUN in the circulation. Decreased GFR will increase the BUN in the circulation. Increase in waste products is called

azotemia. There are three types of azotemia: prerenal, renal, and postrenal.

KIDNEY ENZYMES		
TYPE OF AZOTEMIA	BUN:CR RATIO	CAUSES
Prerenal	BUN rises, Cr remains normal, >20:1	decrease in systemic blood flow (shock, hemorrhage, dehydration), increased protein intake
Renal	BUN and Cr rise at an equal rate, so both will be elevated but the ratio will be normal; 5–20:1	diseases of the kidney resulting in decreased GFR (pyelonephritis, nephrotoxicosis, nephritic syndrome)
Postrenal	same as renal	urinary tract obstruction
Low BUN levels	no protein processing in liver, no conversion of ammonia to urea; <5:1	portosystemic shunts, chronic liver disease

Kidney Function Tests

Kidney function tests assess the ability of the kidneys to concentrate urine. This is under the influence of two hormones: aldosterone and antidiuretic hormone (ADH).

Antidiuretic hormone is produced by the hypothalamus and stored in the posterior pituitary gland. It targets an area in the renal tubules called the distal convoluted tubules and collecting ducts, and increases the resorption of water by those tubules. Failure of antidiuretic hormone can cause polyuria and polydipsia. This can be tested by water deprivation and vasopressin tests.

Aldosterone is a hormone produced by the adrenal cortex. It controls the reabsorption of sodium at the distal convoluted tubule. Water follows sodium, so water is conserved as well. Decreased aldosterone will result in polyuria and polydipsia because sodium is allowed to leave the kidneys. This occurs in hypoadrenocortism.

The best way to measure the ability of the body to concentrate its urine (and retain water) is to measure the specific gravity (s.g.) of the urine. The specific gravity indicates the density (particles per volume) of urine. Large particles such as proteins and glucose have a greater effect on the s.g. than electrolytes. A specific gravity of 1.000 is the s.g. of distilled water. Urine with an s.g. of 1.001–1.012 is considered isosthenuric, which means that the animal is unable to concentrate its urine. An s.g. >1.016 in a dog and >1.030 in a cat means that the animal has the ability to concentrate its urine. Normal concentrating ability means an s.g. >1.030 in the dog and >1.040 in the cat. Urine s.g. should always be considered in the face of TP (hydration status) and urine protein.

Other tests that should be evaluated with kidney problems are phosphorus, calcium, sodium, potassium, chloride, and total CO_2. Since electrolytes are cleared or reabsorbed in the kidneys and the kidneys are responsible for acid–base balance, there may be changes in these levels, especially in severe renal disease.

Electrolytes

Electrolytes are the charged ions that circulate in solution in the plasma. Positively charged ions are called cations (sodium, potassium, calcium, and magnesium) and negatively charged ions are called anions (chloride, bicarbonate, phosphate). Electrolytes may be further broken into groups by whether they are found within the cells (intracellular ions) or in solution in the plasma (extracellular ions). The major intracellular ions are potassium, magnesium, and phosphate. The major extracellular ions are chloride, sodium, and calcium. This is important because, in cases of hemolysis, the intracellular ions may be elevated in the serum tests.

Electrolytes are usually expressed in mmol/L or mEq/L, which are concentrations based on molecular weight (how much individual atoms weigh). Electrolytes function in nerve and muscle activity, as cofactors for enzymes, as acid–base regulators, and in the maintenance of water balance.

Sodium (Na^+). Elevated sodium levels (hypernatremia) are caused by diabetes insipidus (loss of water without sodium loss because of ADH deficiency), excessive sodium supplementation, hyperadrenocorticism (water loss without sodium loss), and dehydration. Hyponatremia (sodium decreases) can be caused by excessive diuretic use (loop diuretics such as furosemide will cause loss of sodium), and chronic vomiting.

Potassium (K^+). 98% of the body's potassium is found within the cell, so the serum levels do not reflect the severity of potassium decreases. Hyperkalemia (elevated potassium) is seen in renal failure, urethral obstruction, hypoadrenocorticism (aldosterone deficiency causing sodium loss and potassium conservation), or due to oversupplementation. Hypokalemia can result from fluid loss, use of loop diuretics such as furosemide, chronic vomiting, and hyperadrenocorticism.

Magnesium (Mg^{+2}). Less than 1% of the total body magnesium is available for testing because 60% is found in the bones and 40% is contained within cells. Of the available 1%, one-third is bound to albumin. Serum must be used for testing. Hypermagnesemia can occur secondary to increased supplementation, decreased renal output, hypoadrenocorticism (aldosterone deficiency), chronic renal failure, and diabetic ketoacidosis. Hypomagnesemia can be caused by anything that causes decreased albumin levels, chronic diarrhea, or poor gastrointestinal absorption. Magnesium absorption is affected by calcium and phosphorus absorption.

Calcium (Ca^{+2}). Calcium is a major component of bone (99% of the body's calcium is bound in the bone). Of the other 1%, over half is bound to albumin. The rest is free in the serum (ionized calcium) and is the active form. Calcium measurement must take into account both the bound and the unbound calcium. The formula for corrected calcium level is as follows:

$$\text{Corrected total calcium} = \text{total serum calcium} - (\text{serum albumin} + 4)$$

This formula is only valid for dogs and should be used if the albumin level is high or low. Calcium measurements should only be performed on serum. Hemolysis will not affect results.

Calcium is regulated by three different mechanisms. Vitamin D is a calcium carrier and facilitates calcium uptake across the intestinal mucosa. Parathyroid hormone (PTH) is required for maintenance of calcium balance. PTH is made in the parathyroid glands and stimulates calcium mobilization from bone, kidney resorption of calcium in the distal convoluted tubule, and gastrointestinal absorption of calcium. All these mechanisms increase serum calcium concentrations. Calcitonin works against PTH by decreasing bone resorption of calcium. Calcitonin does not affect kidney or gastrointestinal uptake of calcium. Calcitonin will decrease serum calcium levels.

		ELECTROLYTES		
ION	INTRA- OR EXTRACELLULAR?	FUNCTION	TEST	AFFECTED BY HEMOLYSIS?
Sodium (Na^+)	extracellular	maintenance of water distribution, osmotic balance	flame spectrophotometry* ion specific electrodes[†]	no
Potassium (K^+)	intracellular	cardiac, nerve, and muscle function	flame spectrophotometry* ion-specific electrodes[†]	yes
Magnesium (Mg^{++})	intracellular	cardiac, muscle function	flame spectrophotometry* ion-specific electrodes[†]	yes (affected by low albumin concentrations)
Calcium (Ca^{++})	extracellular	neuromuscular function, major cofactor in the coagulation cascade, maintains cell membrane integrity		no (affected by low albumin concentrations)
Phosphorus (PO_4^-)	intracellular	muscle and nerve function, nutrient metabolism (ATP), cell membrane integrity (phospholipids), and acid–base balance		yes
Bicarbonate (HCO_3^-)	extracellular	the most important measurable ion in acid–base regulation	measured by arterial blood gases can also be estimated by the total CO_2 level in serum testing (TCO_2), although that is not accurate and is adversely affected by contact with red blood cells during the clotting process; in dogs, arterial HCO_3 levels should be 20–25 mEq/L, in cats it should be 17–21 mEq/L	no
Chloride (Cl^-)	extracellular	water distribution, maintenance of osmotic pressures, acid–base balance, maintains electroneutrality by balancing the charge of sodium		no

*Flame photometry measures the concentration of sodium relative to the plasma volume by analyzing the color of the flame produced by burning the mineral.
[†]The ion-specific electrode test measures the electric impedence (resistance) of the ion.

Hypercalcemia (increased levels of calcium in the serum) can be caused by bone tumors and septic osteomyelitis because it causes osteolysis (bone destruction), which releases calcium. Hyperparathyroidism stimulates the production of PTH, which also causes hypercalcemia. Hypocalcemia (low blood calcium) is usually caused by hypoalbuminemia (low albumin levels).

Phosphate (PO_4^{-2}). Phosphate is the primary anion of intracellular fluid. It is the ionic form of phosphorus. 80% of the phosphorus in the body is found in the bones along with calcium. 14% is found in the muscles and only 1% is found in the serum. Serum should be tested for phosphorus levels. Hyperphosphatemia can occur with renal failure, hypoparathyroidism (decreased PTH) and hemolysis (intracellular anion). Hypophosphatemia can be caused by metabolic alkalosis, neoplasia, and hyperparathyroidism (increased PTH).

Soft-tissue mineralization is a problem that can occur with imbalances of calcium and phosphorus. A calculation that can be used to determine the severity of disease and the likelihood of soft-tissue mineralization is as follows:

$$\text{Total serum calcium} \times \text{serum phosphorus}$$

If the product is greater than 60, there is an increased risk of soft-tissue mineralization.

Chloride (Cl^-). Hyperchloremia (excessive chloride) is caused by dehydration, renal failure, and metabolic acidosis (blood pH <7.35). Hypochloremia is caused by increased sweating (especially in horses), vomiting and diarrhea, and metabolic alkalosis (pH >7.45).

Bicarbonate (HCO_3^-). Metabolic acidosis occurs when bicarbonate levels fall, causing the pH of the blood to drop. This may be caused by renal failure, ketoacidosis, or hyperparathyroidism. Compensation for metabolic acidosis is hyperventilation (the animal is trying to cause respiratory alkalosis). Metabolic alkalosis occurs when the bicarbonate levels increase, causing the blood pH to rise. This may be caused by Addison's disease (hypoadrenocorticism) or anesthesia.

Proteins

Protein levels have been discussed in previous sections. Protein evaluation is performed by use of a refractometer in practice (see Red Blood Cell Indices). If serum is measured, the protein will reflect only the albumin and circulating globulin fractions, not the clotting proteins (fibrinogen). Plasma contains all the proteins. Other methods of protein evaluation include serum electrophoresis. Electrophoresis shows relative concentrations by the molecular weights, sizes, and charges of the proteins and allows evaluation of individual protein types.

Protein levels can be an indicator of hydration in animals and should be evaluated along with PCV, urinalysis, and the chemistry. Hemolysis and lipemia can affect refractometer results.

PROTEINS				
PROTEIN TYPE	MANUFACTURE	CHARACTERISTICS/ FUNCTIONS	TEST	AFFECTED BY HEMOLYSIS?
Albumin	liver (can be used as a measure of liver function)	35–40% of the protein in plasma	colorimetric analysis	yes (will give an apparent increase)
Fibrinogen	liver	forms fibrin in the coagulation cascade elevated in inflammation (especially in cattle)	reference lab	no

(continued)

PROTEINS (continued)				
PROTEIN TYPE	MANUFACTURE	CHARACTERISTICS/ FUNCTIONS	TEST	AFFECTED BY HEMOLYSIS?
Globulins Albumin first peak	liver	forms fibrin in the coagulation cascade	electrophoresis; because of the diversity of the globulins, they should be further evaluated if an abnormality is present	yes
Alpha globulins	liver	elevated in inflammation (especially in cattle)		no
Alpha globulin 1	liver			no
Alpha globulin 2	liver	lipoproteins; carry lipids and other nutrients carrier and transport proteins; carry hormones and act in coagulation cascade		no
Beta globulin	liver			no
Gamma globulin	B lymphocytes	complement, transferrin, and ferritin (iron transport) humoral immunity (may be the largest peak present with hypoproteinemia)		no

Pancreatic Testing

The pancreas acts as both an exocrine and an endocrine gland, which means that it affects both digestion and metabolism. Diseases of the pancreas may affect the liver and vice versa because of the close proximity of the organs. Ascending infections from the gastrointestinal tract may also cause diseases of the pancreas. The cells of the exocrine portion of the pancreas surround ducts. These are called the acinar glands. Between these rows of cells in the pancreas lie the islets of Langerhans, which contain the cells that have endocrine function. Although the cells are not truly mixed together, inflammation of the exocrine cells (pancreatitis) can lead to damage of the endocrine cells (diabetes mellitus). For this reason, the endocrine pancreas is included here rather than in the Hormone Testing section.

Endocrine Testing

The endocrine pancreas regulates glucose metabolism. Two hormones are produced by the islets of Langerhans: glucagon and insulin.

Glucagon is made by the alpha cells in the islets of Langerhans. Glucagon acts on the liver (hepato-cytes) to convert stored glycogen into glucose and stimulates gluconeogenesis (the formation of glucose from amino acids). This has the net effect of raising blood glucose. The secretion of glucagon is stimulated by decreased glucose in the blood.

Insulin is made by the beta cells in the islets of Langerhans. Insulin acts on the cell membranes of all the tissues in the body to increase cell uptake of glucose. This lowers glucose in the blood. The secretion of insulin is stimulated by rising glucose levels. When insulin levels fall, blood glucose rises; when insulin levels rise, blood glucose falls.

Serial Blood Glucose Testing

Blood glucose tests can be performed on either whole blood, serum, or plasma. If plasma is used, it should be collected in a sodium fluoride (gray-top) tube. If serum is used, the blood glucose will be low because blood cells use glucose for metabolism and the cells are in contact with the serum for >30 minutes prior to spinning and separating. If whole blood is used with a glucometer, care must be taken to ensure that the glucometer is calibrated properly for animal blood. Some of the quick glucometers will give falsely low values for canine and feline blood samples. Call the manufacturer to make sure the glucometer you are using is appropriate for your species. Normal blood glucose is usually 70 to 120 mg/dl across species.

Hypoglycemia (low blood glucose) can occur due to technician error, insulinoma (cancer of the beta cells of the pancreas that secrete insulin), insulin therapy, hypoglycemia of toy breeds, liver disease, starvation, and septicemia (bacterial infection in the blood).

Hyperglycemia can occur from diabetes mellitus (most common cause), glucocorticoid usage (prednisone), hyperadrenocorticism (overproduction of glucocorticoids by the adrenal gland), pancreatitis, or administration of glucose-containing fluids.

Serial blood glucose monitoring every 2 hours can establish a glucose curve, which is used for monitoring insulin therapy. A glucose curve is essential for beginning insulin therapy because it explains the way insulin works in a particular animal. The blood glucoses are charted on a graph with the glucose concentration on the vertical axis and the time after insulin on the horizontal axis. A line connects the dots and a curve is established that tells the rise and fall of glucose for that particular animal on that particular form of insulin. If the glucose levels fall and rise within a 6-hour period, the animal will probably need twice-a-day insulin therapy. If the levels fall and rise in a 12- to 14-hour period, once-a-day insulin will be sufficient.

Note: Stressed cats will get a stress-induced hyperglycemia that may increase their blood glucose levels from normal to 400 g/dl, so establishment of glucose curves may be difficult in some cats.

Fructosamine Levels

In animals that have been on insulin therapy and are well controlled, fructosamine assays may be used to monitor glucose levels. Fructosamine is a glycosylated protein (a protein bound to glucose). It is actually albumin bound to glucose in an irreversible bond. This test will establish whether the animal has had adequate glycemic control (control of glucose levels) over a two-

to three-week period. Because the protein binding is irreversible, the levels will not be affected by stress-induced hyperglycemia, so it is a much better monitoring technique than serial blood glucoses in the cat. This test is good as long as blood protein values (TP) is normal. If the animal is hypoproteinemic, the test will show false low values. Serum should be used.

Glycosylated Hemoglobin Levels

Glycosylated hemoglobin is hemoglobin irreversibly bound to glucose. This test has the advantage of being an even longer-term monitor of glucose control (2 to 3 months), so it is good for animals that have been stable on insulin for several months. This test should be performed on EDTA whole blood (purple-top tube).

Exocrine Testing

The exocrine function of the pancreas is digestion. The pancreas secretes many different products into the proximal small intestine including lipase (digests fat), amylase (digests sugars and starches), trypsin (digests proteins), chymotrypsin (also digests proteins), and nucleases (digest RNA and DNA). It also secretes bicarbonate, which makes the pH of the intestines more alkaline (high pH). The action of all these enzymes together is called the *digestive activity*. High levels of the enzymes in the blood mean that the pancreas has become leaky, which could lead to pancreatitis (inflammation of the pancreas). Low enzyme production by the pancreas can lead to *maldigestion*, or inefficient breakdown of food in the intestines. Pancreatic exocrine testing should be performed on serum when available.

Diagnosis of pancreatitis is based on clinical history (consumption of high-fat diet and obesity in dogs, stress in cats), physical exam (vomiting with abdominal discomfort), clinical chemistries (amylase, lipase, PLI), and ultrasound. Damage from pancreatitis may lead to exocrine pancreatic insufficiency (EPI), which causes maldigestion syndrome, or to diabetes mellitus. In dogs, clinical signs are much more severe than in cats, but the damage caused is the same. It is estimated that 40% of cats with diabetes have some evidence of either chronic pancreatitis or damage from acute pancreatitis at necropsy.

EPI is characterized by a normal CBC, normal serum chemistries, and normal urinalysis in an animal with chronic weight loss, diarrhea, and large-volume feces. German Shepherds are predisposed to EPI genetically, but it is possible in any breed. Diagnosis is by clinical signs, TLI, and PLI.

Amylase
Amylase breaks down starches into glucose. The pancreas is the major source for amylase, but the kidneys, liver, and GI tract also contribute to the total. Because it has so many sources, amylase is not a very sensitive indicator of pancreatic function. Amylase testing is usually done by adding a dye to the sample that binds to starches to form a color complex. As amylase reacts with the starches, the color decreases. The color is measured by a spectrophotometer. Because it is a colorimetric test, hemolysis will lead to false elevations while lipemia will lead to falsely low values. Amylase values should be examined along with lipase, kidney, and liver values. If the amylase is elevated and elevations of BUN and Cr are seen, the test is probably a false positive. If lipase is elevated at the same time, it is probably pancreatic in origin.

Lipase
Lipase breaks down fats into fatty acids. Most lipase is derived from the pancreas, so it is a more sensitive indicator of pancreatic activity than amylase. Serum samples are recommended for evaluation. A greater than threefold increase above normal usually indicates pancreatic disease. This test will also be affected by hemolysis and lipemia.

Pancreatic Lipase Immunoreactivity
The pancreatic lipase immunoreactivity (PLI) test is an extremely sensitive test of pancreatic dysfunction. It has an 82% specificity for pancreatitis. The test is actually a test of the lipase specifically derived from the pancreas. Because there is a slight difference in

structure between cat and dog lipase, two different tests have been developed. The cPLI (canine PLI) is actually a tabletop ELISA test. The fPLI (feline PLI) currently still must be sent to the laboratory.

Trypsinlike Immunoreactivity
Trypsin breaks down proteins. Both trypsin and trypsinogen (its precursor) are specifically derived from the pancreas. Like lipase, trypsin is species specific. Trypsinlike immunoreativity (TLI) is a good indicator of functional pancreatic mass, so can be helpful in diagnosing both EPI (low levels) and pancreatitis (high levels). Because trypsin is cleared through the kidneys, levels may be increased with renal disease.

Gastrointestinal Function Tests
The gastrointestinal (GI) system is responsible for final breakdown of food, absorption of nutrients, and excretion of wastes. Intestinal function tests demonstrate the ability of the organs to perform their jobs.

Different things can cause gastrointestinal disease. Maldigestion (as stated in the section on Pancreatic Testing) can occur from a lack of gastric secretions or pancreatic or GI enzymes. Lack of hydrochloric acid release from the stomach prevents the denaturing (unfolding) of the long protein molecules and inhibits the onset of protein digestion. EPI due to pancreatic dysfunction prevents initiation of carbohydrate and lipid and the continuation of protein digestion. Intestinal mucosal disease prevents the secretion of the intestinal enzymes responsible for completion of digestion. Malabsorption is the failure of materials to cross the mucosa into the blood stream. This is usually caused by small intestinal bacterial overgrowth or other diseases that cause thickening of the bowel mucosa. Malassimilation is a combination of maldigestion and malabsorption.

Symptoms associated with gastrointestinal disease are a result of one or more defects in digestion. Steatorrhea is excess fat in the feces caused by a lack of fat digestion or absorption (lipase deficiency). Creatorrhea is undigested muscle fiber in the feces. This may be caused by a failure of protein digestive enzymes. Amylorrhea is undigested starch in the feces caused by lack of carbohydrate digestion. **Melena** (black, tarry stool) indicates upper GI bleeding (digested blood) from the small intestines or stomach. **Hematochezia** (frank, or visible, blood in the stool) indicates lower GI bleeding from the cecum, rectum, or colon.

All animals with GI disease should have a gross, direct, and flotation fecal exam performed. Other fecal evaluations should be performed if the answers are not diagnostic. Ancillary tests include microscopic exam, fecal protease/gelatin digestion, and fecal occult blood. Blood tests should include cobalamin and folate testing as well as assessing exocrine pancreatic function.

Microscopic Examination of the Feces

A number of in-house tests may be used to differentiate diseases and aid in establishing therapy immediately prior to receiving confirmation from the laboratory. They are not highly accurate and should not be used as the sole diagnostic test.

Gross examination of the feces includes recording its color, texture, volume, odor, and consistency. Greasy-looking, foamy stools may indicate excess fat in the stool, for example.

Several microscopic stains can help differentiate the various materials found in the stool. Fats can be stained with Sudan III or IV. If more than 2 to 3 globules of orange-red are present per 40× field, a lipase deficiency is suggested (**maldigestion**). The stained slide is then heated. If there are still globules of orange-red present, free fatty acids are present in the stool indicating malabsorption of fats. High-fat diets may cause false positives.

Carbohydrates can be assessed using Lugol's iodine. Iodine binds with starch, forming blue/black granules. If a lot of granules are present, this suggests amylase deficiency (maldigestion). This test may cause a false positive if the animal is on a low-quality dog food.

No stain is required for muscle fiber visualization, but Diff-Quick may be used to make them more visible (do not stain feces in the same Diff-Quick stain used for cytology). If 2 to 3 fibers are seen per 40× field, it is probably a protease deficiency (may be pepsin, trypsin, or intestinal proteases).

Gelatin Digestion Test

The gelatin digestion test is also called the fecal protease test. This test is diagnostic only for pancreatic proteases (chymotrypsin and trypsin). The feces are mixed with gelatin. If trypsin is present, the gelatin will dissolve. The test can also be performed by mixing the feces with bicarbonate and placing a piece of undeveloped x-ray film (which has gelatin on a plastic base) in it. If the gelatin dissolves (the film clears), trypsin is present and active. This is not a very accurate test.

Cobalamin and Folate

Intestinal bacteria synthesize and secrete vitamins that are absorbed into the systemic circulation. Bacterial overgrowth will increase the levels of these vitamins in the blood.

Cobalamin is vitamin B_{12}. It is normally protein bound and needs a pancreatic enzyme in order to be absorbed in the ileum. Decreased serum cobalamin is seen in distal small intestinal mucosal disease (ileum) and increases are seen with bacterial overgrowth and EPI.

Folate is vitamin B_9. Absorption normally occurs in the proximal small intestine. Decreased levels are seen in small intestinal mucosal disease (proximal small intestine) and increases are seen with bacterial overgrowth and EPI.

Both vitamin levels are checked at the same time. If only cobalamin is decreased, the disease is in the ileum. If folate is decreased, the disease is duodenal/jejunal. If both are increased, bacterial overgrowth or EPI is present.

Other Tests

The fat absorption test may also be a gauge of GI function. The animal is fasted for 12 hours, then a baseline sample is drawn. Triglycerides are measured. Peanut or corn oil is given orally, then hourly blood samples are drawn to check for lipemia. Lipemia should be present by 4 hours after the oil dose. This means that lipid has crossed the intestinal mucosa.

The same type of test may be performed with D-xylose or other carbohydrates. If the blood concentrations increase after 4 hours, there is carbohydrate absorption.

Hormone Testing

The endocrine glands of the body control homeostasis (the ability of the body to maintain proper functions). The endocrine glands all work in concert with each other in a series of feedback loops. Certain hormones raise substances in the body and other hormones will decrease their levels. It is a series of checks and balances.

Thyroid

The thyroid gland is responsible for metabolism and calcium regulation (calcitonin; see Electrolytes). Thyroid hormones cause activation of the mitochondria, which causes increased energy to be produced in the form of ATP. The hormones of the thyroid gland include T_3 (triiodothyronine), T_4 (tetraiodothyronine), and calcitonin.

Thyroid hormone release is under the control of the anterior pituitary gland (thyroid-stimulating hormone, or TSH) and the hypothalamus (thyrotrophin-releasing factor, or TRF). Excessive levels of T_4 will cause feedback inhibition (decreased production) on both the hypothalamus and the anterior pituitary gland.

T_4 and fT_4

T_4 accounts for 80% of the total hormonal output of the thyroid gland. Most (99%) is bound to albumin. The other 1% is called free T_4 (fT_4) and is the form

that can enter cells. T_3 is actually the bioactive form that causes changes in metabolism. A small amount is manufactured by the thyroid gland, but most is converted to T_3 within the cells. This conversion is called deiodination.

Thyroid hormone increases metabolic activity. It is responsible for maintenance of body temperature as well as protein, carbohydrate, and lipid metabolism. It encourages protein synthesis, decreases carbohydrate conversion to fat, and stimulates lipid breakdown. Hypothyroid animals are usually obese while hyperthyroid animals are very thin.

Serum levels of T_4 and fT_4 are measured by radioimmunoassay. The requirements are dependent on the particular laboratory. T_4 can also be checked using an ELISA test. This is not adequate for evaluation of hypothyroidism (decreased T_4, T_3, and/or elevated TSH), but is diagnostic for hyperthyroidism.

T_3 and fT_3 levels are usually produced in such low amounts that they are difficult to measure, so are typically not evaluated.

Thyroid-Stimulating Hormone

TSH is produced by the pituitary gland. High TSH levels usually indicate hypothyroidism. Low TSH numbers can indicate hyperthyroidism because T_4 will cause negative feedback on the pituitary. This test must be run at a reference laboratory.

Adrenal Gland

The adrenal gland is responsible for production of several hormones. The adrenal cortex secretes sex hormones, mineralocorticoids (aldosterone), and glucocorticoids. It is responsible for metabolic hormonal control of glucose utilization (along with insulin and glucagon), and maintenance of mineral balance in the kidneys. It also acts as a secondary source for sex hormones. The adrenal medulla secretes epinephrine which is responsible for flight-or-fight mechanisms and sympathetic responses. The medullary and sex hormones will not be discussed in this section.

HORMONE TESTING		
GLAND	**HORMONES AFFECTING THE GLAND**	**PRODUCTION OF HORMONE**
Thyroid gland	TRH (thyrotropin-releasing hormone) TSH (thyroid-stimulating hormone) T_4 (tetraiodothyronine, or thyroxin) T_3 triiodothyronine	hypothalamus anterior pituitary gland thyroid gland thyroid gland
Adrenal gland	CRF (corticotrophin-releasing factor) ACTH (adrenocorticotrophic hormone) cortisol aldosterone testosterone epinephrine	hypothalamus anterior pituitary gland adrenal cortex adrenal cortex adrenal cortex adrenal medulla
Ovaries	GnRH (gonadotrophin-releasing hormone) FSH (follicle-stimulating hormone) LH (luteinizing hormone) estrogen progesterone	hypothalamus anterior pituitary gland anterior pituitary gland ovary (developing follicle) ovary (corpus luteum)
Mammary glands	progesterone oxytocin polactin	ovary (corpus luteum) hypothalamus (stored in posterior pituitary gland) hypothalamus
Testes	GnRH FSH LH estrogen testosterone	hypothalamus anterior pituitary gland anterior pituitary gland testicles (Sertoli cells) testicles (Leydig cells)
Kidneys	ADH (antidiuretic hormone) vasopressin aldosterone erythropoetin	hypothalamus adrenal cortex kidneys
Pancreas	insulin glucagon cortisol	pancreas pancreas adrenal cortex
Pituitary gland	GnRH TRH CRF FSH LH TSH ACTH ADH/vasopressin T_4 estrogen aldosterone cortisol	hypothalamus hypothalamus hypothalamus anterior pituitary anterior pituitary anterior pituitary anterior pituitary posterior pituitary thyroid gland ovary, testicle adrenal gland adrenal gland

Aldosterone is produced by the zona glomerulosa of the adrenal cortex. It is a mineralocorticoid (a mineral-controlling hormone produced by the adrenal cortex) specific for the control of the retention of sodium in the distal convoluted tubule of the kidney nephron. Sodium is retained in exchange for potassium and hydrogen ion, which helps to maintain the acid–base balance of the kidney. Because water always follows sodium, water is also retained in the body. Retention of water increases blood pressure.

Glucocorticoids are produced by the zona fasciculata of the adrenal cortex. Glucocorticoids are responsible for regulating glucose metabolism. They inhibit protein synthesis and can increase protein breakdown (catabolism). They have an anti-insulin effect and can decrease the animal's response to insulin (insulin-resistant diabetes). Increases in glucocorticoids results in a potbellied appearance due to muscle loss, increased glycogen storage in the liver (which can cause elevations in alkaline phosphatase), and decreased immune competence (because of old, hypersegmented neutrophils in the circulation).

Control of hormone secretion by the adrenal cortex is under hypothalamic (corticotrophin-releasing factor, or CRF) and anterior pituitary gland (adrenocorticotrophic hormone, or ACTH) control. ACTH causes activation of all the hormones of the adrenal cortex (aldosterone, glucocorticoids, and sex hormones). Negative feedback inhibition is caused by excessive levels of glucocorticoids in the circulation. This is important in therapy of animals with corticosteroids such as prednisone. If glucocorticoids are administered, the production of ACTH will be suppressed. Suddenly discontinuing glucocorticoids can result in exceedingly low levels of glucocorticoid and mineralocorticoids being released from the adrenal glands, which may result in life-threatening elevations of potassium. For this reason, the production of glucocorticoids and ACTH are tested as indicators of adrenal cortical function, not aldosterone production.

Baseline Cortisol

Cortisol (glucocorticoid) is the substance tested for all adrenal tests. A baseline cortisol level provides a starting point for adrenal testing, but does not give diagnostic information. Low cortisol levels may indicate Addison's disease (hypoadrenocorticism). High cortisol levels may indicate hyperadrenocorticism, but may also indicate stress.

ACTH Stimulation Test

The ACTH stimulation test is a screening test. It works by stimulating the adrenal gland to produce glucocorticoids (cortisol) by giving an injection of an ACTH analog. Exaggerated elevation of the cortisol level indicates hyperadrenocorticism. Failure to increase the cortisol level indicates hypoadrenocorticism. The procedure for testing is as follows. A baseline cortisol level is taken. ACTH is injected into the animal. The cortisol level is then taken 2 hours after the injection is given.

This test is also used to monitor Lysodren® therapy (0,p' = DDD or mitotane), or trilostane therapy for hyperadrenocorticism.

The ACTH stimulation test should be performed along with a high-dose dexamethasone suppression test to help initially diagnose whether an animal has pituitary-dependent or adrenal-dependent hyperadrenocorticism.

Low-Dose Dexamethasone Suppression Test

The low-dose dexamethasone suppression test (LDDS) is also a screening test for hyperadrenocorticism. In theory, dexamethasone should suppress production of glucocorticoids because of negative feedback inhibition of ACTH. The procedure is similar to the ACTH stimulation test.

Baseline cortisol is obtained and dexamethasone (0.01 mg/kg in dogs, 0.1 mg/kg in cats) is injected into the animal. Postinjection samples are taken at 4 to 6 hours and again at 8 hours post injection. There should be a decrease in the cortisol level after dexamethasone injection.

High-Dose Dexamethasone Suppression Test

The high-dose dexamethasone suppression test (HDDS) is used to distinguish between hyperadrenocorticism of pituitary origin and adrenal origin. The dose of dexamethasone is ten times higher (0.1mg/kg in dogs, 1.0 mg/kg in cats) than in the low-dose test, but the technique is the same. If the post-test cortisol is less than 50% of the pretest value, the animal probably has a pituitary tumor. If it is greater than 50% of the baseline, it is probably an adrenal tumor. Most dogs have pituitary-dependent hyperadrenocorticism. Most ferrets have adrenal-dependent hyperadrenocorticism. Since adrenal tumors can usually be removed, performing the HDDS along with the ACTH stimulation test is important diagnostically.

Reproductive Testing

Reproductive testing is extremely important in production animals and also in breeding stock in small animals. Failure to produce semen or offspring can mean the difference between maintaining that animal in a herd or culling. By evaluating reproductive status, the farmer or breeder can improve the pregnancy rate, milk production, and litter size of the animal and prevent infertile animals from being a drain on valuable resources such as feed. Reproductive testing also allows artificial insemination to be successful, thereby decreasing the numbers of sexually transmitted diseases that occur in companion and production animals.

Female

Control of reproductive status in animals is under the influence of the hypothalamus (GnRH) and the anterior pituitary (FSH and LH), causing ovarian release of either estrogen or progesterone. The release of the various hormones is associated with certain cellular changes on vaginal swabs.

The hormones that are usually tested are estradiol (estrogen) and progestins (progesterone). FSH may also be tested. FSH is produced by the anterior pituitary gland, which causes formation of a follicle on the ovary. This follicle produces estrogen, which rises until the follicle formation is complete (mature follicle). When estrogen is at its peak, LH is released from the anterior pituitary gland. LH causes the follicle to rupture, releasing the egg. The ruptured follicle transforms into a corpus luteum (yellow body) under the influence of LH and begins to produce progesterone. During this time, the estrogen levels are decreasing rapidly. If the animal becomes pregnant, progesterone continues to be produced by the corpus luteum until the end of pregnancy. If the animal does not become pregnant, the corpus luteum dissolves under the influence of prostaglandin F_2 alpha ($PGF_2\alpha$), progesterone levels fall rapidly, and the ovary becomes quiet. Estradiol levels are usually at their peak just prior to ovulation (proestrus). Progestin level elevations are an indicator of pregnancy.

The estrous cycle generally has four phases: proestrus, estrus, diestrus, and anestrus. Specific changes seen on vaginal smears made during each phase are associated with the hormonal, physical, and behavioral changes in the animal. Vaginal smears can be used for timing breeding as well as diagnosis of some pathologies, and are much less expensive than hormonal testing. The animal should be restrained in a standing position and the vulva should be cleaned prior to swabbing. A sterile and lubricated vaginal speculum is then inserted into the vulva and advanced into the vagina. A sterile, moistened cotton swab is then gently rolled against the vaginal wall, removed, and rolled on a clean slide. The slide is then air-dried, Diff-Quick stained, and examined under the microscope at 10× and 40×. The cellular changes will be evaluated and the stage of estrus recorded.

VAGINAL CYTOLOGY				
STAGE OF ESTRUS	HORMONES	PHYSICAL CHANGES	BEHAVIORAL CHANGES	MICROSCOPIC CHANGES
Anestrus (no ovarian activity)	none from either pituitary or ovary	none, normal appearance	normal behavior	parabasal (round cells with round nuclei and open chromatin) and intermediate (slightly flattened cells with open chromatin) epithelial cells
Proestrus (follicle development)	FSH (pituitary) and estrogen (developing follicle)	red, swollen vulva, bloody vaginal discharge; pheromone production (males are interested)	will not stand for breeding	intermediate epithelial cells with cornified superficial epithelial cells (flattened, angular, with pyknotic nuclei), large numbers of RBCs
Estrus (heat)	estrogen at its peak, LH release from pituitary causes follicle to rupture at end of estrus	red, swollen vulva, discharge clears to straw colored; pheromone production at peak	stands for breeding in lordosis (swayback) with tail to the side (flagging)	>95% cornified superficial epithelial cells, occasional RBCs animal should be bred during this phase
Diestrus (pregnancy)	LH surge and follicle rupture is the beginning of diestrus; progesterone production by corpus luteum	swelling and discoloration decrease, discharge stops, pheromone production stops, mammary glands enlarge	no longer interested in males; may exhibit nesting behaviors	sudden drop-off of cornified eptihelial cells, increase in parabasal cells and neutrophils; neutrophils are often seen within epithelial cells
Onset of anestrus	PGF$_2$ alpha destroys corpus luteum	mammary glands become quiescent	none	sudden drop-off of cornified eptihelial cells, increase in parabasal cells and neutrophils; neutrophils are often seen within epithelial cells

Abnormal cytologies can include nonepithelial cell invasion (cancers) and inflammatory cells (neutrophils) in large numbers during anestrus (pyometra).

Male

Semen testing of males is important to limit sexually transmitted diseases, improve genetics of the herd, and increase chances of conception. Some dog and cattle breeds have congenitally low sperm counts or inadequate ejaculate, but the genetics of the animal may be so desirable that they must be used as breeding stock. Artificial insemination can improve conception rates.

Semen is extremely fragile and must be handled carefully when performing laboratory tests. All mate-rials used in semen handling must be dried thoroughly and warmed to body temperature (98.6° Fahrenheit) prior to use to maximize sperm motility and prevent damage. Water and disinfectants will kill sperm quickly. All materials should be assembled prior to sample collection so that the sperm is not exposed to environmental conditions. Materials needed are artificial vagina, collection tubes, slides, coverslips, stains, and diluents.

Sperm evaluation should include all of the categories because each test assesses different attributes of the semen that may be important to fertility of the animal.

The **ejaculate** is the entire semen volume. This may be measured at the time of collection. It consists of three fractions: the sperm-free, sperm-rich, and sperm-poor fractions. The sperm-free fraction is the accessory sex gland secretions. The sperm-rich fraction is mostly sperm cells. The sperm-poor fraction contains sperm and prostatic secretions. The sperm-poor fraction should not be collected in dogs, horses, or pigs because it will dilute and decrease the quality of the sperm in these species. All other species should have all three fractions collected. The gross appearance of sperm should be recorded as color and opacity (thickness). The color is usually white to gray. Blood contamination will change the color. The opacity is usually recorded for those animals with highly concentrated semen (ruminants). Other species have more translucent semen and the opacity may be difficult to evaluate.

Sperm motility is the movement of the sperm in the sample. Motility indicates how much activity is present in the sperm. Strong swimmers make it more likely that the sperm will get to the oviduct of the female and penetrate the egg.

Wave motion is one method of motility assessment. This is performed by placing a drop of semen on a warmed slide and examining on 10× to evaluate the amount of movement present. This activity depends on high sperm concentrations, so it works best on ruminant semen.

A true motility test should be performed in animals with more dilute semen. This tests the motility of individual spermatozoa. A drop of semen is diluted with a drop of warmed physiologic saline (0.9% saline) on a warmed slide and covered with a coverslip. The drop is examined at 100× and individual spermatozoa are examined to see whether they travel. They are classified by the amount of movement, rapidity of movement, and whether they travel in a straight line (linear movement). The percentage of good swimmers is then estimated. This test is subject to poor sample handling, so it should be repeated if bad results are obtained, to rule out error.

Sperm concentration is also an important measure of fertility. This is a quantitative test (not subjective). 0.5 ml of semen is diluted with solution to give a 1:200 dilution and mixed thoroughly. The solution is used to charge the hemocytometer chambers. Wait 10 minutes, then count the spermatozoa in the erythrocyte counting area (large central square) at 400×. Multiply the number by two million. The solution may be either 9g sodium chloride in 1 liter of distilled water mixed with 1 milliliter of formalin, 3% chlorazene or 12.5 g sodium sulfate with 33.3 milliliters of glacial acetic acid in 200 milliliters of water (Gower's solution). The first solution can be made in the clinic.

The live-to-dead ratio allows you to assess the percentage of living versus dead sperm in a sample and can be an indicator of fertility. The sperm is stained with a vital dye (dye that stains only living cells) such as eosin/nigrosin. This stain is prepared by adding 1 g of eosin B to 5 g of nigrosin in 3% sodium citrate dihydrate. The stain and the slide are both warmed and one drop of the dye is added to one drop of semen and allowed to incubate for 3 seconds. A push smear (similar to the blood smear technique) is made and allowed to dry. The slide is examined at 40× and oil immersion. Live sperm will appear white against the dark background, dead sperm will appear pink. 200 spermatozoa will be counted. The number of live versus dead will be counted (use a cell counter) and a percentage is obtained.

Morphology is assessed on the same slide as used for the live-to-dead ratio. 500 spermatozoa are assessed for normal morphology of the head, midpiece, and tail. Morphological abnormalities are broken into primary and secondary abnormalities.

MORPHOLOGY		
Primary abnormalities	occur during development of the sperm (more serious)	two heads two tails abnormally small head abnormally large head pear-shaped head round or elongated head coiled tail bent midpiece
Secondary abnormalities	occur after development of the sperm by movement through the system or capacitation in the epididymis	tailless head droplets on the midpiece droplets on the tail bent tail broken tail

All abnormalities should be noted. It is important also to note that other types of cells should not be seen in the semen. If they are present, their quantity should be recorded. If neutrophils are seen, the semen should be submitted for culture and sensitivity.

Pituitary Testing

The pituitary gland is also known as the *master gland*. It has two components: the anterior pituitary (also called the adenohypophysis) and the posterior pituitary gland (also called the neurohypophysis). The anterior pituitary gland produces hormones that stimulate other glands to produce their hormones (FSH, LH, TSH, ACTH). Problems with the anterior pituitary gland will cause problems with their target glands. Decreases in production of the stimulating hormones may be from primary pituitary dysfunction or secondary to overproduction of hormones from the target glands. Testing for these hormones has been discussed in the previous sections.

The posterior pituitary gland is actually a storage depot for hormones produced by the hypothalamus. These hormones direct milk letdown and parturition (oxytocin) and urine retention/water elimination (ADH). ADH is released in response to a reduction in blood pressure and causes the distal convoluted tubule of the nephron (functional unit of the kidneys) to conserve water. This results in an increase in blood volume, which increases blood pressure.

Failure of ADH will cause diuresis (increased urine production) or **polyuria** (excessive urine production). This can happen due to diabetes insipidus (a pituitary gland dysfunction), nephrogenic diabetes insipidus (a failure of the kidneys to respond to ADH), or a hypothalamus problem where there is no production of ADH. Urine specific gravity, the water deprivation test, and the vasopressin test can be used to determine whether this function is intact.

The specific gravity has been discussed under Kidneys, and will be discussed further under Urinalysis in Chapter 8.

Water Deprivation Test

The water deprivation test is an excellent test of renal tubular function. It should be used only for animals with polyuria/**polydipsia** (PU/PD) or in animals with a specific gravity <1.012. If the animal is azotemic (high BUN and/or Cr), the test should not be performed because it will damage the kidneys even more. Baseline data should be obtained prior to the test including body weight, PCV, TP, SG, and BUN. Food and water should then be withheld. The body weight, PCV, TP, SG, and BUN are monitored every 4 to 6 hours until there is a 5% loss in body weight. Body weight loss indicates fluid loss. The U_{SG} should increase with water deprivation because the urine should concentrate in response to the water loss. A failure to concentrate the urine is due either to a lack of ADH or to an unresponsive kidney.

In some cases a syndrome called *medullary washout* can occur. This occurs when the animal is getting overhydrated by either drinking too much (psychogenic polydipsia) or getting too many fluids. In this case the electrolytes are not at a high enough concentration in the blood or kidneys to cause urine concentration. The urine specific gravity will remain low despite adequate or increased ADH levels. In this case, a gradual water deprivation test should be performed. Water is given in very limited amounts over a 3 to 5 day period. This allows the electrolytes to come back to normal levels. Once the solute levels are normal, the normal water deprivation and vasopressin tests can be performed if they are still indicated. This test should only be performed with close patient monitoring.

Vasopressin Test

The vasopressin test differentiates between unresponsive kidneys and hypothalamic/pituitary disease. The animal is given an injection of vasopressin (synthetic ADH) and the urine concentration (SG) is monitored every hour for 2 to 4 hours. If the urine concentrates (the SG increases), there is a lack of ADH production and the disease is localized to the pituitary or the hypothalamus.

Immunology/Serology

Because immunoglobulins are specific to specific substances (antigens), they can be used by the veterinary practice to diagnose diseases and rapidly identify problems that must be treated immediately. Many tests may be performed in-house (agglutination test, Coombs test, ELISA), but others may need to be sent to a reference laboratory.

Enzyme-Linked Immunosorbent Assay

This testing method allows the practice to rapidly diagnose many diseases in-house with the manufacture of tests like the SNAP® test by IDEXX and other quick-test systems. Some ELISA tests must still be performed in the laboratory because they have not been made into quick-test assays.

Direct Testing

Direct ELISA tests test for the presence of antigen. Direct tests have the specific antibody for the antigen of interest present in the well (filter paper or plastic well). The specimen is then added to the well. Any antigen present in the sample will bind to the antibody and stick to the well. The well is washed to remove any other unbound substances and a second antigen-specific antibody is added to the well. This will bind to the antigen again. An antiantibody (an antibody that binds to that species' antibodies) is added to the well. This antibody has a label that causes a color change. The well is washed again to remove any unbound antibody. The amount of color formed will correlate to the amount of antigen present in the sample.

This test is very specific. False positives are very rare. Examples of direct tests are canine heartworm tests, giardia, feline leukemia, and parvovirus. There are many others.

Indirect Testing

Indirect tests test for the presence of antibody to a specific antigen. In this case, the specific antigen is present in the well. The sample is added and the antigen-specific antibody binds to the well. The sample is washed and an antiantibody with a label is added to the well. This is then washed a second time. Color change correlates to the amount of antibody to the antigen present in the sample.

This test is very sensitive. This means that false negatives are rare. However, animals that have recovered from the disease may still show up positive, so care must be taken when interpreting these tests. Examples of indirect tests are the feline immunodeficiency virus, feline infectious peritonitis, and feline heartworm antibody test.

Agglutination Tests

The theory behind agglutination tests is the formation of insoluble complexes (complexes that cannot be separated by washing with saline) of antibodies and antigen. Because antibodies are specific, they will only react with the substance that is being studied. These complexes can be seen either with the naked eye or by microscopy.

Coombs Test

The Coombs test is used in animals that are suspected of having immune-mediated hemolytic anemia (IMHA), or auto immune hemolytic anemia (AIHA). This disease occurs when the body produces antibodies to the red blood cells, causing clumping and destruction (hemolysis). In many cases, these clumps of red blood cells (autoagglutination) are seen when examining the CBC. In other cases, Coombs testing is necessary.

The patient's cells are washed with saline after separating them from the plasma to remove any free-floating antibodies. Coombs serum containing anticanine antibody (antibody specific for dog antibodies) is then added to the sample. If **agglutination** (clumping) occurs, that indicates that the red blood cells have antierythrocyte antibody attached to them. This is called a Coombs positive test, and the animal should be treated for IMHA.

Blood Typing

Blood typing is also a serologic test based on the formation of antibody:antigen complexes. In dogs, DEA (dog erythrocyte antigen) is the most important test. Animals that are DEA$^-$ will have life-threatening transfusion reactions to DEA$^+$ blood. In cats, type A blood will cause life-threatening reactions when given to type B cats.

Blood testing for both breeds involves mixing blood with the antibodies located on the test card surface. Positive agglutination will occur in dogs with DEA$^+$ blood. Cats have one well with type A antibody and one well with type B antibody. All animals should be tested prior to receiving a blood transfusion.

Brucellosis Testing

Brucellosis testing is the reaction of Brucellosis organisms with the antibodies in the serum to form complexes that clump on the card. It is commonly performed in canine fertility testing (both males and females) and on milk from dairy cattle.

Polymerase Chain Reaction

Polymerase chain reaction (PCR) is not really an immunologic test, but it can increase the amount of protein available for immunologic testing. It is the formation of multiple copies of a piece of DNA in order to amplify the ability to detect it in a sample. This will allow the formation of protein by reverse transcription that may be analyzed by immunology or serology. It has become very common to use PCR for viral testing and hereditary diseases.

Agar Gel Immunodiffusion

Agar gel immunodiffusion (AGID) uses the same principles as agglutination testing. The antibody: antigen complex is seen as a line in the agar between the sample (patient antibody) and the test antigen. The test antigen is placed in a well in the center of the plate. The patient's serum and positive and negative controls are placed in wells surrounding the center well. Since agar is porous, the serum and antigen will diffuse through it. Where they meet, a white line of precipitate is formed.

This test is used for equine infectious anemia (EIA) in horses, pseudorabies virus, bovine leukemia virus (BLV), and Johne's disease in ruminants.

Fluorescent Antibody Testing

Fluorescent antibody testing (FAB) can be used both as a diagnostic test for disease and as a protein labeling test in the pathology laboratory. An antibody specific to the protein or organism to be identified is labeled with a fluorescent marker that will glow yellow or green under black light. This is added to the specimen and examined under the fluorescent microscope. It can be used to identify certain viruses and bacteria. This is called immunohistochemistry because it uses immune complexes to find things in the tissues.

Titers

Serologic titers measure the concentration of a specific antibody in the serum. Serial dilution is performed by continuing to dilute the serum until there are no complexes formed with the antigen to be tested.

Serum titers can be very important in vaccination. A higher titer means that there is more antibody available to fight off a specific infection. Vaccines that cause higher titers are generally more effective at protecting the animal from disease.

Titers measure only humoral immunity (immunity from antibodies), not cellular immunity, so a low titer does not necessarily mean low immunity. Some vaccines stimulate humoral immunity better, some stimulate cellular immunity. It is difficult to measure cellular immunity in the laboratory.

Practice Questions

1. Which of the following blood tubes should be used for coagulation studies?
   a. gray-top
   b. blue-top
   c. lavender-top
   d. green-top

2. What is the anticoagulant in a lavender-top tube?
   a. heparin
   b. sodium citrate
   c. calcium EDTA
   d. calcium oxalate

3. Which blood tube should be used for glucose studies?
   a. gray-top
   b. blue-top
   c. lavender-top
   d. green-top

4. Which blood tube contains heparin?
   a. gray-top
   b. blue-top
   c. lavender-top
   d. green-top

5. Which zone of the blood smear is used to identify cell morphology?
   a. monolayer
   b. feathered edge
   c. body
   d. buffy coat

6. The red blood cell count of Gunther, a white boxer mix, is 1.4×10^6 ml with a total protein of 8 g/dl. This indicates
   a. absolute polycythemia
   b. hypoproteinemia
   c. relative polycythemia
   d. anemia

7. Holly, a golden retriever, has a PCV of 14 and a red blood cell count of 2.3×10^6 ml. Her total protein was within normal limits. Which of the following describes Holly's anemia?
   a. normocytic, normochromic
   b. microcytic, hypochromic
   c. macrocytic, hypochromic
   d. microcytic, normochromic

8. Freakazoid has been living in a house built in the 1950s. He tends to chew wallboard and wooden banisters. He has been on fipronyl (Frontline®) and Heartgard® Plus monthly. He comes in with a PCV of 12. If paint ingestion is causing his anemia, you would expect to see:
   a. Basophilic stippling on his red blood cells.
   b. He will have Heinz bodies present on his red blood cells.
   c. He will have morula present in his white blood cells.
   d. He has autoimmune hemolytic anemia.

9. Fifi, a Persian cat, comes into the clinic with pale mm. She is FeLV positive. Her hemoglobin is 5 g/dl, PCV 20%, RBC count 4.7×10^6 ml, and there were 70 reticulocytes per 1,000 RBCs. Which of the following is true?
   a. She has a strongly regenerative anemia.
   b. She will have polychromasia on her Diff-Quick® stained slide.
   c. She is microcytic.
   d. She has aplastic anemia.

10. Sunshine, a 6-year-old female Shih Tzu, presents with a fever. The veterinarian orders blood work. The hematologic indices are normal and there is no anemia. The white blood cell count is 23,000 ml. The differential is 85% neutrophils, 1% bands, 10% lymphocytes, 4% monocytes, 1% eosinophils. There are 5 nRBCs present on the count. Which of the following is true?
    a. This is an inflammatory leukogram.
    b. This is a physiologic leukogram.
    c. This is a stress leukogram.
    d. This is a reverse stress leukogram.

11. The veterinarian prescribes antibiotics. Twenty-four hours later, the owner brings Sunshine into the clinic again. The fever is still present and the veterinarian again orders blood work. The WBC count is up to 24,000 ml. The differential is 75% neutrophils, 5% bands, 12% lymphocytes, 4% monocytes, and 1% eosinophils. There are 7 nRBCs present on the count. Which of the following is true?
    a. The bone marrow is keeping up with the demand for neutrophils.
    b. The bone marrow is not keeping up with the demand for neutrophils.
    c. This is a stress leukogram.
    d. This is a reverse stress leukogram.

12. A 4-month-old puppy comes into the clinic with fever, dehydration, and nasal and ocular discharge. It has been diagnosed with distemper. Which of the following would be consistent with distemper infection?
    a. intranuclear inclusions in all blood cells
    b. intracytoplasmic inclusions in all blood cells
    c. intracytoplasmic inclusions only in the red blood cells
    d. intranuclear inclusions only in the neutrophils

13. Fred, a 10-year-old miniature poodle, has bad skin. He is getting some preoperative blood work for dentistry. His PCV, TP, and indices are fine. His WBC count is 25,000/ml with segs 70% (with moderate hypersegmentation), eosinophils 25%, monocytes 10%, and lymphocytes 5%. No basophils or bands are present. Which of the following is true?
   a. This is an inflammatory leukogram.
   b. This is a physiologic leukogram.
   c. This is a stress leukogram.
   d. This is a reverse stress leukogram.

14. The bone marrow on a cat is hypocellular and has an M:E ratio of 2:1. He has decreased hemosiderin and 4 megakaryocytes per low power field. Which of the following is possible?
   a. nonregenerative anemia
   b. myeloid leukemia
   c. thrombocytopenia
   d. erythroid leukemia

15. Which of the following is NOT a potential cause of aplastic anemia?
   a. estrogen toxicity
   b. renal failure
   c. chemotherapy
   d. parasitism

16. Which of the following is a good site for bone marrow aspiration in the cow?
   a. dorsal ribs
   b. sternum
   c. proximal humerus
   d. proximal femur

17. Which of the following is true of the myeloid series with Diff-Quick® stain?
   a. The cytoplasm is dark blue.
   b. The nucleus stains pink/purple.
   c. The cytoplasm contains vacuoles.
   d. Both agranulocytes and granulocyte precursors should be counted.

18. Which of the following is true of the megakaryocyte?
   a. It becomes a macrophage on maturation.
   b. It is the smallest cell in the bone marrow.
   c. It is easily confused with a monocyte.
   d. It has multiple nuclei.

19. Which of the following is false of the lymphocyte?
   a. It can live in the tissues for long periods.
   b. The highest number of circulating lymphocytes are B cells.
   c. B cells secrete immunoglobulins.
   d. T cells are labeled in the thymus.

20. Which of the following is true of *Dipetalonema reconditum*?
   a. It is a filariid parasite.
   b. It is a protozoan.
   c. It is often confused with *Trypanosoma*.
   d. It is pathogenic.

21. Which of the following is true of *Cytauxzoon* in the housecat?
   a. Its definitive host is the housecat.
   b. It causes massive hemolysis that is almost always fatal.
   c. It can be treated with tetracyclines.
   d. It is confused with *Haemobartonella*.

22. Which of the following statements is correct about preparing a cytological sample?

　a. On a fine needle aspirate, negative pressure should be released prior to removing the needle.

　b. On a touch prep, the site must be cleaned well prior to the sample touching the slide to avoid artifact.

　c. A swab is the best method for obtaining a cytological sample from a moist superficial skin ulceration.

　d. On a fine-needle aspirate, with grainy material, it is important to choose a smaller syringe and needle in order to get an adequate sample.

23. Cases of immune mediated arthritis will usually have elevations of which type of inflammatory cell?

　a. neutrophils

　b. monocytes

　c. eosinophils

　d. basophils

24. The ability of joint fluid to form a string is called

　a. viscosity

　b. lubrication

　c. extension

　d. turbidity

25. The hallmarks of cancer include all of the following *except*

　a. increased nuclear-to-cytoplasmic ratio

　b. increased nucleoli

　c. increased mitotic figures

　d. condensed chromatin

26. Normal cell types found on trachea wash include all of the following *except*

　a. ciliated columnar epithelium

　b. cuboidal epithelium

　c. mesothelial cells

　d. macrophages

27. Romanowsky stains have all of the following characteristics *except*

　a. water based

　b. excellent cytoplasmic detail

　d. ease of use

　d. quickness of stain

28. A sample of abdominal fluid is brought to the lab. The cell count is $15,000/mm^3$, the sample is greenish and turbid, and the total protein is 7.5 g/dl. On cytology, 80% of the cells were neutrophils and bacteria were seen. What is the sample?

　a. a septic inflammatory exudate

　b. a nonseptic inflammatory exudate

　c. a noninflammatory exudate

　d. a modified transudate

29. A sample of pleural fluid from a cat is brought to the lab. The fluid is milky. The cell count is $4,000/mm^3$ and the total protein is 5 g/dl. Lymphocytes, mesothelial cells, and occasional neutrophils are seen on cytology. What other tests should be run on this sample?

　a. BUN

　b. Cr

　c. triglycerides

　d. SG

30. Gerard, a black-and-tan coonhound, presents with bleeding and bruising. His PCV and platelet count are normal. His buccal mucosal bleeding time is prolonged. His PT and APTT are normal. Which of the following is possible?
a. He probably has a vitamin K deficiency.
b. He probably has liver disease.
c. He may have vWF.
d. He probably has DIC.

31. Hammer, a pit bull, comes in after being hit by a car. His PCV and platelet count are normal. About 4 hours after the accident, he starts bleeding from the anus and the nose. The veterinarian determines that he has DIC. Which of the following tests is the *best* indicator of disseminated intravascular coagulation?
a. BMBT
b. PT
c. APTT
d. FSP

32. Which of the following does NOT cause hypoalbuminemia?
a. anemia
b. protein losing enteropathy
c. liver failure
d. protein losing nephropathy

33. Which of the following electrolytes is decreased in animals with hypoalbuminemia?
a. sodium
b. potassium
c. phosphate
d. calcium

34. An animal has metabolic acidosis. How does he compensate for this?
a. increased respiratory rate (hyperventilation)
b. decreased respiratory rate (hypoventilation)
c. increased urination
d. increased defecation

35. Which of the following is elevated in a hyperthyroid cat?
a. TSH
b. T_4
c. triglycerides
d. blood glucose

36. Which of the following tests should be performed in a dog with PU/PD, low specific gravity, normal blood glucose, and an elevated BUN?
a. vasopressin test
b. water deprivation test
c. gradual water deprivation test
d. none of the above

37. Which of the following tests is NOT needed to establish a diagnosis of portosystemic shunt disease?
a. bile acids
b. Cr
c. blood glucose
d. ammonia

38. A German shepherd presents with vomiting and large-volume stools. The cPLI is normal, the TLI is low, and the cobalamin and folate levels are both high. What is the problem?
a. pancreatic insufficiency
b. upper intestinal disease
c. lower intestinal disease
d. further testing is needed to diagnose this case

39. Which of the following is seen in a case of malabsorption of fats?
a. positive muscle fibers in the stool
b. positive on iodine staining of the stool
c. positive Sudan IV test (heated)
d. positive Sudan IV test (unheated)

40. A 10-year-old cat comes into the clinic for testing for diabetes. He has been on insulin therapy for one year and has been well maintained. He tends to get stressed with testing. His last evaluation was 3 months ago. Which of the following would be the best test to use?
   a. glucose curve with hospitalization
   b. fructosamine level
   c. glycosylated hemoglobin level
   d. insulin response test

41. An 8-year-old female spayed miniature schnauzer comes into the clinic with what appears to be a bladder infection (urinating all over the house). As an excellent technician, you recommend blood work and urinalysis to the client. The dog has a blood glucose of 220 mg/dl, elevated amylase and lipase, TNTC bacterial rods, and 10 WBC/hpf in the urine. Her urine glucose is +1. She has been diagnosed with diabetes mellitus. Which of the following is true?
   a. Her symptoms are inconsistent with diabetes mellitus.
   b. The next step in diagnostics is a vasopressin test.
   c. Pancreatitis is common in miniature schnauzers and may have caused the diabetes.
   d. The periodontal disease has nothing to do with the diabetes.

42. An 8-year-old black-and-tan coonhound presents for lethargy, depression, and subcutaneous edema. His PCV is 45%, BUN 8.5 mg/dl, Cr 1.0 mg/dl, TP 3.3 g/dl, albumin 1.3 g/dl, ALT 200 U/L, AST 100 U/L, Alk Phos 250 U/L, GGT 20 IU/L, cholesterol 116 mg/dl, calcium 10 mg/dl, phosphorus 5 mg/dl, sodium 150 mg/dl, potassium 5 mg/dl, chloride 100 mEq/L, bicarbonate 14 mEq/L (low). Urinalysis shows 2+ bilirubin and a specific gravity of 1.012. The edema is due to
   a. hyponatremia.
   b. hypocalcemia.
   c. hypoglobulinemia.
   d. hypoalbuminemia.

43. The dog in question 42 also has
   a. respiratory acidosis.
   b. respiratory alkalosis.
   c. metabolic acidosis.
   d. metabolic alkalosis.

44. A 6-year-old male cat presents on emergency. He is recumbent and semicomatose. His BUN is 125 mg/dl, Cr is 8 mg/dl, TP is 8 mg/dl, ALT 50 U/L, AST 35 U/L, Alk Phos 50 U/L, bicarbonate 27 mEq/L, total bilirubin is 0.2 mg/dl, calcium 10 mg/dl, chloride 130 mEq/L, cholesterol 150 mg/dl, CPK 400 U/L, glucose 80 mg/dl, potassium 7 mEq/L, sodium 159 mEq/L. Urine SG 1.050, protein 3$^+$, pH 8, TNTC RBC, occasional struvite crystals (cystocentesis sample). Which of the following is likely?
   a. This is prerenal azotemia due to liver failure.
   b. This is renal azotemia due to glomerular disease.
   c. This is renal azotemia due to renal tubular disease.
   d. This is postrenal azotemia due to obstruction.

45. A 5-year-old dog presents with polyuria and polydipsia of 4 weeks' duration. Which of the following is a differential for polyuria and polydipsia?
   a. diabetes insipidus
   b. liver failure
   c. psychogenic water drinking
   d. all of the above

46. A 10-month-old Yorkie puppy presents with abdominal distention, panting, and weight loss. The owners say he has been having a real problem with potty training and seems dull. His PCV is 43%, BUN 5.5 mg/dl, TP 5 g/dl, albumin 1.5 g/dl, ALT 23 U/L, Alk Phos 22 U/L, bile acids preprandial 13 μmol/L, postprandial 50 μmol/L, glucose 70 mg/dl, calcium 8.0 mg/dl, sodium 146 mEq/L, potassium 4.7 mEq/L, chloride 107 mEq/L. This puppy has
   a. cholestasis.
   b. hepatocellular abnormalities.
   c. azotemia.
   d. liver function abnormalities.

47. Which of this Yorkie's test abnormalities can be explained by his low albumin levels?
   a. BUN
   b. glucose
   c. calcium
   d. bile acids

48. Which hormone *decreases* blood calcium levels?
   a. insulin
   b. parathyroid hormone
   c. aldosterone
   d. calcitonin

49. Which of the following hormones increases gluconeogenesis?
   a. cortisol
   b. insulin
   c. glucagon
   d. aldosterone

50. Which of the following is *incorrect* for the parvovirus SNAP® test?
   a. It is a direct test.
   b. It is an agglutination test.
   c. It is an antigen test.
   d. It is an ELISA test.

Answers and Explanations

1. b. Blue-top tubes are used for PT and APTT. The gray-top tube with diatomaceous earth is used for ACT only. The lavender- and green-top tubes are not used for coagulation studies.

2. c. Calcium EDTA is the anticoagulant found in lavender-top tubes. Heparin is in green-top, sodium citrate is in blue-top, and calcium oxalate is in gray-top tubes.

3. a. Gray-top tubes contain sodium fluoride, which is the best for glucose studies since it stabilizes flucose in the plasma.

4. d. The green-top tube contains heparin.

5. a. The monolayer should be used to identify blood cell morphology. The feathered edge is used to identify large extracellular organisms and to analyze for platelet clumping. The body should not be used.

6. d. Gunther is severely anemic. The total protein is elevated, which may mean dehydration. If he is anemic in the face of dehydration, that means that his anemia would be even worse when he was hydrated.

7. a. She is anemic. Her $HGBest = \frac{PCV}{3} = \frac{14}{3} = 4.7$ g/dl, $MCV = PCV \times \frac{10}{RBC} = 14 \times \frac{10}{2.3} = 61$ fl which means normocytic. $MCH = HGB \times \frac{10}{RBC} = 4.7 \times \frac{10}{2.3} = 20.4$ pg. $MCHC = HGB \times \frac{100}{PCV} = 4.7 \times \frac{100}{14} = 33.6$ g/dl which is normochromic.

8. a. Basophilic stippling is common in lead poisoning. Heinz bodies are common with zinc, maple leaf, onion, and acetaminopen toxicity. Morula are seen with *Ehrlichia* infections, and autoimmune hemolytic anemia shows agglutination of red blood cells.

9. b. She will have polychromatophils on her Diff-Quick® stained slide because she has reticulocytes. She is not microcytic because her MCV is 42.5 fl. She does not have aplastic anemia because reticulocytes are being made by the bone marrow. This is not a strongly regenerative anemia.

10. c. This is a stress leukogram because the eosinophils and lymphocytes are low and there is a neutrophilia without significant bands. Cortisol decreases the numbers of lymphocytes and eosinophils present in the blood and increases the longevity of the neutrophils. An inflammatory leukogram will have increased bands, and a physiologic leukogram will have all white blood cells (WBCs) increased, not just the neutrophils.

11. a. The bone marrow is keeping up with the demand for neutrophils. There is still a mature neutrophilia, but the bands have increased. It has become an inflammatory leukogram.

12. b. Pink, intracytoplasmic inclusions may be seen with distemper virus infection in all blood cells and mucosal epithelia.

13. c. Elevated white blood cell counts with hypersegmented neutrophils and no bands are called a stress leukogram.

14. a. Nonregenerative anemia. There should be a 1:1 ratio of myeloid to erythroid cells and normal iron levels. Since the megakaryocytes are normal, it is not a thrombcytopenia; decreased hemosiderin means it is probably an iron deficiency anemia.

15. b. Renal failure would only influence the red blood cell line because erythropoietin only affects RBC formation. Estrogen and chemotherapy affect all cell lines, and some parasites (such as *Ehrlichia*) can affect all cell lines.

16. a. The dorsal ribs are the bone marrow collection site of choice in the cow. The sternum is the site of choice in the horse and the other two sites in the dog and cat.

17. b. The nucleus of the myeloid series stains pink/purple. The cytoplasm stains pale blue; granules are usually present within the cytoplasm; only the granulocytes are counted on bone marrow evaluation.

18. d. The megakaryocyte is the largest cell in the bone marrow and has multiple nuclei. Monocytes become macrophages when they mature and move into tissues. Megakaryocytes never leave the bone marrow.

19. b. The highest numbers of circulating lymphocytes are actually T cells. All lymphocytes live in the tissues for long periods of time. This allows animals to develop long-lasting immunity. B cells secrete immunoglobulins and are labeled in the bone marrow. T cells are involved with cellular immunity and are labeled in the thymus.

20. a. *Dipetalonema* is a nonpathogenic filariid parasite that is often confused with *Dirofilaria immitis*.

21. b. *Cytauxzoon* causes massive hemolytic anemia in the cat, which is almost always fatal. Its definitive host is the bobcat. There is no treatment. *Hemobartonella* is rarely confused with *Cytauxzoon*.

22. a. On a fine-needle aspirate, negative pressure should always be released prior to removing the needle. Touch preps should be performed before and after cleaning. The best method for obtaining a cytological sample from a moist lesion is touch prep. With grainy material, a larger syringe and needle are needed for FNA.

23. a. Neutrophils are often elevated in cases of immune mediated arthritis.

24. a. Viscosity is the ability of material to form a string. It is a measure of how gooey a substance is.

25. d. Condensed chromatin means that the nucleus is quiet and not dividing. Increased size of the nucleus, numbers of nucleoli, and mitotic figures all indicate rapid cell division.

26. c. Mesothelial cells will be seen in body cavity aspirates. Ciliated columnar epithelium is seen from the trachea, cuboidal epithelium from the bronchioles, and macrophages from the alveoli and bronchioles.

27. a. Romanowsky stains are alcohol based, which allows better penetration of the stain into the cytoplasm. They are very easy to use and fast.

28. a. Septic inflammatory exudate, because there were a lot of neutrophils, the total protein and cell count were elevated, and there were bacteria seen.

29. c. This is a chylous effusion. Pleural samples should be run for triglycerides and cholesterol. BUN and Cr should be run on abdominal fluid.

30. c. A deficiency of vWF is common in black and tan breeds. This is obviously a problem with the formation of the initial platelet plug (prolonged BMBT), but his platelet count was normal. It is not a problem with the clotting cascade because the PT and APTT were normal, so liver disease and vitamin K deficiency are ruled out. DIC is unlikely with a normal PT and APTT because thrombin formation is not affected.

31. d. FSPs are a good indicator of DIC. The other tests will also be affected, but FSP elevations are diagnostic.

32. a. Anemia will not cause hypoalbuminemia. Protein losing enteropathy and nephropathy will cause decreased albumin due to leakage, and liver failure will cause decreased albumin manufacture.

33. d. Calcium is carried on the albumin molecule. The most common cause of calcium decreases on serum testing is hypoalbuminemia.

34. a. Increasing the respiratory rate will decrease the CO_2 levels in the blood and make the animal more alkalotic.

35. b. The T_4 levels will be elevated in hyperthyroidism. The TSH levels should be decreased as should the triglycerides.

36. d. None of the above. Azotemic animals should not have any water deprivation tests because these will make the situation worse.

37. b. Cr has nothing to do with liver function. Bile acids and ammonia are primary liver function tests and blood glucose is a secondary liver function test.

38. a. This is probably EPI. CPLI works best when diagnosing pancreatitis. TLI is the best indicator of EPI.

39. c. Positive Sudan IV test (heated) is a test of the ability of the body to absorb free fatty acids. The unheated test tests the ability of the body to break down whole fats. Iodine tests for the presence of amylase (sugar) and the muscle fibers tests the ability of the body to break down proteins (trypsin).

40. c. Glycosylated hemoglobin level is a test for control of glucose over a 3-month period. Fructosamine only tests for a few weeks. The glucose curve would cause undue stress to the cat. Glycosylated hemoglobin and fructosamine are not affected by stress-induced hyperglycemia.

41. c. Pancreatitis can lead to diabetes. Her symptoms are consistent with diabetes mellitus. Vasopressin testing is unwarranted in this case. Periodontal disease can lead to pancreatitis but could also be caused by the hyperglycemia.

42. d. Hypoalbuminemia often leads to edema because of a loss of oncotic pressure, which holds the water in the vasculature. In this case, it is probably due to liver disease.

43. c. Metabolic acidosis.

44. d. Both the Cr and the BUN are elevated together (the BUN:Cr ratio is 15), the liver values are WNL (within normal limits), the urine SG is normal for a cat, so renal azotemia is unlikely.

45. d. All of the answers will cause polyuria and polydipsia. The first step is a urinalysis and blood chemistry.

46. d. This is probably portosystemic shunt disease. The BUN is low, indicating failure to form urea from ammonia; the blood glucose and albumin are low, indicating failure to process glucose or manufacture proteins; and the postprandial bile acids are high. Since all liver enzymes are low, a probable bypass of the portal circulation is occurring.

47. c. His calcium is low because he is hypoalbuminemic. Albumin is the calcium carrier in the blood.

48. d. Calcitonin decreases blood calcium by increasing the deposition of calcium in the bones. Parathyroid hormone increases blood calcium by increasing osteoclast activity (bone reabsorption) and increasing the amount of calcium coming across the intestinal mucosa. Insulin and aldosterone have no effect on blood calcium.

49. c. Glucagon increases blood sugar by increasing gluconeogenesis and glycogenolysis. Cortisol increases glycogenolysis only, insulin decreases glucose by increasing cellular uptake, and aldosterone does not affect glucose levels.

50. b. The parvovirus SNAP® test is a direct ELISA test because it tests for the presence of antigen by adsorbing the antibodies onto an immunosorbent paper and looking for serum antigen to bind. Examples of agglutination tests are the Coggins and Coombs tests.

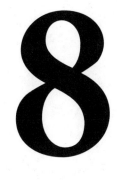

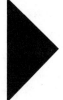

LABORATORY PROCEDURES PART 2

CHAPTER OVERVIEW

Laboratory procedures is such a significant topic and so central to any veterinary practice that we were forced to divide it into two chapters. Chapter 7 covered blood issues and testing as well as cell structure and function and allied subjects. This chapter discusses the second half of lab work, namely parasitology, urinalysis, and microbiology.

U rinalysis is one of the most common ways of discovering disease processes in different organs. These tests are simple and easy to perform and inexpensive, which is why urine testing is one of the mainstays of any veterinary practice.

Key Terms

alpha hemolysis
arachnid
bacillus
beta hemolysis

cast

cestode

definitive host

differentiating medium

ectoparasite

endoparasite

facultative parasite

gram-negative

gram-positive

hemoglobinuria

hydatid cyst

intermediate host

isosthenuria

larva

microfilaria

myiasis

nematode

nit

obligate parasite

ovum

parasite

paratenic host

proglottids

protozoa

pupa

renal epithelial cell

selective media

specific gravity

spirochete

squamous epithelium

supernatant

symbiote

transitional epithelial cell

trematode

turbidity

urine sediment

vector

zone of inhibition

Concepts and Skills

This chapter will include questions that focus on the second part of laboratory procedures, covering three primary concepts:

- parasitology
- urinalysis
- microbiology

Parasitology

Parasite infestation is one of the top causes of disease in animals. From fleas to nematodes, parasites are responsible for symptoms ranging from itching to anemia, to death. Diagnosis and treatment of parasites will benefit the animal and the community. Knowledge of life cycles will allow better environmental control of parasites and prevent reinfection. Parasites are divided into those that live outside the body (ectoparasites) and those that occur inside the body (endoparasites).

Ectoparasites

Ectoparasites are the parasitic insects and **arachnids** that live outside the body and infect the host organism on its surface. These two classes of animals are the largest in the animal kingdom. They are invertebrates, having chitinous (hard) exoskeletons and jointed bodies. Insects and arachnids may fill several categories in parasitic diseases, including acting as the parasite, the vector (the animal carrier that transfers a parasite from one host to another), the intermediate host (the animal in which the asexual stage of the parasite occurs), and the definitive host (the animal in which the sexual stage of the parasite occurs). Insect parasites include flies, fleas, and lice. Arachnid parasites include mites and ticks.

Flies

The order Diptera contains the flies with wings. In some flies only the female takes a blood meal in order to complete its life cycle and lay eggs. Others require an animal host to complete the larval phase of development (**obligate parasites**) and still others will only infect an animal that has a break in the skin (**facultative parasites**). Flies that complete their larval phase in the host animal are called myiasis producers. Flies that require a blood meal to make eggs may act as vectors and carry diseases to the animal. In general, flies may be treated with topical insecticides and repellents.

Myiasis Producers

Myiasis producers are the flies that complete their larval phase within the host. This group includes the only reportable insect (*Cochliomyia hominivorax*), as well as facultative parasites and obligate parasites. The government (either state or national) requires that certain diseases be reported in order to protect the food supply. These are called reportable diseases.

Obligate Myiasis Producers

These are the flies that require a mammalian host for the larval stage of development (see Figure 8.1). The life cycle is as follows.

The adult fly lays eggs on the animal's coat where the larva hatches and burrows into the skin

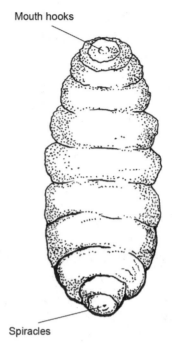

Mouth hooks

Spiracles

Figure 8.1 *Third Stage Bot Fly Larva*

or the oral mucosa; the larva then migrates to the infectious site (this varies with the species of fly) and continues to develop until the fourth shed (instar stage) when it drops from the animal or is excreted through the feces as a pupa. The adult emerges from the pupal stage and begins the life cycle again. Prevention of myiasis by the use of insect repellents and grooming as well as topical insecticides may be helpful.

OBLIGATE MYIASIS PRODUCERS				
SPECIES	**APPEARANCE**	**SITE OF INFECTION (LARVA)**	**SITE OF EGG LAYING**	**REPORTABLE?**
Cochliomyia hominivorax (primary screwworm)	red head and eyes (looks similar to housefly)	skin and deeper tissues of cattle	intact skin (burrow into other tissues)	yes
Cuterebra (rodent fly)	large and bee-like	skin epidermis of any mammal species; most common in rabbits and rodents	intact skin (maggot stays where it is laid)	no
Gasterophilus (bot fly)	very small fly	mouth, pharynx, and esophagus of horses	on hair on the backs of the forelegs of the horse	no
Hypoderma (warbles)	fly looks like a honeybee	subcutaneous tissues of cattle (migrates through the tissues to get to the skin)	superficial skin	no

Some flies, such as *Cuterebra* and *Hypoderma*, invade the upper layer of the skin, forming a cyst with a breathing pore. When it has completed its molt, the pore enlarges and the maggot falls to the ground and pupates. Maggots may be removed by enlarging the breathing pore and removing the **larva** with forceps. Care should be taken to avoid crushing the larva to prevent anaphylaxis of the patient.

These fly species generally complete their life cycle in decaying matter, including fecal material and carcasses. They only cause infestation in animals with an open wound and generally will not complete their life cycle on the animal. Problems associated with facultative myiasis are usually from the secondary bacterial infections and toxicity reactions associated with maggot debris. Symptoms can include shock, fever, renal failure, and death.

FACULTATIVE MYIASIS PRODUCERS				
SPECIES	APPEARANCE	SITE OF INFECTION	SITE OF EGG LAYING	VECTOR
Calliphora vomitoria (blue bottle fly)	shiny blue or green body, hairy legs	open, suppurating wound	open, suppurating wound	
Musca domesticus (house fly)	black, hairy body, red eyes, black face	open, infected wound, also act as irritants	open, infected wound	*Habronema, Thelazia, Moraxella bovis*

Vectors

Vectors are the carriers of parastics, for example, the biting insects. They can also be grouped into two categories depending on whether only the adult female or both sexes take a blood meal. There are two types of vectors: mechanical and biological. Mechanical vectors transmit the parasite to the host without its developing in the carrier. Biological vectors actually serve as intermediate hosts and the parasite has part of its life cycle within the vector.

VECTORS					
GENUS/ SPECIES	APPEARANCE	EGG-LAYING ENVIRONMENT	FEMALE (F) OR BOTH (B) PARASITIC	DISEASES INFLICTED BY THE FLY	VECTOR BIOLOGICAL (B) OR MECHANICAL (M)
Lutzomyia (sand fly)	hairy wings, mothlike appearance	burrows in the sand, Gulf Coast beaches	F—feed after dusk	powerful bite; pruritis and inflammation	(B) *Leishmania* in dogs and humans (B) *Trypanosoma* in all species
Simulium (black fly)	tiny, black	swiftly moving streams and rivers	F—feed in the morning	powerful bite, may cause stampedes, hypersensitivity, and anaphylaxis	(B) *Leukocytozoon* in birds (B) *Onchocerciasis* in horses

(continued)

					VECTORS (continued)			

GENUS/ SPECIES	APPEARANCE	EGG-LAYING ENVIRONMENT	FEMALE (F) OR BOTH (B) PARASITIC	DISEASES INFLICTED BY THE FLY	VECTOR BIOLOGICAL (B) OR MECHANICAL (M)
Stomoxys (stable fly)	resembles *Musca domesticus*	feces near stagnant water	F	irritation and biting (has lancet-type mouthparts, laps up blood)	(B) *Habronema* in cattle
Tabanus and *Chrysops* (horse flies)	very large flies with brown bodies and green or brown eyes	feces	F—feed during the day	discomfort and agitation so severe that animals will not be able to graze; decreased milk production and weight loss; wounds tend to bleed after the fly finishes feeding, so other flies congregate	(M) *Anaplasma* (cattle) (M) anthrax (M) tularemia (M) equine infectious anemia (EIA) (B) *Trypanosoma*
Culex anopheles (mosquitoes)	thin, long-legged flies with hunched backs	stagnant water (puddles)	F—feed at dawn and dusk	discomfort, agitation, hypersensitivity, anemia	(M) equine encephalitis (viral) (M) West Nile (viral) (M) myxomatosis in rabbits (M) fowl pox (viral) (B) Dirofilaria immitis definitive host for *Plasmodium* (malaria)
Culicoides (biting gnats, no-see-ums)	tiny gnats with brown or tan bodies	fresh or salt water, depending on species	F—feed at dawn or dusk	severe pruritis, hypersensitivity (summer itch in horses)	(M) bluetongue in cattle (M) African horse sickness (B) onchocerciasis in horses (B) *Haemoproteus* in birds (B) *Leucocytozoon* in birds

Lice

Lice are host-specific insect parasites that spend their entire life cycle on the host (see Figure 8.2). There are two basic types of lice: Anoplura and Mallophaga. Lice produce a characteristic egg, called a **nit**, that is cemented onto the hair of the animal. It is extremely difficult to remove and resistant to insecticides. Treat-ment may take several weeks in order to kill all phases of the life cycle. The nymph and adult forms are easily killed with insecticides including fipronil, pyrethrins, and permethrins.

All lice have the same life cycle:

egg/nit > nymph > adult

LICE				
GENUS/SPECIES	APPEARANCE	DISEASE CAUSED BY PARASITE	VECTORS (B) BIOLOGICAL (M) MECHANICAL	OTHER FACTS
Anoplura (sucking lice)	head narrower than thorax, grey to black in color	blood suckers: anemia and death	(B) and (M) for many blood-borne parasites and pathogens	
Mallophaga (chewing lice)	head wider than thorax, brown to yellow in color	eat skin debris: severe pruritis (no anemia)	(B) the dog louse serves as an intermediate host for *Diplydium caninum*	all bird lice belong to this group

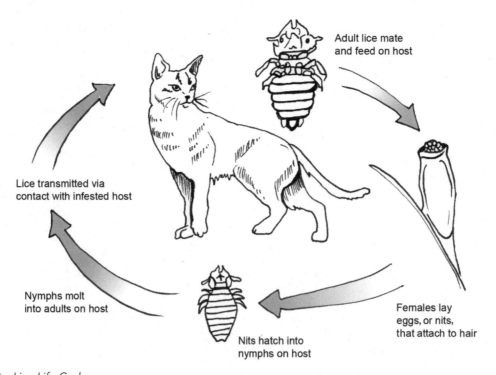

Adult lice mate and feed on host

Lice transmitted via contact with infested host

Nymphs molt into adults on host

Nits hatch into nymphs on host

Females lay eggs, or nits, that attach to hair

Figure 8.2 *Lice Life Cycle*

Fleas

Fleas are wingless insects with a laterally flattened body. Both males and females feed on blood. They have a complex life cycle including free-living larval forms and a pupal form that is extremely resistant to insecticides and may remain patent in the environment for months (see Figure 8.3). Fleas can cause hypersensitivity reactions in many species (flea allergic dermatitis). Fleas also act as efficient arthropod vectors for plague (*Yersinia pestis*), *Rickettsia typhi* of mice, myxomatosis of rabbits, and feline panleukopenia. They also may act as intermediate hosts for *Diplydium caninum* (flea tapeworm) and *Dipetalonema reconditum* (a filarial worm whose microfilariae are often mistaken for *Dirofilaria immitis* (heartworm).

It is important to understand the flea life cycle because it is key to flea control. The egg of the flea is laid on the coat of the animal and may either stay on the host or be dropped into the environment. The egg hatches into a larva that feeds on skin debris and flea feces/flea dirt (digested blood) in the environment. After molting twice, the L_3 larva then forms a cocoon and becomes a pupa. The pupa may remain in this form for a few months waiting for the correct stimulus (vibration and heat). It hatches into the adult form, which is parasitic. Flea control is geared toward controlling the larvae and the adults with insecticides or dehydrating products. Adults can live up to two months without food.

The flea life cycle is as follows:

egg > larvae > pupa > adult

Flea control products such as fipronil (affects the neurotransmitter GABA) and imidacloprid (affects acetylcholinesterase) kill adult fleas. Lufenuron and methoprene prevent development of the larvae. Organophosphates, pyrethrins, and permethrins cause seizures and death of the adult flea. All adulticides have the potential for toxicity in mammals. Organophosphates have been replaced with the second and third generation flea control products because of the more selective toxicities. Permethrins are highly toxic to cats and fipronil is highly toxic to rabbits, so care should be taken with selection of insecticides. Appropriate personal protective equipment (PPE) must be worn when applying insecticides because of the potential for human toxicity reactions.

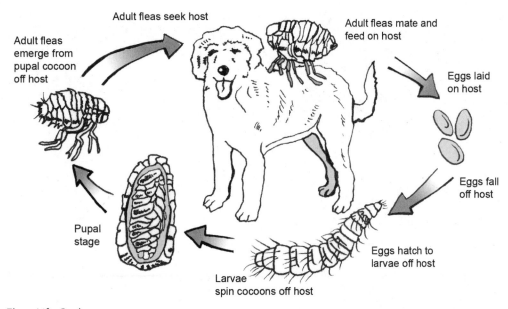

Adult fleas seek host

Adult fleas emerge from pupal cocoon off host

Adult fleas mate and feed on host

Eggs laid on host

Eggs fall off host

Pupal stage

Larvae spin cocoons off host

Eggs hatch to larvae off host

Figure 8.3 *Fleas Life Cycle*

FLEAS		
GENUS/SPECIES	PREFERRED HOST	VECTOR
Ctenocephalides felis (cat flea)	dog, but will feed on any warm-blooded animal if dogs are not available	(B) *Diplydium caninum* (B) *Dipetalonema reconditum*
Ctenocephalides canis (dog flea)	dog, relatively rare, will feed on any warm-blooded animal if dogs are not available	(B) *Diplydium caninum* (B) *Dipetalonema reconditum*
Echidnophaga (sticktight flea)	birds, will feed on any warm-blooded host	
Xenopsylla and *Pulex*	rodents and humans, but will feed on any warm-blooded host	(B) *Yersinia pestis* (bubonic plague)

Miscellaneous Insects

There are several insects parasites that are associated with various diseases but do not have a great deal in common; they are merely grouped together for convenience.

MISCELLANEOUS INSECTS				
GENUS/SPECIES	APPEARANCE	DISEASES CAUSED BY INSECT	VECTOR	INTERMEDIATE HOSTS
Hippoboscids (keds)	look like lice, may have rudimentary wings	anemia (spend entire life cycle on the host like lice)	(B) trypanosomes in sheep	no
Reduviid bugs	large, winged insects with cone-shaped beaks	anemia (feed on blood at night)	(B) trypanosomes of animals and humans (Chaga's disease) (M) equine encephalomyelitis	no
Cockroaches	flattened dorsoventral body, large wings	no	no	*Hymenolepis* (rodent tapeworm—zoonotic) *Spirura, oxyspirura, gongylonema*
Beetles	flattened dorsoventral body, hard shell	some species contain cantharadin, which causes blisters in the mouth and GI tract of herbivores, which can lead to death	no	hymenolepis (rodent tapeworm—zoonotic) *Physaloptera* (cause of stomach granulomas in cats and dogs), *Oxyspirura, Gongylonema*

Mites

Mites are arachnids. All mites are parasitic but not all cause disease. Generally, their entire life cycle is spent on the host (see Figure 8.4). Mites are usually identified by their body type as either sarcoptoid (round) or miscellaneous (other shapes) and by their pedicles which may be long, short, jointed, or ornamented.

Sarcoptoid Mites

Sarcoptoid (scabies) mites have round bodies and defined pedicles. They generally burrow into the skin and cause severe pruritis, hyperkeratosis, edema, and lichenification. Some animals can actually die from the stress of infestation. Some sarcoptoid mites are zoonotic; in other words, they can transmit diseases from animals to humans. Diagnosis of mites is based on deep skin scrapes in multiple sites for microscopic exam. A negative test does not necessarily mean a negative diagnosis. Treatment for sarcoptoid mites is generally two doses of ivermectin/avermectin 2 weeks apart.

Miscellaneous Mites

These mites have different body types than the sarcoptoid mites and include *Demodex canis* and *Demodex cati/gatoi* and *chyletiella*.

Demodex mites are all host-specific (they only infect one species) and are a normal part of the body fauna in all species. Demodecosis is commonly seen in animals at the time of teething and vaccination, although old dogs with systemic illness (cancer, hyperadrenocorticism, diabetes mellitus, etc.) may also

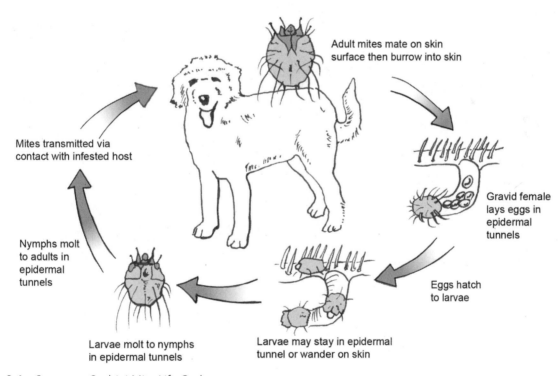

Figure 8.4 *Sarcoptes Scabiei Mite Life Cycle*

Adult mites mate on skin surface then burrow into skin

Gravid female lays eggs in epidermal tunnels

Eggs hatch to larvae

Larvae may stay in epidermal tunnel or wander on skin

Larvae molt to nymphs in epidermal tunnels

Nymphs molt to adults in epidermal tunnels

Mites transmitted via contact with infested host

develop mange. The puppy or kitten receives the demodectic mite from the dam and lesions usually begin on the face, progress and fade over time. *Demodex* mites live in the hair follicles. (See Figure 8.5.)

SARCOPTOID MITES				
GENUS/SPECIES	**SPECIES AFFECTED**	**SYMPTOMS**	**DIAGNOSIS**	**TREATMENT**
Cnemidocoptes (scaly leg mite)	birds	severe pruritis, hyperkeratosis on the legs, face, and anus	skin scraping	ivermectin 2 doses 2 weeks apart
Notoedres (cat scabies)	cats (zoonotic)	severe pruritis, miliary dermatitis of face and neck	skin scraping	ivermectin 2 doses, 2 weeks apart, or weekly Lym Dip
Psoroptes ovis Chorioptes	cattle, horse, sheep	wool damage, pruritis, alopecia	skin scraping	ivermectin or insecticide spray
Psoroptes cuniculi (rabbit scabies)	rabbit (zoonotic)	severe pruritis, hyperkeratosis		ivermectin, Lym Dip
Sarcoptes (scabies) several species	multiple species (zoonotic)	severe pruritis, hyperkeratosis, edema	skin scraping	same as above
Otodectes cynotis (ear mite)	dog and cat	pruritis of ears, coffee-ground discharge in ears, may cause miliary dermatitis of face and neck in cats	microscopic examination of ear discharge with mineral oil	treat with topical avermectin; all animals in environment should be treated simultaneously
Pneumonyssus (lung mite)	macaques	coughing; lesions may be confused with tuberculosis on radiographs	tracheal wash	ivermectin
Pneumonyssoides (nasal mite)	dogs	chronic sneezing, nasal discharge, epistaxis	nasal flush	
Sternostoma (tracheal mite)	birds	coughing	transillumination of trachea	ivermectin

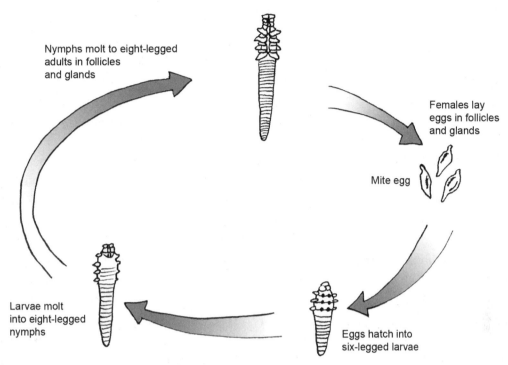

Nymphs molt to eight-legged adults in follicles and glands

Females lay eggs in follicles and glands

Mite egg

Eggs hatch into six-legged larvae

Larvae molt into eight-legged nymphs

Figure 8.5 *Demodex Canis Mite Life Cycle*

MISCELLANEOUS MITES				
GENUS/SPECIES	**SPECIES AFFECTED**	**SYMPTOMS**	**DIAGNOSIS**	**TREATMENT**
Demodex canis (red mange)	dog	alopecia and secondary pyoderma/folliculitis in immunocompromised animals or at puberty; generally not pruritic, usually self-limiting, generalized cases must be treated aggressively	multiple deep skin scrapings; see long, cigar-shaped mites with 8 legs	amitraz dips weekly until 2 negative skin scrapes (no live or dead mites are seen); minimum 6 weeks of treatment; ivermectin or selamectin daily may also be effective
Demodex cati *Demodex gatoi*	cat	intense pruritis, skin lesions (miliary dermatitis)	multiple deep skin scrapings; mites are shorter and stouter than *Demodex canis* mites	ivermectin 2 doses 2 weeks apart (similar to scabies treatment)
Chyletiella (walking dandruff)	rabbit, although any mammal may be affected	increased scale, moderate pruritis, greasy coat, may be asymptomatic	superficial skin scraping; mites have very large mouthparts and saddle-shaped backs	topical insecticides (fipronil, imidacloprid, pyrethrins)

Ticks

Ticks are arachnids, and all species are parasitic. Ticks are vectors for a wide range of diseases including parasitic, bacterial, and viral diseases. Certain ticks may also be responsible for toxicity reactions resulting in paralysis of the host animal. This usually occurs in ticks from the genus *Dermacentor*. Gravid (pregnant) female ticks secrete a neurotoxin in their saliva that will cause neuromuscular blockade (paralysis). Treatment is removal of the gravid female from the animal. Complete recovery is usually within 48 hours.

Tick identification may lead to diagnosis of specific diseases prior to obtaining laboratory results. The best treatment for ticks is prevention. Some tick-borne diseases require 24 to 48 hours of feeding time in order to be transmitted; some require less. Amitraz collars will cause paralysis of the tick and prevent feeding in most cases. Fipronil will cause death of ticks, but will not cause the tick to release from the host prior to transmission of disease-causing organisms. Permethrins will also kill ticks, but must not be used on cats. Most tick-borne diseases are rickettsial organisms that can be treated with tetracycline/doxycycline antibiotics. Ticks are not host specific, and humans can become infested with ticks. Humans are susceptible to most tick-borne diseases, so control of ticks is necessary to prevent human disease. All stages of the life cycle are parasitic. Ticks only eat once per life stage. A blood meal is required for molting to next stage. (See Figure 8.6.)

In the *Amblyomma*, *Ixodes*, and *Dermacentor* species life cycle, the ticks are on different animals for each life stage. This makes it difficult to eradicate infestations because the larval/nymph stages are in the environment rather than on one host. Rhipicephalus also falls into this category because it also drops off the host between feedings, although it only attacks dogs and, occasionally, humans. These ticks may all act as transstadial vectors, which means that the organisms that they carry will be transmitted between the various life stages of the tick. *Boophilus* is a one-host tick of cattle which means it spends all of its time on the same host. Disease is transmitted from the adult to the nymph via transovarian transmission.

Tick life cycle:

egg > first stage nymph attaches to small mammal/bird/reptile > second stage nymph another small mammal or definitive host > adult on definitive host

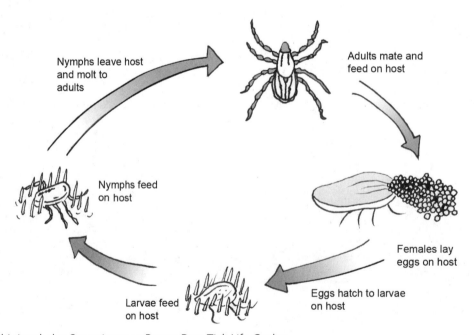

Nymphs leave host and molt to adults

Adults mate and feed on host

Nymphs feed on host

Females lay eggs on host

Larvae feed on host

Eggs hatch to larvae on host

Figure 8.6 *Rhipicephalus Sanguineus or Brown Dog Tick Life Cycles*

		TICKS		
GENUS/SPECIES	**PREFERRED HOST FOR ADULT**	**INTERMEDIATE HOST**	**VECTOR**	**TICK PARALYSIS (Y/N) AND OTHER DISEASES?**
Ixodes	white-tailed deer; may feed on other hosts including humans, dogs, and cats	white-footed mouse and other small rodents	(B) *Borrelia burgdorferi*—Lyme disease (humans and dogs) (B) *Babesia microti*—microtinic piroplasmosis (cattle) (B) *Anaplasma phagocytophilum* (horses)	**no** Lyme disease is zoonotic organisms are not found on blood smears (tissue infection); acute phase is 2 to 6 months; *Babesia microti* and *Anaplasma phagocytophilum* are also zoonotic; *Babesia* may be seen on RBCs, *Anaplasma* may be seen on neutrophils
Rhipicephalus sanguineus (brown dog tick)	dog, cattle (common in veterinary and kennel facilities), will also infect humans	dogs	(B) *Babesia canis* (canine piroplasmosis) (B) *Ehrlichia canis* (tropical canine pancytopenia) (B) *Babesia bigemina* (bovine piroplasmosis) (B) *Theileria parva* (East Coast fever of cattle—Africa)	**no** *Babesia canis* is common in racing greyhounds *Babesia bigemina* is one of the highest causes of bovine production losses; *Ehrlichia canis* is very common and can cause mortality
Boophilus	cattle only (one-host tick)	cattle	(B) *Babesia bigemina* (bovine piroplasmosis)	see above
Dermacentor	not host specific, but	any warm-blooded animal, usually small rodents		**yes** *D. albipictus* can cause increased winter mortality in cervid species such as deer, elk, and moose by causing hair loss prior to the onset of the snowy season. The animals waste so much energy keeping warm that they are unable to meet their energy demand and die before spring
D. variabilis	dog (American dog tick)		(M) Rocky Mountain spotted fever (B) *Francisella tularensis* (tularemia)	
D. andersoni	dog and rodents (Rocky Mountain wood tick)		same as *D. variabilis* plus Colorado tick fever and Q fever	
D. nitens	horse (tropical horse tick)		(B) *Babesia caballi* (equine piroplasmosis)	
D. albipictus	deer and elk (winter tick)			
Amblyomma	many species	many species	Rocky Mountain spotted fever, Q fever, tularemia, *Cowdria ruminatum* (heartwater), blood parasites of reptiles and amphibians	**yes**

Endoparasites

As the name implies, **endoparasites** are parasites that occur within the body, such as in the internal organs. They contain a huge number and diversity of different families, genera, and species varying from single-celled organisms such as protozoa to complex species such as worms. They can (and do) infect hosts internally, affecting every system in the body. Endoparasitism is responsible for huge direct economic losses to farmers, threats to the food supply, and zoonotic disease in humans (especially in low-income areas and Third World countries due to lack of health care and hygiene).

Types of Endoparasites

Endoparasites may be divided into two groups: the protozoa (single-celled organisms) and the helminths (various types of worms or wormlike organisms).

Protozoa

Protozoa are single-celled eukaryotic (have a true nucleus) organisms that may or may not be motile, may or may not have a complex life cycle, and may or may not be zoonotic. Some are transmitted directly and some use intermediate hosts.

Sporozoa are also called apicomplexans. They have a complicated life cycle that includes sexual and asexual stages. Apicomplexans include the coccidians and the hemosporidians.

Enteric coccidia live in the gastrointestinal system and include the genera *Isospora* and *Eimeria*. In general, these species tend to be relatively host spe-

cific and may or may not cause symptoms. Disease usually affects the GI tract, causing chronic diarrhea (scours), but may infect the nervous system in some animals. Treatment of these species is by the use of coccidiostats (antibiotics that control replication) such as sulfa drugs and monensin.

The life cycle of the coccidians is as follows:

Sporulated oocyst ingested by host (either definitive or intermediate host) > hatch into a sporozoite > enter a cell to form a trophozoite > mature into a schizont/meront > asexual fission > multiple merozoites > burst the host cell > invade new cells as schizonts/meronts > develop into a male or female gametocyte > undergoes repeated nuclear division to form microgametes which fertilize a macrogamete to form a zygote (this only happens in the definitive host) > zygote encysts to form an oocyst > host cell ruptures > oocyst is released from the body > fission occurs to form a sporulated oocyst containing sporozoites

Diagnosis is based on clinical signs or seeing sporulated or unsporulated oocysts on the flotation of the feces of the definitive host. Histologic examination of infected tissues may also be helpful in diagnosis. PCR may be available. Toxoplasma and cryptosporidium have very small oocysts. It may be beneficial to stain cryptosporidium oocysts with acid-fast stain prior to microscopic exam.

SPECIES/GENUS	DEFINITIVE HOST	SYMPTOMS IN DEFINITIVE HOST	INTERMEDIATE HOST	SYMPTOMS IN INTERMEDIATE HOST	DIAGNOSIS (DX) TREATMENT (TX)
COCCIDIANS					
Sarcocystis	carnivore	asymptomatic	herbivore	neurological disease	(Tx) Pyrimethamine with
Sarcocystis neurona	canine	asymptomatic	equine	equine protozoal myelitis	Trimethoprim/Sulfadiazine (neurological damage may be permanent)

(continued)

		COCCIDIANS (continued)			
SPECIES/ GENUS	DEFINITIVE HOST	SYMPTOMS IN DEFINITIVE HOST	INTERMEDIATE HOST	SYMPTOMS IN INTERMEDIATE HOST	DIAGNOSIS (DX) TREATMENT (TX)
Toxoplasma gondii	feline	asymptomatic or mild fever for 3 to 4 days	multiple species, including humans	myalgia, lymphadenopathy, flu-like symptoms; infection during pregnancy can cause mental retardation, malformation, abortion, and death of the fetus	(Dx) if serum titers are present, the intermediate host will be resistant to the infection (Tx) clindamycin in the definitive host is curative
Neospora caninum	canine (can be transmitted transplacentally without an intermediate host)	neurologic and hepatic disease in adult dogs, polyradiculoneuritis in puppies (paralysis)	cattle	abortions	none
Cryptosporidium	multiple species; cattle are commonly affected	severe diarrhea, kidney, and/or liver damage	multiple species	severe diarrhea, kidney and/or liver damage	none; the entire life cycle takes place in the intestines

Hemosporidia. These sporozoan parasites enter the body through arthropod vectors (such as insects) and can be very difficult to treat.

Malarial Hemosporidia. These parasites invade the red blood cell and while some species are relatively nonpathogenic, they may be easily confused with pathogenic forms on blood smears.

Their life cycle is as follows:

Sporozoites enter via blood meal from arthropod vector > enter somatic cells (usually the liver) and become trophozoites (schizogony) in the definitive host > merozoites are formed by asexual fission > hepatocyte ruptures and merozoites enter the red blood cells and undergo asexual fission again (schizogony) > develop into micro and macrogametes which invade another mosquito (this only happens in the definitive host) > fuse to form a zygote > form a motile ookinete which invades the mosquito's gut > develop into an oocyst > oocyst ruptures and sporozoites are released which infect the arthropod vector's salivary glands.

MALARIAL HEMOSPORIDIA				
GENUS/SPECIES	**INTERMEDIATE HOST**	**DEFINITIVE HOST**	**SYMPTOMS**	**DX**
Plasmodium (malaria)	Mosquitoes (*Anopheles* and *Culex spp.*)	primates (including man), birds, and reptiles	cyclical fever (associated with RBC rupture due to schizogony), fatalities with brain infection; release of hemoglobin from ruptured RBCs causes renal failure	visualization of small, round basophilic organisms in the red blood cells (Wright's Giemsa stain)
Haemoproteus	biting gnats, horseflies	birds, reptiles	nonpathogenic	horseshoe-shaped, basophilic, cytoplasmic inclusions that do not displace the nucleus of the RBC
Leucocytozoon	*Simulium* (black flies)	birds	intravascular hemolysis, acute death	inclusions completely occupy the cell and cause displacement of the nucleus and bizarre cell shapes in WBC and RBC
Hepatocystis	*Culicoides* (gnats)	lower primates, rodents	liver abnormalities	
Hepatozoon canis	*Rhipicephalus* tick (via ingestion, not bite)	dog	subclinical in US, chronic GI disease overseas	intracytoplasmic inclusions in WBC
Hepatozoon americanum	ingestion of *Rhipicephalus*	dog	neutrophilic leukocytosis, joint pain, myositis	muscle biopsy with intracytoplasmic inclusions

Piroplasms. These diseases are red blood cell parasites that are carried by ticks. In large animals, anemia and hemoglobinuria are usually the cause of illness and death; in small animals, organisms released in large numbers may cause pulmonary vessel occlusion and death. No effective treatment regimens are approved in the United States, but imidocarb may be effective for *Babesia*.

		PIROPLASMS		
GENUS/SPECIES	**INTERMEDIATE HOST**	**DEFINITIVE HOST**	**SYMPTOMS**	**DX/TX**
Cytauxzoon felis	*Dermacentor* tick	bobcat, feline	subclinical in bobcat; in domestic cats, high fever, anemia, icterus, dehydration; usually fatal	signet ring appearance of intracytoplasmic inclusion in the RBC
Babesia bigemina (bovine piroplasmosis)	*Boophilus* tick	cattle	acute disease: fever, hemoglobinuria, anemia, icterus, splenomegaly; can cause death	paired trophozoites in cytoplasm of RBC; titers
Babesia canis/ Babesia gibsonii (canine piroplasmosis)	all ticks	dogs (especially greyhounds)		
Babesia caballi/ Babesia equi (equine piroplasmosis)	all ticks	horses		
Babesia ovis	all ticks	sheep		
Babesia trautmanii	all ticks	swine		
Theileria (East Coast fever)	*Rhipicephalus* ticks	cattle	dyspnea, emaciation, weakness, melena, high mortality	trophozoites in all blood cells including lymphocytes

Ciliates. Ciliates are protozoal organisms with tiny hairlike projections that allow motility. The only pathogenic form is *Balantidium coli*. This organism has a fairly simple life cycle and is nonpathogenic in its definitive host, the pig, but may cause disease in infected humans (diarrhea, tenesmus/straining, colitis symptoms). Diagnosis is by visualization of trophozoites on a direct smear or by fecal flotation to visualize the large cysts.

The direct lifecycle is as follows:

Cyst is ingested by host > trophozoite hatches in large intestine > encysts and is passed in stool

Flagellates. Flagellates are protozoa with whip-like appendages called flagella in the trophozoite form that are used for movement. There are several parasitic forms that invade various tissues and have differing life cycles.

Mucosal Flagellates. These protozoa all attach to mucosal surfaces where they cause disease. They can include organisms spread by venereal (sexual) transmission or fecal-oral transmission. There are some species of nonpathogenic mucosal flagellates that may be confused with disease-causing forms. Care must be taken to identify the species correctly.

Giardia. Giardia is a zoonotic flagellate parasite of the small intestine. It can be subclinical or cause severe enteritis and diarrhea. Cysts containing two trophozoites are passed in feces and may contaminate the water supply. Cyst shedding may be intermittent. This is a direct life cycle with fecal oral contamination (cysts in feces > water or directly eaten > hatch into trophozoites in the small intestine > encyst). Diagnosis is based on seeing the pear-shaped, motile trophozoites on direct smear or seeing the oval cyst on flotation with zinc sulfate solution. Sheather's solution flotation will rupture the cysts and sodium nitrate will distort them and may not have a high enough specific gravity to float the cysts adequately (see section on Parasite Testing). ELISA is also an effective method of diagnosis with high sensitivity and specificity (few false positives and false negatives). See section on Immunology and Serology.

Trichomonads. Trichomonads include a number of different pathogenic species. They are named by the number of flagella in the trophozoites (*Tritrichomonas*, *Tetratrichomonas*, etc.). These species do not form cysts and are diagnosed by direct smear.

GENUS/SPECIES	INTERMEDIATE HOST	DEFINITIVE HOST	DISEASE	DX/PREVENTION/ TX
Tritrichomonas foetus	none	cattle, also affects cats	venereal disease causing abortion, infertility, and fetal mummification; infection of the bull is subclinical	vaginal swab for diagnosis; semen should be collected by artificial insemination; infected bulls should be culled; infected females should be treated with metronidazole and sexual rest
Trichomonas gallinae	none	chickens, turkeys, quail, pigeons	GI ulcerations of the crop and esophagus	cull infected birds
Histomonas meleagridis (black head)	earthworms carrying *Heterakis gallinarum* eggs	chickens and turkeys	necrosis of the cecum and liver, acute death	raised enclosures; cull infected birds

Hemoflagellates. Hemoflagellates live in the blood stream for all or part of their life cycle. They have a flagellum and an undulating membrane. They have arthropod intermediate hosts.

The amastigote stage generally causes disease in animals. Some of the trypanosomes are able to infect multiple species, including humans. Wildlife serves as reservoirs of infection.

Amebiasis rarely occurs in animals. Occasional infections of *Entamoeba histolytica* will occur in dogs. Diagnosis is based on observation of the trophozoite in direct smears or the cyst on fecal flotation.

TRYPANOSOMES				
GENUS/SPECIES	INTERMEDIATE HOST	DEFINITIVE HOST	SYMPTOMS	DX
Trypanosoma cruzi (Chagas' disease)	mosquito	dogs, humans	myocarditis, CNS disorders, can infect any tissue	tissue biopsy
Trypanosoma equiperdum (dourine)	none	horses	venereal disease in horses (discharge, abortion)	vaginal wash; this is a reportable disease
Leishmania donovani (visceral leishmaniasis)	*Lutzomyia* (sand fly), usually found on the Gulf Coast	dogs, humans	disease of any organ including spleen and liver	found in the macrophages of spleen and liver and skin on biopsy
Leishmania tropica (cutaneous leishmaniasis)		dogs and humans	cutaneous lesions only (swelling and fibrosis)	found in the macrophages of the skin on biopsy (Langerhans cells)

Helminths

Helminths are worms. All species of helminth are complex, multicellular organisms. Only a fraction of helminths are parasitic. The helminths can be divided into the flat worms (trematodes and cestodes) and the round worms (nematodes and acanthocephalids)

Cestodes are the tapeworms. They are flat, segmented worms. The segments are called proglottids.

Proglottids are the hermaphroditic (containing both sexes) reproductive elements. Cestodes have complex life cycles involving at least one intermediate host. The proglottids form from a holdfast organ, or scolex, that attaches the worm to the host. The chain of proglottids can grow very long and, in some cases, can even cause obstruction of the digestive tract. Proglottids only form in the definitive host. (See Figure 8.7.)

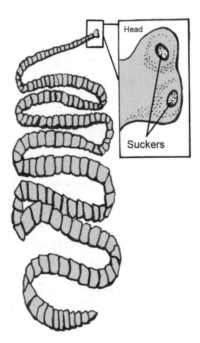

Figure 8.7 *Taenia Pisiforms or Tapeworm*

				ECHINOCOCCUS		
GENUS/SPECIES	INTERMEDIATE HOST	DEFINITIVE HOST	SYMPTOMS IN DEFINITIVE HOST	CYSTICERCOID (C) OR HYDATID CYST (H)
Taenia saginata	cattle	humans, dogs	GI obstruction, pernicious anemia (vitamin B_{12} deficiency), or asymptomatic	C
Taenia solium	pigs	humans		
Taenia taniaeformis	rodents	cats		
Taenia pisiformis	cattle	dogs		
Diplydium caninum	fleas	dogs, cats	asymptomatic, possible itching of the anus	C
Echinococcus granulosus	sheep, deer, humans	canids (wolves, coyotes, dogs)	GI obstruction, pernicious anemia (vitamin B_{12} deficiency), or asymptomatic	H
Echinococcus multilocularis	rodents, lagomorphs	cats, dogs, humans		
Hymenolepis	fleas, beetles	rodents, humans	GI obstruction, pernicious anemia (vitamin B_{12} deficiency), or asymptomatic	C

The pseudophyllidean tapeworms have bothria (sucking lips) rather than hooks on the scolex. The egg (oncosphere) of the pseudophyllidean tapeworm looks similar to a fluke egg in that it has an operculum (lid) and is oval with a pointy end (similar to a trematode egg). Pseudophyllideans require two intermediate hosts: the first intermediate host is a copepod (a tiny, water-dwelling insect), the second is a vertebrate (usually a fish or a rodent). Inappropriate consumption of the first intermediate host may result in a disease called sparganosis, which is an infection of the subcutaneous fascia and other tissues by the plerocercoid stage. (See Figure 8.8.)

The life cycle of the pseudophyllidean tapeworm is as follows:

The first stage (procercoid) develops in copepods which are then eaten by fish > the procercoid develops into a plerocercoid (sparganum) in the muscles of the fish which is then eaten by the mammal > the scolex attaches to the intestinal wall and proglottids are formed > the proglottids die and discharge the eggs into the feces > fecal contamination of water releases the larval form which is eaten by a copepod and the cycle continues.

Diphyllobothrium latum is also called the fish tapeworm. It can cause disease in all carnivorous mammals including humans. Prevention is by avoiding raw fish products.

The cyclophyllidean tapeworms have a scolex containing a number of hooks with which they attach to the intestinal wall. These worms have only one intermediate host. The eggs are called hexacanth oncospheres because they are round, relatively thick walled,

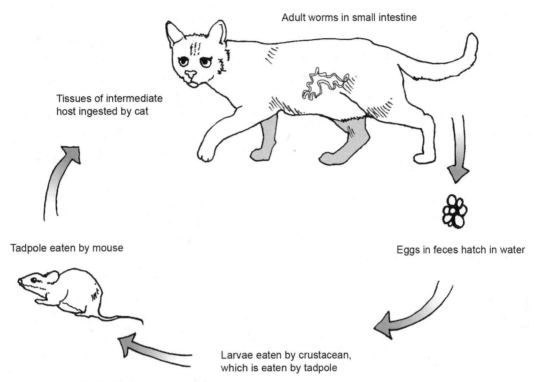

Adult worms in small intestine

Tissues of intermediate host ingested by cat

Tadpole eaten by mouse

Eggs in feces hatch in water

Larvae eaten by crustacean, which is eaten by tadpole

Figure 8.8 *Tapeworm Life Cycle*

and contain six teeth. Species cannot be differentiated by examining the eggs on fecal exam. The eggs have a high specific gravity (1.2251) and may be missed with some fecal flotation solutions. They can be broken into groups based on life cycles.

The taeniid type tapeworms (including *Diplydium caninum*) have similar life cycles but different intermediate and definitive hosts:

Oncosphere is shed in feces > intermediate host ingests oncosphere > oncosphere hatches into a cysticercus > cysticercus develops into a coenurus/bladderworm > definitive host ingests intermediate host > scolex attaches to intestinal wall > proglottids form and produce oncospheres which are shed in the feces individually. Proglottids may also be shed.

It is possible for cysticercus formation to occur in the definitive host if the infective oncosphere is ingested. This can result in hepatitis, cardiac disease, and skeletal muscle inflammation. This may also happen by direct fecal oral contamination in humans and carnivores who act as the definitive host. Prevention is by maintaining good hygiene and avoiding eating raw or undercooked meat. Treatment of the definitive host is with praziquantel.

The flea tapeworm of dogs and cats (*Diplydium caninum*) is of huge economic impact in veterinary medicine. Because the life cycle is wrapped up with the flea life cycle, control of both parasites is key to treatment and prevention. The interval between eating the infected flea and onset of segments in the stool is very short (2 to 3 weeks) so owners may not see the benefit from treatment of the tapeworm unless the flea problem is also controlled. Diagnosis of this tapeworm is possible because eggs are generally shed in packets of 10 to 13 oncospheres per packet. Both proglottids and packets are shed in the feces.

Echinococcus is an important tapeworm because it can be so devastating to the intermediate host. In these species, instead of forming a coenurus or bladder worm, the parasite forms a **hydatid cyst**. This thin-walled cyst can contain hundreds or thousands of infective scolices. Cysts can form anywhere in the body including the brain, but are usually found in the liver, spleen, and peritoneum. It is usually endemic in the wildlife population and domestic animals, so it can be extremely difficult to control.

The **trematodes** are the flukes. They are flat, unsegmented, hermaphroditic worms. They have complex life cycles involving at least one intermediate host:

Egg falls into the water > hatches into a ciliated miracidium > swims until it finds a snail, loses the cilia and migrates to the liver of the snail > forms a sporocyst > becomes a redia, which eats through the snail and divides into multiple cercaria, which leave the snail and swim freely in the environment > cercaria swim to target (may be plant material or a fish or crustacean depending on species) and encyst into a metacercaria > definitive host eats metacercaria > metacercaria becomes a marita, which migrates through the definitive host until it gets to its target organ and becomes a breeding adult

Most trematodes require snails or copepods as intermediate hosts, so most are more common near bodies of water. Treatment includes prevention of infection (avoidance of low-lying land; cooking fish and meat) and treating with praziquantel or fenbendazole.

Fluke eggs are pigmented and oval with a pointed end and a blunt end with an operculum. They look very similar to pseudophyllidean tapeworm ova.

TREMATODES				
GENUS/SPECIES	**FIRST INTERMEDIATE HOST**	**SECOND INTERMEDIATE HOST**	**DEFINITIVE HOST**	**SYMPTOMS AND DX**
Fasciola hepatica *Fasciola magna* *Fasciola gigantica*	snail	none; metacercaria are encysted on plants	ruminants, humans (liver)	acute: hepatic necrosis, abdominal pain, inflammation, and death; no adults, so cannot diagnose by fecal chronic: cholestasis, jaundice, weakness, anemia, hypoproteinemia, liver failure; diagnoses by ova in fecal

(continued)

	FIRST INTERMEDIATE HOST	SECOND INTERMEDIATE HOST	DEFINITIVE HOST	SYMPTOMS AND DX
TREMATODES (*continued*)				
GENUS/SPECIES				
Opisthorchis	snail	freshwater fish, roaches	carnivores, humans (liver)	severe liver disease
Nanophyetus salminicola (salmon poisoning fluke)	snail	trout or salmon	carnivores (liver)	usually asymptomatic unless have secondary infection with *Neorickettsia helminthoeca*—severe lymphadenopathy and hemorrhagic enteritis (may be fatal); treat with praziquantel and tetracyclines; diagnose by ova in feces
Platynosmum fastosum	snail	lizard or amphibian	cat (bile duct)	cholestasis, pancreatitis
Paragonimus kellicotti	snail	crayfish	carnivores, humans (lungs)	coughing, bronchitis; lesions may be seen radiographically; diagnosis by tracheal wash and seeing ova in sputum or feces

The **nematodes** contain most of the parasitic worms. Nematodes are vastly different between genera, although within genera, life cycles are similar. Control of nematode infections requires a knowledge of the life cycle of each worm.

Filarial worms all have an arthropod vector for transmission and a complex life cycle. These are long and thin worms that may be found in the blood vessels, lymphatic tissues, and body cavities of animals. The general life cycle is as follows:

Microfilaria are picked up by the biting insect (intermediate host) from an infected animal > microfilaria transform into infective larvae in the insect > insect bites the definitive host and transmits the L_3 larva by injection into the subcutaneous tissues where they develop into L_4 larvae > the L_4 larvae migrate to the target tissues and become adults (there are two different sexes) > microfilaria are formed (there are no eggs) and released into the bloodstream or lymphatics where they are available for pickup by the insect.

SPIRURIDS AND FILARIAL WORMS

GENUS/SPECIES	INTERMEDIATE HOST	DEFINITIVE HOST	SYMPTOMS	DX AND TX
Onchocerca gutterosa *Onchocerca cervicalis*	flies flies and gnats	cattle horses	adults: asymptomatic microfilaria: pruritis (summer mange in horses)	microfilaria are seen on conjunctival scraping and skin biopsy; treat with avermectin
Dirofilaria immitis (heartworm)	mosquitoes (all species)	dogs (cats, ferrets, and humans may act as aberrant hosts)	dogs and ferrets: inverted *D* sign of the heart, thickened, torturous pulmonary vessels, pulmonary edema cats: *hard* coughing, gagging, and vomiting, bronchial pattern on radiographs humans: granuloma formation in the lungs	prepatent period (before antigen or microfilaria are seen in the blood) is 6 to 9 months Dx microfilaria: direct visualization of microfilaria in blood film, concentration tests (Knott's and Difil-Test®); dogs only Dx Adults: direct antigen ELISA for canine and feline, indirect antibody ELISA for felines
Dipetalonema reconditum	fleas	dogs	nonpathogenic	Dx microfilaria testing (concentration methods such as Knott's and Difil-Test® only); this parasite is easily confused with *Dirofilaria immitis* (see Hematology parasite section)
Physaloptera	beetles, cockroaches	dogs, cats	ulcerative granulomas in the stomach and esophagus of cats; they may become so severe that they cause obstruction and death; melena, hemoptysis, vomiting	Dx endoscopy, fecal flotation Tx fenbendazole
Thelazia (eyeworm)	*musca* (face flies)	all domestic animals	conjunctivitis, corneal ulceration	Dx direct visualization Tx removal of the worm from the conjunctival sac

Adult heartworms in dogs are treated with arsenic-containing compounds such as melarsomine dihydrochloride (Immiticide®). This is given as a series of two injections deep into the epaxial (lower back) musculature 2 weeks apart. The adult worms will slowly die over 4 to 6 weeks. The complications of adulticide therapy are thrombus (clot) formation in the pulmonary vessels and acute death. The incidence of these complications are increased in animals that are not kept quiet after therapy. Adulticide treatment may be followed by microfilaricidal therapy with ivermectin to reduce circulating microfilaria in the blood. Ferrets and cats do not respond well to adulticide therapy (death). (See Figure 8.9.)

Hookworms/strongyles have no true intermediate hosts, but many animals may act as paratenic hosts. Transmission may be transplacental or transmammary. Larvae infest the lungs, resulting in coughing and gagging symptoms. The adult lives in the small intestine or abomasum of the primary host, attaches to the mucosa, and sucks blood. Anemia is the result of adult parasites in the intestine, which cause melena, vomiting, and di-

arrhea. Adults are very small and not visible on fecal or vomitus examination without magnification. Adults pass ova in their feces, which larvate within 48 hours. If conditions are good, ova may remain viable for months in the soil. They are very resistant to chemicals. Under appropriate conditions, larvae hatch and migrate to the tips of grass where they are either consumed by the host or penetrate the skin. They migrate to the lungs, transform into the next stage larvae, and are coughed up and swallowed. They become adults in the small intestine. Diagnosis is based on visualization of ova on fecal flotation. Ova are thin walled, clear, oval, and contain multiple-celled embryos. (See Figure 8.10.)

Treatment of these parasites is difficult because of large egg numbers, ability of the ova to lie dormant in the soil if conditions are not favorable, and arrested larval stages that can occur in the tissues and are not susceptible to anthelminthics. Most of the available anthelminthics are effective against the adult stages, however. In ruminants more than one of these species may infect a single host, resulting in severe anemia and death.

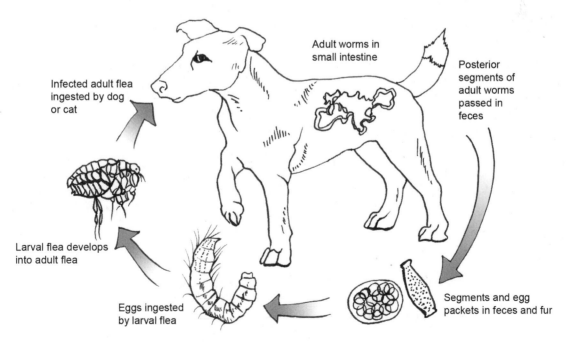

Infected adult flea ingested by dog or cat

Adult worms in small intestine

Posterior segments of adult worms passed in feces

Larval flea develops into adult flea

Eggs ingested by larval flea

Segments and egg packets in feces and fur

Figure 8.9 *Dirofilaria Immitis or Heartworm Life Cycle*

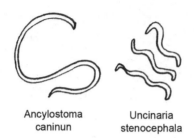

Ancylostoma
caninun

Uncinaria
stenocephala

Figure 8.10 *Hookworms/Strongyles and Hairworms*

HOOKWORMS/STRONGYLES AND HAIRWORMS

GENUS/ SPECIES	DEFINITIVE HOST	ROUTE OF INFECTION	SYMPTOMS FROM ADULTS	SYMPTOMS FROM LARVAE
Ancylostoma caninum	dogs (humans occasionally)	cutaneous penetration by or ingestion of larvae, transmammary infection in puppies less than 6 weeks of age	anemia, gastritis, diarrhea, melena	coughing from migrating larvae during prepatent period
Ancylostoma tubaeformae	cats		peracute; in puppies, the adult worms will not be passing ova until the animal is dead	creeping eruption; dermatitis from cutaneous penetration of larvae
Ancylostoma braziliense	dogs, cats			
Uncinaria stenocephala	dogs, cats	cutaneous penetration by or ingestion of larvae	see above	see above
Ollulanus tricuspis (strongyloid)	cats	ingestion of infected vomit	in cats, chronic gastritis that can lead to death	none
Ostertagia ostertagii (trichostrongylus)	ruminants	ingestion of larvae	submaxillary edema, emaciation, abomasitis, watery diarrhea, anemia, hypoproteinemia	none
Haemonchus contortus (trichostrongylus)			severe nonregenerative anemia, hypoproteinemia, death	
Strongylus vulgaris	horses	ingestion of larvae	severe anemia, large intestinal disease, death	thrombi in the mesenteric arteries, colic, death (not easily treatable)
Strongylus edentatus				
Strongylus equinus				
Dictyocaulus (lungworm)	ruminants and horses	ingestion of larvae	cough, bronchitis; treat with febendazole	none

Ascarids have a direct life cycle but may also have transmammary transmission. (See Figure 8.11.) Many animals may act as **paratenic**, or temporary, hosts. This may result in visceral larval migrans in which the larval stages burrow through the tissues of the paratenic host (eyes, brain, liver, and lungs primarily) and cause damage. The larval stage in the primary host lives in the lungs and may result in coughing and gagging. The adult phase resides in the target organ of the primary host. Most ascarids are host specific.

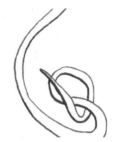

Figure 8.11   *Ascarids (Roundworms)*

ASCARIDS (ROUNDWORMS)					
GENUS/ SPECIES	DEFINITIVE HOST	ROUTE OF INFECTION	SYMPTOMS FROM ADULTS	SYMPTOMS FROM LARVAE	OVA
Ascaris suum	pigs	fecal, oral	diarrhea, vomiting, gastrointestinal obstruction; Tx with Pyrantel	coughing, liver disease; respiratory distress in piglets	pigmented
Parascaris equorum	horses	fecal, oral	diarrhea, vomiting, GI obstruction; in foals, bowel perforation and death	coughing, liver disease	pigmented
Toxascaris leonina	dogs, cats	fecal oral, ingestion of paratenic host (rodent), transmammary, transplacental	diarrhea, vomiting, GI obstruction	coughing, liver disease; larval migrations will occur in humans	clear, smooth shell
Toxocara canis	dogs	fecal oral, ingestion of paratenic host (rodent), transmammary, transplacental	see above	see above; larvae will migrate through the CNS and the eye; larval migration will occur in humans	pigmented
Toxocara cati	cats	as above, but no transplacental			
Baylisascaris	skunks, raccoons, woodchucks	fecal oral	see above	larvae will migrate through the CNS and the eye; larval migration will occur in humans; the larvae will grow in the tissues and cause severe damage and death	pigmented

The parasites primarily target organs in the intestines (*Ascaris*, *Parascaris*, *Toxocara*, *Toxascaris*, *Baylisascaris*) or the stomach (*Physaloptera*). In intestinal ascarids, the worms are large and may appear as moving spaghetti in the vomit or the diarrhea of affected animals. In small animals, large infestations may result in intestinal blockage or intussusception due to the size of the worms. In stomach ascarids, the worms make granulomas in the stomach or esophagus and may cause severe ulcerations or blockage by granulomatous inflammation.

Ova are generally round and thick walled. Individual species may have different coloration and textures, but they are generally brown with a golden pitted shell and are virtually indistiguishable from each other on fecal examination. Ova may remain viable in the soil for years if conditions are good.

Pinworms have a direct life cycle:

gravid female lays eggs > contaminate water > ingested > hatch in small intestine and mature in colon

The eggs tend to cause itching in the perineum but the adults are generally nonpathogenic otherwise. Infections respond to most anthelminthics. Species are host specific. *Oxyuris equi* (horse) is the only important species in this group.

These parasites all have interesting life cycles which are very individual for the species. They contain the largest and some of the smallest parasitic worms and can cause significant human health problems. (See Figure 8.12.)

Life cycle of *Trichinella*:

female lays eggs in intestinal crypts > eggs release larvae, which migrate through the intestinal wall to the muscles > larvae encyst in muscles > host eats encysted larvae

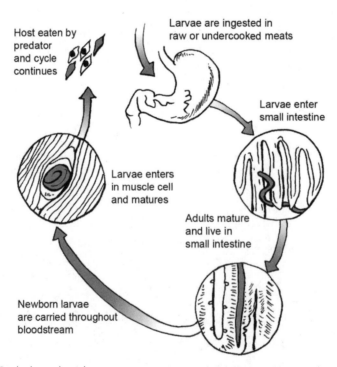

Figure 8.12 *Trichinella Life Cycledenophorides*

ADENOPHOREA				
GENUS/SPECIES	INTERMEDIATE HOST	DEFINITIVE HOST	SYMPTOMS	DX AND TX
Trichinella	pigs	omnivores, carnivores, and humans	fever, malaise, eosinophilia, muscle pain	muscle biopsy
Trichuris vulpis (whipworm)	none	dogs	severe diarrhea with blood and mucus; prepatent period is 3 months	Dx visualization of pigmented, football-shaped ova with thick, golden shell and two clear polar plugs. Tx febendazole, repeat in 3 months
Capillaria plica (bladder worm)	earthworm	dogs, cats	may be asymptomatic	Dx visualization of ova in the urine (look exactly the same as *Trichuris*) Tx febendazole
Capillaria felis cati (bladder worm)		cats only		
Eucoleus aerophila (lungworm)	earthworm	dogs, cats	coughing, wheezing, bronchitis	Dx visualization of ova in the feces or tracheal wash (look exactly the same as *Trichuris*) Tx fenbendazole
Dioctyphema renale (giant kidney worm)	first intermediate host: earthworms; second intermediate host: fish or frogs	carnivores, pigs, humans	asymptomatic	Dx usually at necropsy in the left kidney; cause significant damage to kidney, but function is compensated by the other kidney in infections with both sexes in the same kidney, visualize large, lemon-shaped ova, yellow pigmented with very rough shell and two polar plugs

Parasite Testing

Testing for parasites is a large component of the veterinary technician's job. From a public health aspect, it helps to control the environmental concentration of potential zoonotic disease organisms, increases yield in production animals, and increases the health and well-being of the animal population.

When testing for flies, visualization of the adult fly on the animal may not be practical. Often the testing involves visualization of the larval form in cases of myiasis or diagnosing the diseases transmitted by the fly. In cases of startling, stampeding, or restlessness, time of day or location (breeding sites, preferred habitat) may be key to the diagnosis of a specific fly species.

Lice and keds (sheepticks) are diagnosed by direct visualization of nits (eggs) on hair or adults on hair or skin.

Fleas are diagnosed by direct visualization of adults or flea dirt (digested blood) in the animal's coat.

Mites are diagnosed by microscopic examination of a skin scraping. Skin scrapings are made by moistening a #10 scalpel blade and scraping it along the surface of the skin to remove scale and hair. This must be done until capillary bleeding is seen at the surface. The scraping is then transferred to a drop of mineral oil on a slide, coverslipped, and examined using the 10× objective. Multiple sites should be scraped to ensure a better chance of diagnosis. *Chyletiella* may be visualized by direct exam because of its size.

Ticks may be diagnosed by direct visualization. Species identification may be important in helping diagnose transmission of tick-related illness. Speciation may be performed by examining the patterns on the back of the tick.

Most endoparasites are diagnosed by a combination of fecal techniques including direct, flotation, sedimentation, and Baermann apparatus. Blood parasites were discussed separately in the Hematology section in Chapter 7.

The direct fecal exam is a good screening test, but should not be performed without a fecal flotation to confirm. A fecal smear should be made with saline (water may be used, but saline is preferable), mixed thoroughly, coverslipped, and examined at 10× to 40× objectives. Direct fecal exams can help diagnose trophozoite (motile) forms of protozoal organisms such as *giardia* or *balantidium*, which are very fragile and will not be seen with flotation or sedimentation techniques. Clostridial organisms and bacterial overgrowth may also be seen on direct exam of feces.

The fecal flotation is the mainstay of the fecal exam in most practices. The theory behind flotation is simple. Distilled water has a specific gravity (SG) of 1.000. Parasite ova have specific gravities >1.000 and <1.245, so, if we use a solution with a specific gravity higher than the densest ova (>1.245), the ova should float to the surface of the solution and stick to the slide. The various solutions used in veterinary medicine for flotation vary in SG and other characteristics. In general, the fecal sample should be roughly the size

of a quarter for maximum accuracy. Fecal solutions should be tested frequently with a hygrometer (instrument that measures the SG of a fluid) to assure quality control in practice.

Zinc sulfate is commonly used in veterinary practices for floation. The SG is usually between 1.180 and 1.200. This is well below the SG needed for flotation of some of the heavier eggs, such as those of *Taenia* and *Physaloptera*. The advantages of zinc sulfate are that crystals do not form until the solution has been sitting for about 20 minutes, and it does not distort eggs. It is the solution of choice for *Giardia* cyst recovery.

Sodium nitrate has an SG of 1.200, but it tends to distort fragile eggs and crystallizes readily. The advantage is that it is very inexpensive.

Sheather's solution (simple saturated sugar solution) has an SG of 1.270 and will recover more parasitic ova and oocysts than any other solution. It does not distort most ova, but will destroy *Giardia* cysts. It will not crystallize. Care must be taken to avoid spilling this solution because of vermin attraction (ants and roaches). It is cheaper than any other flotation solution.

Saturated sodium chloride has a low SG and will distort ova and oocysts as well as increase corrosion of equipment, which is why it is not generally used even though it is inexpensive.

The passive flotation technique is most commonly used in clinical practice although it may give many false negatives (low egg yield). With this technique, the stool sample is mixed thoroughly with the flotation solution, strained into a tube, filled to form a positive meniscus, covered with a slide or coverslip and allowed to sit for 10 to 20 minutes. The coverslip is then lifted straight up and placed liquid side down onto a slide and examined under the microscope from 10× to 40×.

The centrifugal flotation technique is the preferred method because it increases yield of ova/oocysts and gives fewer false negatives. The flotation solution is prepared as above, except instead of allowing it to sit, it is placed in a centrifuge at 1200–1800 rpm for 5 minutes, allowed to sit for 10 minutes, and then read as above. Be sure to balance the tubes.

The sedimentation technique may be used for very heavy ova, such as fluke eggs, as well as for larvae visualization. In this technique, the feces is mixed thoroughly with water, filtered with cheesecloth, and centrifuged at 1200 to 1800 rpm without a coverslip. Because the density of water is lower than that of the eggs, the eggs will sink to the bottom along with the debris. The **supernatant** (liquid portion of tube contents) is poured off and the resulting pellet is resuspended. A drop of the solution is placed on a slide with a coverslip and examined at 10 to 40× on the microscope. Because the material has a great deal of debris, it may be difficult to see the ova.

This technique is a dilution one, which gives a minimum estimate of the number of ova in a given fecal sample, unlike the concentration procedure, which gives a maximum. The procedure is as follows:

> 10 gm feces is mixed with 150 ml of water and mixed thoroughly > 0.3 ml of Sheather's solution is added to the counting chamber along with 0.3 ml of fecal solution > mix solution and feces with a needle > allow 15 minutes to stand > count all eggs in each pool on low power

The Baermann apparatus is the technique of choice for visualizing larval forms of nematodes. The fecal slurry with water or normal saline is placed in a cheesecloth-lined funnel connected to a rubber tube with a stopcock attached. This is allowed to sit for 12 to 24 hours and the stopcock is opened and a small amount of fluid is released and examined for larvae. This is important for *Filaroides* and other nematodes as well as some worms which lay larvated eggs.

The lung worms and flukes may be diagnosed by either fecal flotation or sputum flotation. The technique for both is the same. In some cases, the adult organisms may be seen via bronchoscopy with an endoscope.

Ova may be seen on urinalysis in cases of *Capillaria* and *Dioctyphema*. Techniques for urinalysis will be discussed in the Urinalysis section.

Hemosporidia, hemoflagellates, and filarial nematodes are all diagnosed via hematologic testing. These techniques were discussed under Hematologic Testing in Chapter 7.

Ectoparasite treatment and prevention was discussed in the section on Ectoparasites. Endoparasite treatment is more varied. Most of the protozoal organisms can be treated with some type of antibiotic (metronidazole, clindamycin, sulfadimethoxine, etc.). Most of the nematodes may be treated by anthelminthics, but the drug required will vary by the species. Special consideration must be given to the treatment of food animals. Drug residues can cause meat products to be condemned. A complete listing of drugs to avoid in food animals is available from FARAD (Food Animal Residue Avoidance Database) and the USDA (U.S. Department of Agriculture).

Urinalysis

Urinalysis is evaluated along with the CBC and clinical chemistries in order to evaluate the health of the animal. A complete urinalysis can give information on hydration status, kidney health, liver function, and glucose metabolism. Complete urinalysis involves specific gravity, chemical analysis, and microscopic analysis of the sediment. All three components of the urinalysis should be performed in practice. Failure to perform the urine sediment may cause valuable information about the function of the kidney to be missed.

Urine should be obtained in a sterile container. All urine samples should be analyzed as quickly as possible after collection, preferably within 30 minutes. If they cannot be read within 30 minutes, samples may be refrigerated for as long as 6 to 12 hours. Samples should be at room temperature prior to analysis. If a specimen needs to be shipped, 1 drop of formalin may be added to preserve it. Samples should be protected from light because most of the pigments that give urine color are light sensitive. Early morning specimens will yield the maximum urine concentration. Collect in a clean, dry container or a Ziploc® baggie. Used pickle jars will not work! Of the three collection methods that may be used, each has drawbacks.

The most commonly used method is the free catch. Drawbacks to free catch sampling are the high possibility of contamination from the environment and also from preputial or vulval contaminants. Animals that are in estrus will have blood contamination that may cause misdiagnosis. Care must be taken to avoid contamination during collection. Getting a midstream catch gives the best sample. The advantage of this method is that it is the least stressful to the patient.

Cystocenthesis is the second most common method of collection. A needle and syringe are introduced percutaneously into the urinary bladder and a quantity of urine is removed. The advantages of this method are sterility of the sample; assurance of no sperm, vaginal epithelial, or preputial cells present in the sample; no anesthesia is required; and it is easy to collect by this method. This is the best method to use if sediment analysis is required. Cells and bacteria seen on cystocenthesis are guaranteed to originate in the urinary tract. The drawbacks of cystocenthesis is that blood contamination may occur, it requires restraint of the animal, and the animal must have a moderately full bladder in order to obtain a sample.

Catheterization is the third method. This method has many drawbacks. It requires sedation in the cat and in the bitch. Asepsis is a must. In animals that already have cystitis or bladder infections, catheterization may make it worse. It is uncomfortable, and there still may be some contamination of the sample. The advantages of the method are that the sample can still be used for culture and sensitivity and there will not be as high a possibility of blood contamination as there is with cystocenthesis.

The urine should be examined grossly for color, clarity, **turbidity** (particles suspended in the sample), and odor. The color of urine comes from cytochrome pigments. Urine should be slightly yellow to amber in color (urochrome). Red urine may indicate blood or hemoglobin, brown urine may indicate myoglobin or bilirubin, green urine might indicate biliverdin or some bacterial infections, and clear, colorless urine could indicate a problem with concentrating ability.

Clarity and turbidity come from the amount of material present in the urine. Urine should be clear, but cloudiness can occur with increased protein concentration or suspended cells, fats, or crystals.

Specific Gravity

As previously stated, the urine specific gravity (SG) gives information on the concentrating ability of the kidney. It is the measurement of the density of urine compared to distilled water by a refractometer (the same instrument used to measure the total protein level). There is an SG pad on the urine chemistry dipstick, but this is completely unreliable in veterinary medicine. Very dilute urine may indicate failure of the renal tubules in the kidney nephron to recycle water (osmotic diuresis). Osmotic diuresis occurs in diabetes mellitus when there is increased sugar in the bloodstream due to insulin deficiency. The glucose must be diluted and the animal increases its water intake and its urination quantity and frequency. Because water follows the glucose, the urine is dilute. Normal SG in the dog is >1.030, in the cat it is >1.035. Glucose in the urine will increase the SG. A glucosuria of 1+ on the urine chemistry strip will increase the specific gravity by 0.001. A proteinuria of 3+ will also increase the SG by 0.001.

Isosthenuria is defined as an SG of 1.008–1.012 (distilled water has an SG of 1.000). It may be normal in animals drinking large volumes of water. If the animal is dehydrated (this can be assessed by looking at the serum protein level) or azotemic (high BUN) with isosthenuria, there is an inability of the kidney to concentrate the urine.

Polyuria is formation and elimination of large quantities of urine. It may be due to increased fluid intake (physiologic polyuria). In this case, control of water consumption will improve the symptoms. If it is pathologic polyuria, it will be due either to a lack of ADH or to impaired ability of the renal tubules to re-absorb electrolytes. The first situation is diabetes insipidus, which we have already discussed. The second is due to nephrosis (disease affecting the renal tubules), hypoadrenocorticism, or diabetes mellitus. These problems will usually result in azotemia as well as in reduced SG.

Oliguria is a state that results in decreased urine formation or elimination of urine caused by the body. This can be from urinary obstruction, dehydration, or shock.

Anuria is the absence of urine formation.

For the above reasons, serum chemistry results (BUN and Cr) should be interpreted along with SG in order to determine whether the azotemia is prerenal, renal, or postrenal.

Chemical Analysis

Chemical analysis of urine is usually tested by doing a Chemstrip®, which is a plastic strip with paper pads containing various chemicals that change color in contact with urine. The color of the pad should be measured against the color chart on the bottle. This measure is semiquantitative, which means that the degree of color change indicates the approximate concentration of the test substance in the urine. There are also incubation times listed for the various chemicals. This is the amount of time that the pad must be exposed to the urine prior to being read. Failure to read the strip at the appropriate times can cause error. Urine must be at room temperature to use these trips because some of the reagents are temperature sensitive.

The strips must be used correctly to prevent errors. The strip should be completely submerged in the sample quickly, then blotted. Adequate lighting is important to ensure proper color analysis. Errors can occur if the sample has been contaminated or if there is unusual color in the urine from hemoglobin, blood, or other pigments.

pH

The pH measures the amount of hydrogen ion in the sample. The pH of urine is generally acidic (<7.0) in carnivores and alkaline (>7.0) in herbivores. The urine pH is a crude index of the acid–base balance because the kidney participates in maintenance of proper pH in the body by excreting hydrogen ions, ammonium ions, and phosphates. The kidney is responsible for maintaining metabolic acid–base balance. Corresponding to this is the action of the respiratory system, which regulates pH by adjusting the bicarbonate levels; this is called respiratory acid–base balance.

Aciduria can result from starvation, diabetes mellitus, and high-protein diets and some respiratory diseases (pneumonia). Akalinuria can result from increased lactate (lactated Ringer's fluid therapy or muscle soreness), vegetarian diets, bicarbonate or bacterial infection, or contamination. Many types of bacteria produce a substance called urease, which is an enzyme that breaks down urea into ammonia. Since ammonia is a strong base, it will drive up the pH of the urine. Storage of samples at room temperature will also cause loss of carbon dioxide from the sample, which will drive up the pH. Detergent residues can also increase pH.

The pH indicators are usually methyl red and bromthymol blue. They can measure pH in a range from 5 to 9.

Although urine pH is not a very sensitive indicator of systemic pH, it can be used along with TCO_2 (total CO_2 content) and arterial blood gases to complete the picture. A better use of urine pH is in interpreting the urine sediment. Certain crystals are only formed in acidic urine and others are only seen in alkaline urine. Knowing the urine pH can help in both diagnosis and treatment of crystalluria.

Urine Protein

Urine protein should be interpreted along with the SG and the urine pH because alkaline urine may give a false positive on the protein pad. The SG should be increased if the urine protein is increased. A sulfosalicylic acid test is a more sensitive indicator of urine protein and should be used as confirmation if there is any doubt about the accuracy of the dipstick result. The dipstick is more sensitive to albumin than to the other proteins. Contamination of the urine sample with chlorhexidine or Roccal-D® can give false negatives on protein levels.

Urine protein is used to evaluate the glomeruli of the nephron. The glomeruli usually only allow water and small molecules (such as electrolytes, glucose, BUN, and Cr) to pass into the urine. Proteins should not pass through the blood vessels of the glomeruli. Preglomerular proteinuria (before the glomerulus) is caused by problems such as inflammation, exercise, and seizures (can cause muscle damage and release of proteins), which can cause increases in urine protein levels. If proteinuria is seen in the absence of inflammation, blood, or pigment increases, it is probably due to a problem with the glomerulus (glomerular proteinuria). Inflammation of the bladder or the genital tract can also cause proteinuria (postglomerular), although this is not as common.

Urine Glucose

Urine glucose should be negative on the urine dipstick unless the blood glucose levels are >200 mg/dl. This value is called the renal threshold. Glucosuria occurs with diabetes mellitus, renal tubular disease, shock, glucose-containing fluids, and anesthesia. Glucosuria with hyperglycemia is the definition of diabetes mellitus. False negatives on the test strip may occur with vitamin C supplementation.

Urine Ketones

Urine ketones indicate fat mobilization (starvation) or anaerobic glycolysis (breakdown of sugars without oxygen) caused by diabetes mellitus or shock. The urine ketone pad only reacts with acetoacetic acid, not acetone or hydroxybutyric acid, so the problem may be worse than is measured with the dipstick.

Blood

The blood strip will react with either hemoglobin, myoglobin, or erythrocytes. Pigments (hemoglobin and myoglobin) will cause a diffuse color change in the strip. Erythrocytes will cause spotty color changes. False positives can occur in bacterial urinary tract infections.

Hematuria (whole blood cells in the urine) generally indicate disease of the lower urinary (bladder) or genital tract.

Hemoglobinuria (hemoglobin in the urine) can occur if the pH is very alkaline (high pH), or if intravascular hemolysis (red blood cell destruction in the vasculature) has occurred.

Myoglobinuria (myoglobin in the urine) can occur if muscle damage has occurred. The dipstick cannot differentiate between hemoglobin and myoglobin. If the serum is icteric (yellow) or hemolyzed (red) along with a positive urine blood dipstick, think hemoglobin.

Bilirubin

Bilirubin is a breakdown product of hemoglobin. Bilirubin may be increased in animals with cholestasis (bile duct blockage or diffuse liver damage) or extravascular hemolysis (red blood cell destruction in the liver or spleen). Small amounts of bilirubin in the urine are normal in canines, but not in felines.

Urobilinogen

Urobilinogen is usually not important in veterinary medicine, although increased levels will confirm extravascular hemolysis because urobilinogen is also made as a breakdown product of hemoglobin.

Other Test Pad Concerns

Leukocyte test pads were developed for humans and are not useful in veterinary medicine because false positives occur in cats and false negatives in dogs. The same is true of nitrites in animal tests. The sediment should always be examined for the presence of white blood cells in the sample.

Sediment and Microscopic Analysis

The **urine sediment** can give the technician invaluable information and should be part of every urinalysis. It can give information on every part of the urinary tract including the kidneys. Proper technique for performing sediment analysis begins with sample collection. In order to ensure that the cells seen on the sediment are truly from the urinary tract and not the genital tract, the urine should be collected by cystocenthesis. Sediment should also be evaluated at room temperature as quickly as possible after collection. Refrigeration will increase crystal formation and heating will decrease crystals. Sediment should be evaluated along with SG and pH. High SG will tend to increase the number of cells, crystals, and casts present. For this reason, if any crystals or cells are seen in a low SG specimen, it is considered significant.

Sediments are examined by centrifugation of the sample at low speed for 5 minutes and pouring off the supernatant (liquid portion). The pellet is resuspended and a drop is placed on the slide. A drop of stain (urine sedi-stain or new methylene blue) is added to the remaining pellet and a drop of that is also placed on a slide for viewing. Both a stained and an unstained sample should be evaluated because the stain may be contaminated or have crystal formation that can interfere with results. Comparison is the key.

The slide(s) should be examined at low power (10×) to identify casts and crytals. These should be reported as number of casts or crystals per low power field (LPF). The magnification should then be increased to 40× and examined for bacteria and cell morphology. Epithelial and blood cells should be counted and recorded as number of cells per high power field (HPF).

Cells

Cells that are normally seen in urine are epithelial cells. The most common epthelial cell is transitional epithelium. These cells are variable in size and shape and are specially adapted to allow stretching of the bladder wall. They are larger than white blood cells, but smaller than squamous cells. **Transitional epithelial cells** are found in the bladder, the ureter, and the renal pelvis. They may be increased in number with urinary tract inflammation.

Squamous epithelial cells may be seen in free catch samples because of contamination from the genital tract. These cells are more angular and very flat with darker staining cytoplasm than the transitional epithelium.

The **renal epithelial cell** is also called the *caudate cell*. This is a triangular or egg-shaped cell that normally lines the renal tubules. The nucleus is at the base of the triangle. Caudate cells are generally smaller than transitional epithelial cells and slightly larger than white blood cells. They are rarely seen and when present may indicate kidney tubule disease (nephrosis).

Normal urine should have very few red blood cells (<2–3/HPF). Red blood cells cannot cross the normal glomerulus. Red blood cells appear on urinalysis as colorless disks. In alkaline urine, the red blood cells lyse. Hematuria may occur from bladder irritation, bleeding disorders, or trauma (even from cystocenthesis).

In normal urine, white blood cells should be <1/HPF. White blood cells indicate urinary tract inflammation if >5 cells/40× field. This is called pyuria and can be caused by inflammation, infection, or neoplasia. Presence of bacteria along with white blood cells in a cystocenthesis sample means infection. If the sample was obtained by cystocenthesis, it indicates a problem either in the urinary tract or in the prostate. Patients with diabetes mellitus have a higher incidence of urinary tract infections.

Sperm may occasionally be seen in the urine of intact males. Sperm should not be present if the sample was obtained by cystocenthesis.

Other cells that may be seen in the sediment include neoplastic cells. These may arise from any tissue. Primary cancers of the urinary tract are usually transitional epithelial tumors.

Crystals

Crystals occur in all animals when urine concentration of a particular material becomes higher than what is referred to as the saturation point. The saturation point of a substance is the concentration at which it comes out of solution and forms a solid. The saturation point depends on many factors including the pH of the urine, temperature, certain drugs, and diet. When crystals form, they often come together and form seeds for further crystal formation. Over time these seeds will grow larger and larger and eventually form uroliths or urinary stones. Uroliths can cause obstruction of the urinary tract and may occur anywhere from the renal pelvis to the urethra.

Evaluation of crystals can help detect problems in metabolism, estimate the type of crystals that have made up a bladder stone, and evaluate the effectiveness of diet change in the treatment of stones. Sediment analysis is performed to evaluate crystals. The urine should be as fresh as possible because many factors can cause crystal formation that have nothing to do with the patient. If a urine sample is kept in a hot car, crystals will dissolve because heat will increase the saturation point. If it is cold, more crystals will form because the saturation point decreases. For these reasons, samples should be at room temperature for evaluation. If part of the sample evaporates, the concentration of the urine will increase, causing crystals to form. Therefore, sediment should be analyzed as quickly as possible.

The pH affects which crystals will form because some substances have a lower saturation point in acid urine than in alkaline urine and vice versa. Most carnivores have acid pH urine, so will have crystals that have a low saturation point in acid urine (urates, calcium oxalate, bilirubin, cysteine, cholesterol). Herbivores have alkaline urine and form crystals that have a low saturation point in alkaline urine (calcium carbonate, struvite, amorphous phosphate). It is important to remember that changes in pH caused by disease or diet will change which crystals are formed. Dietary change may be all that is required to treat an animal with certain types of stones.

Struvite Crystals

Although struvite (magnesium ammonium triple phosphate) crystals are more common in alkaline urine, they are the most common crystal seen in dogs and cats. This is probably because the commercial diets available for both dogs and cats are very high in grains and tend to alkalinize the urine. Bacterial infection by bacteria that produce urease (an enzyme that breaks down urea into ammonia) will also increase urine pH.

Struvite crystals look like coffin lids. They are colorless and have very sharp edges. They are the most common urolith (bladder stone). They may or may not be radiodense on x-ray, so contrast studies (injection of dye or air into the bladder) may be required to visualize the stones.

Calcium Oxalate Crystals

Calcium oxalate crystals can form in any pH, but are more common in acidic urine. They are completely square with a double pyramid top and bottom. On microscopy, they look like a box with an x in it. This is also called a Maltese cross pattern. They vary in size and can occur in aggregates (clumps). They occur in two types: calcium oxalate dihydrate and calcium oxalate monohydrate. Stones from calcium oxalate are radiodense.

The calcium oxalate dihydrate is the most common form and has the shape discussed above. It can occur in clinically normal animals and is the most common bladder stone seen in cats and miniature schnauzers. It may be seen in animals with ethylene glycol toxicity.

The calcium oxalate monohydrate form is most common in ethylene glycol toxicity. These crystals look like spears with points on both ends and may aggregate to form sheaves of crystals (they look like sheaves of wheat).

Calcium Carbonate Crystals

Calcium carbonate crystals are found in alkaline urine. Horses, rabbits, guinea pigs, and goats have these crystals in large numbers. Dogs and cats do not make calcium carbonate crystals. Rabbits and guinea pigs make so many of these crystals that it may cause a kind of sludge in the bladder that is visible on radiographs because these crystals are radiodense. The crystals are sphere shaped and usually yellow to yellow brown.

Bilirubin Crystals

Bilirubin crystals form in acid urine only, so should never be seen in herbivores. Bilirubin crystals are brownish red and very thin. They may be seen in very highly concentrated urine in normal dogs at low numbers. If large numbers of bilirubin crystals are seen, a problem with cholestasis (bile duct blockage) should be suspected.

Urate Crystals

Although amorphous urates are occasionally found in normal highly acidic urine, they are not common. They only form in acid urine. Refrigeration will in-

crease these crystals, so they may be seen in normal urine that has not been warmed to room temperature prior to sediment analysis. They are commonly seen in dalmatians and English bulldogs because of a defect in metabolism. In these breeds, stones may occur. They are also common in dogs with portosystemic shunts (bypass of the liver by the portal circulation). Amorphous urates are small, yellow-brown granules that may be pinkish-orange on microscopy.

Uric acid crystals also form in acid urine and are common in dalmatians and English bulldogs as well. They come in a variety of shapes and have the same significance as amorphous urates.

Ammonium biurate crystals form in neutral and alkaline urine. They may occur in normal dogs and cats in small numbers, but if found in large numbers may indicate portosystemic shunts. In appearance, these crystals are round and spiky and look like World War II naval mines.

Cystine Crystals

Cystine crystals occur in acidic urine. If seen, they usually indicate a problem with the breakdown of nucleic acids or a problem with the renal tubules (nephrosis).

Drug Crystals

Some drugs will cause precipitation of crystals in the urine. Sulfur-containing drugs (sulfonamides) may appear like angel wings in alkaline urine.

Organisms

Free catch samples are not adequate to assess urine for the presence of bacteria because of the possibility of contamination from the environment, the genital area, and the skin. Cystocenthesis is the preferred method of collection, although catheterization will also give an adequate sample.

Bacteria

Bacteria will multiply quickly, so the sample must be read as soon as possible after collection. Bacteria can be confused with stain precipitate, so fresh stain should be used and comparison between stained and unstained samples should be made. Cocci are round bacteria, spirochetes are spiral shaped, and bacilli are rod shaped. Bacteria in the presence of increased white blood cells indicate a bacterial infection. Samples should be further analyzed by culture and sensitivity to confirm choice of the correct antibiotic for treatment.

Fungi

Fungal infection of the urinary tract is rare. Presence of yeast is usually from contamination in free-catch samples or environmental contamination. Exceptions may occur with pathogenic yeast such as blastomycosis. Yeast will generally be budding or the fungus may develop filaments called hyphae. If present, fungal culture will be needed.

Parasites

Ova from several parasites may be seen in the urine. Most of the urinary parasites do not cause severe pathology.

Dioctophema renale is the largest known nematode and can infect most mammals. The male can be 45 cm and the female 103 cm in length. Its intermediate host is the earthworm. *D. renale* usually infects the left kidney and can destroy the entire kidney on that side. Because the other kidney is rarely infected, clinical signs are minimal and it is usually diagnosed at necropsy. On urinalysis a large, brownish-yellow, lemon-shaped egg with two polar plugs is seen. Prepatent period (time from infection to production of eggs) is 3 to 6 months. Single sex infections will not produce ova.

Capillaria plica and *Capillaria felis* are the bladder worms of carnivores. They also have the earthworm as the intermediate host. They are very small worms. The eggs have polar plugs and look very similar to *Trichuris vulpis* (seen in feces) and *Eucoleus aerophila* (seen in feces or sputum) ova.

Casts

Casts are tube-shaped cylinders found in the urine; they are made from proteins that are secreted in the renal tubules. This mucoprotein is called Tamm-Horsfall protein. Cells may be embedded in the cast. High numbers of casts can indicate renal tubular disease (nephrosis).

Hyaline Casts

Hyaline casts are only the mucoprotein matrix. They generally have rounded ends and parallel sides and stain uniformly pink with sedi-stain. They may be missed if evaluating unstained slides. It is normal to see up to one hyaline cast/HPF. Hyaline casts are increased in fevers, exercise, and mild renal tubular disease. They will dissolve in low-SG urine.

Cellular Casts

Cellular casts can include epithelial, white blood cell, and red blood cell casts. No cellular casts should be seen in normal animals.

Epithelial cell casts are renal epithelial cells stuck in the mucoprotein. They are the earliest indicator of renal tubular damage and may indicate toxicity of drugs that can damage the kidney (gentamycin, tetracyclines, etc.).

White blood cell casts form with inflammation of the renal tubules. They are generally neutrophils. They are seen in diseases causing bacterial pyelonephritis (kidney infections).

Red blood cell casts indicate renal hemmorhage.

Granular Casts

Granular casts are degenerated cellular casts. As the name suggests, they appear grainy on microscopic exam. Similar to epithelial cell casts, if seen in large numbers, they indicate renal tubular disease. A few (0–1/HPF) may occur in normal animals.

Waxy Casts

Waxy casts are usually associated with chronic renal disease. They are believed to be the result of granular cast degeneration in the kidney. They are clear casts with sharp, broken-off ends. None are seen in normal animals.

Microbiology

Microbiology is very important in diagnosis and in the choice of treatment for patients. In some cases, a gram stain may be adequate for identification of bacteria, but most often culture (growth of the bacteria in a sterile medium) is needed for identification. Luckily, many types of media are available for growth of bacteria and some of them allow differentiation of microbes into groups based on their metabolism of certain products. This allows rapid identification and helps to narrow down the choice of medications.

Sensitivity testing of organisms should also be performed. Sensitivity refers to how effective an antibiotic is against a particular organism. This helps the veterinarian to make a better choice of antibiotic for treatment.

Cultures may be obtained by a sterile swab in a transport medium or by sending a liquid (or solid) sample in a sterile container. It is important to avoid contamination of the sample by environmental contaminants. It is also important to avoid contamination of the technician by the sample, because many bacteria and fungi are zoonotic. Samples should arrive at the laboratory for processing as quickly as possible. This will reduce the chance that contaminating bacteria or fungus will divide and overgrow the pathogenic organism.

When the specimen arrives, the first test to perform is a gram stain to determine whether the organism is gram positive or gram negative and whether it is a bacillus (rod) or a coccus. The culture medium is then inoculated (specimen is added to the medium) and incubated in an incubator at body temperature for 18 to 24 hours. If there is growth, that is termed a positive plate. Growth is usually small, separated, round colonies on a plate of agar or cloudiness in a broth. The colonies are then selected from the plate, gram-stained again, and replated on a differentiating medium that will allow the technician to check the metabolic properties of the organism. The new plates are again incubated.

The gram stain is used to differentiate organisms based on cell wall structure. **Gram-positive** bacteria have sugars in their cell wall. **Gram-negative** bacteria have a lipid (fat) coating. After the sample or colony is collected with a sterile loop (a thin wire that has been sterilized in a flame), it is smeared onto a slide and allowed to dry. The slide is then passed through a flame quickly 3 to 4 times to heat fix, specimen-side up. This will kill the bacteria, allow stain to penetrate, and cause the bacteria to stick to the slide. The slide should be placed on a staining rack. All the staining materials should be available prior to beginning the stain because timing is important. Gram's crystal violet is flooded onto the slide and allowed to sit for 30 seconds. The slide is rinsed with water and flooded with Gram's iodine for 30 seconds, then rinsed again. Decolorizer (methyl alcohol) is then poured on quickly and rinsed off immediately. The slide is rinsed again with water. Safranin is then poured onto the slide and rinsed off after 30 seconds. The slide is allowed to air dry.

The iodine step is the reason that the gram stain works. The crystal violet penetrates the sugar cell wall of both gram-positive and gram-negative bacteria. The iodine complexes with the crystal violet and makes it too big to leave the cell in gram-positive bacteria. The decolorizer dissolves the leftover crystal violet that is not complexed and rinses away, leaving the gram-positive bacteria purple and the gram-negative bacteria clear. The safranin binds to fats, so it sticks to the gram-negative bacteria, making them red.

The bacteria are then examined on oil immersion (100×) to assess their shape. Rods may be gram positive or gram negative. Most gram-negative bacteria are either enteric bacteria (live in the guts or respiratory tract) or external contaminants. Gram-negative bacteria can be pathogenic. Some gram-negative rods move on a wet prep. This is called motility. Gram-negative rods can be further differentiated by growth on Mac-Conkey agar, oxidase activity, and oxidation or fermentation testing.

Most gram-positive bacilli are nonpathogenic and are seen as contaminants. Important species of gram-positive bacteria that can cause disease include *Listeria, Corynebacterium, Erysipelothrix, Actinomyces, Nocardia*, some *Bacillus*, and *Clostridium*. Some gram-positive rods form spores, which are difficult-to-kill structures that can survive in the environment for long periods of time. Important spore formers are *Clostridium* and *Bacillus*. Further differentiation can be made by catalase, oxidase, and oxidation/fermentation testing.

Cocci are spherical and are rarely motile (*Listeria* is one exception). Most cocci are gram-positive. The only gram-negative cocci of interest in veterinary medicine include *Neisseria* spp. *Neisseria gonorrhea* causes gonorrhea in humans. Other *Neisseria* species occur in the mouths and the vaginal tracts of animals. Gram-positive cocci may be further differentiated by catalase testing and coagulase testing.

Spirochetes are spiral-shaped, motile bacteria. The most important spirochete is *Leptospira*.

Growth Media

Growth media are substances that can be inoculated with bacteria or other organisms and support their growth. They may be either pure-growth media, differentiating media, or selective media. Growth media are generally used for single-colony incubation in preparation for sensitivity testing.

Differentiating media have substances added on which the bacteria act, causing a color change either in the colony or in the agar.

Selective media have substances added that can either be inhibitory to growth (cause reduced growth) of sensitive bacteria or kill them outright. Some media are both differentiating and selective.

Agar

Agar is made from seaweed. It is actually a long-chain sugar molecule. It comes in powder form, to be mixed with water, heated, and poured onto plates or into tubes where it solidifies. It provides a solid surface for bacterial growth and can be mixed with many substances to make selective or differentiating media prior to solidifying. Bacterial colonies can be examined for color, size, and texture on agar.

Plain agar will not support growth for many organisms, so an enrichment medium such as nutrient broth is often added.

Nutrient Broth

Nutrient broth contains beef extract and peptone, which provide nutrition for many species of bacteria. More bacterial types can grow in nutrient broth than on agar gel. Evidence of bacterial growth is seen as increased turbidity (cloudiness) of the sample. The drawbacks to nutrient broth are that colony characteristics cannot be seen or evaluated. It is usually used for single-colony incubation.

Blood Agar

Blood agar is agar mixed with mammal blood (usually from sheep). Blood agar is used for diagnosis of gram-positive organisms. The concentration of blood is 5% in the total agar volume. Colonies that cause hemolysis will destroy the red blood cells in the agar. Beta-hemolytic (β hemolysis) organisms completely lyse the red blood cells, leaving a clear zone around the colony. *Streptococcus hemolyticus* (causes strep throat) is an example of a beta hemolytic organism. Alpha hemolysis (α hemolysis) causes partial red blood cell destruction and will leave a greenish zone around the colony (*Streptococcus viridans*). Beta-hemolytic organisms are usually much more pathogenic. This means that blood agar is a differentiating medium.

Chocolate agar is agar with lysed red blood cells added. This gives it a brown color. This may be used to grow some bacteria that are difficult to grow, such as *Neisseria*.

MacConkey Agar

MacConkey agar is both selective and differential. This means that it will only grow specific bacteria and the bacteria that will grow can be told apart by the characteristics of the colony. MacConkey agar contains bile salts and crystal violet, which inhibit the growth of gram-positive bacteria. Lactose is added to the agar along with a color indicator (neutral red). Colonies that can ferment lactose show up as pink colonies. Most of the lactose fermenters are enteric bacteria.

Brilliant Green Agar

This agar is highly selective for *Salmonella*, *Escherechia*, and *Pseudomonas*. It will inhibit the growth of gram-positive bacteria and most other gram-negative rods. The normal color of the agar is orange-brown. Growth of lactose or sucrose fermenters (see MacConkey Agar) will cause the agar to turn yellow. The *Salmonella* colonies will be white to red with a red zone in the agar. *Escherechia* colonies will be yellow surrounded by green zones in the agar. *Pseudomonas* will have red colonies with yellow zones in the agar. Because all three of these organisms are pathogenic, this is a great differentiating medium for gram-negative organisms.

Saboraud's Dextrose Agar

Saboraud's dextrose agar (SDA) is used to culture fungi. It contains gentamicin and chloramphenicol to inhibit gram-negative bacteria and is very acid, which inhibits gram-positive bacteria. This is the best medium to use for culturing dermatophytes (ringworm).

In dermatophyte testing, SDA may be plated on one side with a differentiating medium (SDA plus cyclohexamide and phenol red as a color indicator) on the other side. The cyclohexamide inhibits fungal contamination from the environment. In the differentiating medium, dermatophytes will cause a red color change in the agar surrounding the colony.

In either case, the colony should be checked by performing a lactophenol blue stain for definitive identification of fungus. Fungal identification is based on the fruiting bodies and the hyphae. The fruiting bodies are the spores of the fungus and have definite shapes based on the fungus. The hyphae may be septate (segmented) or aseptate (no segments); this fact can be used for further differentiation. The most common species are *Microsporum canis* (cats and dogs), *Microsporum gypsum* (cats and dogs), *Trichophyton mentagrophytes* (rabbits and cats), and *Trichophyton equinum* (horses). All species are zoonotic.

Testing

Further testing of colonies is important because differentiating media may not be enough to discover the species. Testing can also help to determine which antibiotics will be necessary for treatment.

Differentiating Tests

The following tests will enable the technician to narrow down the species of the bacteria.

Catalase Test

The catalase test should be performed on any gram-positive organism. Catalase breaks peroxide into hydrogen and oxygen. Since hydrogen and oxygen are gases at room temperature, if the bacteria are placed on a slide with a drop of peroxide, bubbles will form. If bubbles form, the bacteria is catalase positive. The technician must be sure to obtain isolated colonies. The colonies should not come from blood agar plates because blood will also cause a catalase reaction with peroxide. If there is more than one type of bacterium in the sample, the results will be inconclusive. Catalase-positive cocci are *Staphylococcus* species.

Coagulase Test

Coagulase testing is used only for gram-positive organisms that are also catalase positive. Coagulase causes coagulation of the clotting factors. The bacterium is added to plasma. If the plasma proteins coagulate, it is called coagulase positive. *Staphylococcus aureus* and *Staphylococcus intermedius* are coagulase positive. Coagulase negative, catalase positive, gram-positive cocci are either *Staphylococcus epidermidis* or *Staphylococcus saprophyticus*.

Oxidase Test

Oxidase testing is typically performed on gram-negative bacteria. In a positive test, a purple color change will be seen on the test strip. The strip contains tetramethyl-p-phenylenediamine, which tests the ability of the bacteria to produce the enzyme oxidase.

Oxidation-Fermentation Test

Oxidation-fermentation testing tests the ability of a bacteria to ferment or to oxidize carbohydrates (glucose). Enteric bacteria, *Pseudomonas* and *Aeromonas*, will grow in the media. The media will either be covered with oil or left open to the air. Organisms that ferment glucose (enteric bacteria and *Aeromonas*) will cause a color change of the entire tube from green to yellow in both the oil-covered and the open tubes. Organisms that will only oxidize glucose (Pseudomonas) will not cause a color change in the tube with oil.

Antibiotic Testing

The choice of the correct antibiotic is extremely important in veterinary medicine. Antibiotic drug residues can enter the food supply or the water table, causing bacteria to become antibiotic resistant and even more highly pathogenic. Formation of super bugs resistant to most antibiotics makes treating both animal and human diseases more difficult and can create a huge public health issue. The choice of the appropriate antibiotic for the appropriate bacteria is much better for the patient as well.

Kirby-Bauer Testing

The Kirby-Bauer test uses disks containing known concentrations of antibiotic to test the bacterial response. The colony of bacteria mixed with enrichment broth is smeared onto the agar plate and the disks are placed onto the agar. The plate is incubated for 18 hours and examined. Antibiotic sensitivity (the ability of the antibiotic to kill the bacteria) is seen by examining the *zone of inhibition* around the disk. This is a clear area surrounding the disk that indicates lack of bacterial growth. The size of the zone in millimeters indicates the effectiveness of the antibiotic.

Minimum Inhibitory Concentration (MIC)

The minimum inhibitory concentration is the lowest concentration of an antibiotic that will stop the growth of a bacteria after incubation. It may be performed on either broth or agar. This technique not only evaluates the choice of antibiotic, but can also tell the veterinarian the dosage of antibiotic needed to fight the infection.

Practice Questions

1. Which statement is true of Mallophaga?
   a. They suck blood.
   b. The environment must be treated with insecticides in order to control them.
   c. They live in hair follicles.
   d. Their heads are wider than their thorax.

2. Which of the following is true of Cochliomyia?
   a. It can invade living tissue.
   b. It is a facultative parasite.
   c. It carries malaria.
   d. It can cause stomach ulceration.

3. Which of the following is true of Simulium?
  a. They lay their eggs in rapidly moving water such as streams and brooks.
  b. They lay their eggs in puddles.
  c. They lay their eggs in slow-moving water such as rivers.
  d. They lay their eggs on the animal's hair.

4. Which of the following does NOT have a life cycle similar to that of the other three?
  a. *Hypoderma*
  b. *Gasterophilus*
  c. *Cuterebra*
  d. *Musca*

5. Which of the following about flea infestation is *false*?
  a. Flea allergy symptoms are generally seen on the rump and tail head.
  b. *Ctenocephalides canis* is the causative agent in most cases of canine flea infestation.
  c. Pulex irritans can carry bubonic plague.
  d. The flea pupa cannot be killed by ordinary means.

6. A dog comes into the clinic with signs of nonspecific lameness, mild fever, and a rash. He was on vacation in West Virginia three weeks ago at a campsite with his family in the mountains. The owners said he had a few ticks and fleas when he came back home, so they applied tick control two weeks ago. He has been otherwise normal. They saw a lot of animals on their trip including white-tailed deer, bear, and bobcats. The SNAP® test was positive for *Borrelia burgdorferi*. What type of tick is the most likely?
  a. *Dermacentor*
  b. *Rhipicephalus*
  c. *Amblyomma*
  d. *Ixodes*

7. A hunting dog is brought into the clinic with hind-end paralysis. Which of the following ticks may cause these symptoms?
  a. *Dermacentor*
  b. *Ixodes*
  c. *Rhipicephalus*
  d. *Amblyomma*

8. A rabbit is brought into the clinic with severe dandruff. On physical exam, the dandruff appears to be moving around. What is it?
  a. *Chyletiella*
  b. *Otodectes*
  c. *Sarcoptes*
  d. *Psoroptes*

9. Which stage of the protozoal life cycle is resistant to disinfection?
  a. trophozoite
  b. cyst
  c. sporozoite
  d. tachyzoite

10. You have performed a fecal exam on a kitten that has come from the humane society in your area. You find very small, unsporulated oocysts on the direct exam. The kitten has a mild fever but is otherwise fine. Which of the following is *most* likely?
  a. *Isospora*
  b. *Eimeria*
  c. *Cryptosporidium*
  d. *Toxoplasma*

11. Which of the following would NOT be appropriate for testing a dog with giardia?
  a. direct fecal exam
  b. centrifugal float with Sheather's solution (saturated sugar)
  c. ELISA test
  d. passive flotation with zinc sulfate solution

12. Which of the following is NOT zoonotic?
   a. *Cryptosporidium*
   b. *Eimeria*
   c. *Balantidium*
   d. *Giardia*

13. Which of the following does NOT live in the intestines of the definitive host as an adult?
   a. *Ancylostoma*
   b. *Trichuris*
   c. *Paragonimus*
   d. *Toxascaris*

14. Which of the following does NOT have similar-looking ova?
   a. *Eucoleus*
   b. *Trichuris*
   c. *Dioctyphema*
   d. *Capillaria*

15. An 8-week-old puppy presents with coughing and mild diarrhea. A fecal sample is run and roundworm ova are seen. Which of the following is a roundworm found in dogs?
   a. *Toxocara*
   b. *Toxascaris*
   c. *Strongyles*
   d. both **a** and **b**

16. What can the eggs of cestodes also be called?
   a. hexacanth
   b. oncospheres
   c. embryos
   d. all of the above

17. Which of the following will not cause anemia and dark, tarry stools (melena)?
   a. *Diplydium*
   b. *Spirocerca*
   c. *Physaloptera*
   d. *Ancylostoma*

18. Which of the following is true for hookworm and roundworm infestations?
   a. Stools should be buried in the ground. The eggs will not be infective after one week.
   b. Spraying the yard with bleach is a great way to control infestations.
   c. Picking up all stool in the yard will control the infestation within two to three weeks.
   d. They are difficult to control with normal means.

19. What is diagnosis of *Spirometra* (a fluke) based on?
   a. Finding an oval ovum with multiple cells inside it.
   b. Finding a golden-colored ovum with a pointy end and an operculum.
   c. Finding a golden-colored ovum with 2 polar plugs and a thick shell.
   d. Finding a round ovum with a yellow shell and a heavily pigmented center.

20. A puppy mill consistently sells puppies that come to the pet store with roundworms and coccidia. What do you tell the owner of the puppy mill?
   a. Explain proper stool disposal and disinfection of the environment with 10% bleach for the coccidian.
   b. Explain transmammary infection.
   c. Explain that treatment must include all the animals in the puppy mill with two different medications.
   d. All of the above.

21. How many intermediate hosts do flukes have?
   a. 0
   b. 1 to 2
   c. 2 to 3
   d. 3 to 4

22. What does *Echinococcus* in the intermediate host cause?
   a. hydatid cyst disease
   b. sparganosis
   c. diarrhea
   d. pernicious anemia

23. What is the reproductive element of the tapeworm?
   a. the scolex
   b. the bothria
   c. the proglottid
   d. the hydatid cyst

24. Which of the following has the highest specific gravity?
   a. Sheather's solution
   b. zinc sulfate
   c. sodium nitrate
   d. saturated sodium chloride

25. Which of the following would be best retrieved from a sedimentation procedure?
   a. *Toxocara*
   b. *Spirometra*
   c. *Paragonimus*
   d. *Trichuris*

26. A cat comes into the clinic for polyuria/ polydipsia of three weeks duration. She is BAR (bright, alert, and responsive). Urinalysis showed an SG of 1.012 with no other abnormalities on either the dipstick or the sediment. Her PCV was 45 and her TP was 7.2. BUN and Cr were within normal range. What should be on the list of differentials for this cat?
   a. renal failure due to glomerular disease
   b. renal failure due to tubular disease
   c. severe cystitis
   d. none of the above

27. A rabbit presents with a urolith. Which of the following crystal types is the likeliest cause of bladder stones in this species?
   a. struvite
   b. calcium oxalate
   c. calcium carbonate
   d. ammonium biurate

28. A 6-month-old miniature schnauzer puppy presents with seizures three hours after eating. You do not have an in-house lab, so the blood work (CBC and blood chemistry panel) was sent to a reference laboratory. In the meantime, you run a urinalysis. The urine shows low SG, pH of 6, ammonium biurate, and uric acid crystals. Which of the following blood tests should be run in addition to the ones listed above?
   a. ammonia
   b. cortisol
   c. amylase
   d. estradiol

29. A 24-year-old cat has an SG of 1.012 and granular casts are seen on the sediment. The urine protein is within normal limits and the serum TP is normal. The BUN and Cr are slightly elevated. What, if anything, is the problem?
   a. glomerular disease
   b. renal tubular disease
   c. liver disease
   d. nothing (this is normal for an old cat)

30. What does turbidity of urine indicate?
   a. increased bilirubin
   b. increased fat
   c. increased protein
   d. increased glucose

31. Which of the following would NOT cause increased urine pH?
   a. a high-protein diet
   b. a urease producing bacteria
   c. urine exposed to room air for more than 30 minutes
   d. metabolic alkalosis

32. A urine glucose of 2+ will cause what increase in the urine's SG?
   a. 0.000
   b. 0.001
   c. 0.002
   d. 0.003

33. A cat has an SG of 1.050. How was the measurement performed?
   a. urine dipstick reading
   b. refractometer
   c. urinometer
   d. none of the above can read a specific gravity that high

34. Which of the following will cause the destruction of hyaline casts?
   a. high specific gravity
   b. high pH
   c. both of the above
   d. neither of the above

35. A dog has an SG of 1.012 and a TP of 5 g/dl. His urine protein is negative. Which of the following is true?
   a. he has renal tubular disease
   b. his low SG is due to overhydration
   c. he has glomerular disease
   d. he has diabetes mellitus

36. A dog has an SG of 1.040 and a TP of 8 g/dl. His urine protein was 3+. Which of the following is probable?
   a. he has renal tubular disease
   b. he has glomerular disease
   c. he is dehydrated
   d. his tubules and glomeruli are in disorder

37. A cat has an SG of 1.020 and a TP of 6 g/dl. Her urine protein is negative and she has a urine glucose of +2 and a urine ketone of +1. What is her disease?
   a. renal tubular disease
   b. low specific gravity due to overhydration
   c. glomerular disease
   d. diabetes mellitus

38. A dog has a urine pH of 8.5. Which of the following crystals will form in that pH urine in the dog?
   a. calcium carbonate
   b. uric acid/urate
   c. bilirubin
   d. calcium oxalate

39. A dog has a urine pH of 6. Which of the following crystals will form in that pH?
   a. calcium carbonate
   b. magnesium ammonium triple phosphate
   c. amorphous phosphate
   d. ammonium biurate

40. Which type of cell is contained in an epithelial cell cast?
   a. caudate (renal) cell
   b. transitional cell
   c. squamous cell
   d. white blood cell

41. Which type of cell will NOT be seen in a cystocenthesis sample?
a. caudate cell
b. transitional cell
c. squamous cell
d. white blood cell

42. Which of the following is NOT common in cats with renal failure?
a. polyuria
b. stranguria
c. proteinuria
d. isosthenuria

43. Which pigment is associated with brown urine color?
a. hemoglobin
b. myoglobin
c. urochrome
d. urobilinogen

44. Which of the following pads should NOT be used on the urine dipstick in animals?
a. leukocytes
b. ketones
c. pH
d. blood

45. Which is true of catheterization in the bitch?
a. The urethral papilla is located on the most ventral portion of the vestibule.
b. The vaginal speculum should be sterile.
c. The vagina should be flushed with chlorhexidine solution to minimize bacteria.
d. The catheter should be measured from the vulva to the umbilicus for proper length.

46. Why are enteric bacteria the most common causes of kidney and bladder infections?
a. They tend to leave the intestines through the blood stream and lodge in the capillaries of the kidneys.
b. They tend to transmit them when sniffing each other.
c. They tend to cause ascending infections that come from bacteria from the external genitalia.
d. They are the most common causes of skin disease.

47. Ketonuria is NOT caused by which of the following?
a. breakdown of fats and proteins by anaerobic metabolism
b. starvation
c. diabetes mellitus
d. hypoadrenocorticism

48. Which of the following is a breakdown product of hemoglobin?
a. urobilinogen
b. chromogen
c. myoglobin
d. porphyrin

49. Bilirubinuria will NOT result from which of the following?
a. extravascular hemolysis
b. severe liver disease
c. dilute urine
d. cholestasis

50. What is the renal threshold?
   a. The concentration of blood glucose that is too high for the kidneys to reabsorb.
   b. The concentration of bilirubin that exceeds the kidneys' ability to control.
   c. The highest blood pH that the kidneys can compensate for.
   d. The maximum amount of damage the kidneys can sustain before spilling protein into the urine.

Answers and Explanations

1. d. Mallophaga have heads that are wider than their thorax. They cause itchiness and remain on the surface of their host, so they do not need to have environmental treatment, just treatment on the animal.

2. a. Cochliomyia can invade living tissue, which makes it a very dangerous parasite. Most other myiasis producers live only in the epidermis of the animal. Cochliomyia is an obligate parasite, so it requires an animal host for part of its life cycle. It does not invade the gastrointestinal system. Mosquitoes carry malaria; Cochliomyia does not.

3. a. Simulium prefers to lay its eggs in rapidly moving water. Most of the other flies prefer either stagnant water, feces, or the animal's hair.

4. d. *Musca domestica* is a facultative myiasis producer. The other three are obligate myiasis producers.

5. b. *Ctenocephalides canis* is the more common cause of flea infestation in the dog and actually prefers the dog to the cat as a host. Flea allergy is usually seen on the rump and tail head. Pulex irritans is the human flea and does carry bubonic plague. The pupa is the only phase of the flea life cycle that is difficult to kill.

6. d. *Ixodes scapularis*, the deer tick, is the most common tick associated with Lyme disease. The other ticks on the list are not carriers of Lyme disease.

7. a. Gravid (pregnant) *Dermacentor* ticks are most commonly associated with tick paralysis in dogs. The symptoms can include paralysis leading to respiratory paralysis and possible death, but will resolve within 48 hours if the tick is removed.

8. a. *Chyletiella* is the mite associated with walking dandruff. *Otodectes* is the ear mite, *Sarcoptes* and *Psoroptes* are both scabies mites.

9. b. The cyst is the stage that is resistant to disinfection. The trophozoite and tachyzoite are within the host and the sporozoite is susceptible to disinfection.

10. d. *Toxoplasma* is the most probable. *Eimeria* does not infect cats, *Cryptosporidium* is rare in cats, and *Isospora* have large oocysts.

11. b. Sheather's solution would burst the cysts of giardia. Zinc sulfate solution is the preferred float for giardia cysts. The trophozoites may be seen on a direct fecal and the ELISA test for giardia is excellent and may be done in house.

12. b. *Eimeria* is not zoonotic because it is host specific. *Cryptosporidium*, *Balantidium*, and *Giardia* have all been diagnosed in humans.

13. c. *Paragonimus kellicotti* is a liver fluke. *Ancylostoma*, *Trichuris*, and *Toxascaris* all infect the GI system of the definitive host.

14. c. *Dioctyphema renale* has a lemon-shaped, bumpy, yellow, double-polar-plugged large egg. *Eucoleus*, *Trichuris*, and *Capillaria* all have smooth, football-shaped shells with double polar plugs.

15. d. *Toxocara* and *Toxascaris* will both infect dogs. *Strongyles* are seen in equines.

16. d. Cestode ova can also be called hexacanth, oncospheres, or embryos.

17. a. *Diplydium caninum* is the only one that does not cause some type of gastrointestinal ulceration. *Spirocerca* and *Physaloptera* infect the stomach and esophagus causing ulceration. *Ancylostoma* sucks blood in the intestines.

18. d. These ova and larvae are difficult to control with ordinary means. Burying the stool in the ground will not work because roundworm eggs stay patent in the soil for months to years. Hookworms will also stay in the soil for extended periods of time. Roundworm ova are resistant to most disinfectants.

19. b. All fluke eggs have a golden color, a pointy end, and an operculum. Polar plugs are seen on *Trichuris*, *Capillaria*, and *Eucoleus*. A round ovum with a pigmented center is *Toxocara* species and an oval ovum with multiple cells inside is generally a hookworm.

20. d. All of the above. Roundworms are transmitted by transmammary infection as well as by fecal-oral contamination. Treatment for rounds should be with pyrantel or febantel; treatment for coccidia should be with sulfa drugs.

21. b. Flukes have 1 to 2 intermediate hosts, one of which is generally either a snail or copepod.

22. a. *Echinococcus* causes hydatid cyst disease in the intermediate host. Sparganosis is caused by *Diphylobothrium*. Diarrhea and pernicious anemia may be seen in the definitive host.

23. c. The reproductive element (sexual form) is the proglottid. The scolex and the bothria are the head pieces and the hydatid cyst is the asexual form of the parasite.

24. a. Sheather's solution has the highest specific gravity of all the listed solutions. Sodium nitrate has the lowest.

25. c. *Paragonimus* is a trematode. Most trematodes, other than *Spirometra*, are best retrieved by sedimentation. *Toxocara* and *Trichuris* are best retrieved by centrifugal flotation.

26. b. Renal failure due to tubular disease will cause a decrease in specific gravity. Normally, cat urine is very concentrated (>1.035). Glomerular disease results in increased protein. Cystitis will cause sediment changes in the urine.

27. c. Calcium carbonate is the most common crystal found in herbivores with high pH urine. The other crystals are either seen in acid pH (ammonium biurate) or more frequently in carnivores (struvite, calcium oxalate).

28. a. Ammonium biurate and uric acid crystals are commonly seen in animals with portosystemic shunts. The history of eating-related seizures and acid pH urine leads us to this possible differential. Ammonia levels can be an indicator of liver bypass by the portal circulation. Cortisol would test for adrenal gland dysfunction, amylase for pancreas dysfunction, and estradiol is a reproductive hormone.

29. b. This is probably renal tubular disease because the specific gravity is low, granular casts were present, and the BUN and Cr were elevated, indicating renal azotemia. If the urine protein were elevated, glomerular disease would also be a possibility.

30. c. Protein levels cause turbidity. Although fat droplets also increase the cloudiness of the urine, they will separate out on centrifugation. Bilirubin changes the color of the urine.

31. a. A high-protein diet decreases urine pH. Urease producing bacteria, metabolic alkalosis, and exposure to room air for >30 minutes all increase urine pH.

32. c. Urine glucose increases SG by 0.001 for every +1 glucose on the stick. Urine protein increases SG by the same amount for every +3 protein on the stick.

33. c. The urinometer must be used if the urine SG on the refractometer is over 1.040. The urine dipstick for SG should never be used for animal urine.

34. b. High pH and low specific gravity will both dissolve hyaline casts.

35. b. He has a low SG due to overhydration because his total protein was low, and his urine protein was negative. If his urine protein were elevated, there would be the possibility of protein-losing nephropathy (glomerular disease).

36. c. He is probably dehydrated. His specific gravity and total protein were both elevated and this can also increase the concentration of protein in his urine.

37. d. This cat has diabetes mellitus: glycosuria, ketonuria, low SG. The glucose causes an osmotic diuresis, which decreases the specific gravity of the urine without renal tubular disease.

38. d. Calcium oxalate crystals can form in any pH urine. Calcium carbonate crystals are only seen in herbivores and urate and bilirubin crystals are only seen in acid urine.

39. d. Ammonium biurate crystals form in acid urine. Magnesium ammonium triple phosphate (struvite) and amorphous phosphate crystals only form in alkaline urine and calcium carbonate crystals are seen in herbivores.

40. a. Caudate cells are the cells lining the renal tubules and are seen with epithelial cell casts. Transitional cells line the bladder and the urethra, squamous cells are from the genital tract, and white blood cells are indicators of inflammation.

41. c. Squamous cells would not be seen on cystocenthesis samples because they are from the genital tract, not the urinary tract.

42. b. Stranguria is straining to urinate. This is most commonly seen with cystitis. Polyuria, proteinuria (glomerular disease), and isosthenuria (tubular disease) are commonly seen with renal failure.

43. b. Myoglobin is commonly associated with brown urine. Hemoglobin turns the urine red, urochrome turns it yellow, and urobilinogen turns it greenish yellow.

44. a. The leukocyte pad on the urine dipstick should not be used for animal urine because it is not accurate. The ketone, pH, and blood pads are very useful.

45. b. All materials used for catheterization of the bitch should be sterile, including the gloved hands. The urethral papilla is located on the floor of the vagina at the intersection of the vestibule with the vagina. Flushing with chlorhexidine could cause irritation. The catheter should be measured from the vulva to just cranial to the pubis.

46. c. Enteric bacteria tend to cause ascending infections first to the bladder and then to the kidneys. It is rare to have intestinal bacteria come through the bloodstream to the kidneys, and they do not usually cause skin disease.

47. d. Ketonuria is caused by the breakdown of fats and proteins due to starvation and diabetes mellitus (perceived starvation). Hypoadrenocorticism does not cause ketones.

48. a. Urobilinogen is the end product of hemoglobin metabolism. Myoglobin is similar to hemoglobin and broken down in a similar fashion. Porphyrin is a precursor to hemoglobin and myoglobin. A chromogen is any substance that can be converted into a pigment or dye.

49. c. Dilute urine will not cause bilirubinuria. Bilirubinuria results from the breakdown of red blood cells (hemoglobin metabolism) or cholestatic diseases (including diffuse liver disease).

50. a. The renal threshold is the concentration of blood glucose that causes spillover into the urine. This occurs because it overwhelms the body's ability to reabsorb it.

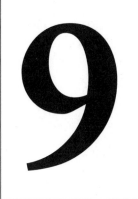

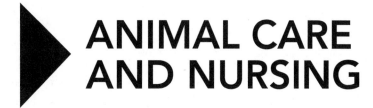

ANIMAL CARE AND NURSING

CHAPTER OVERVIEW

The veterinary technician has a moral and ethical duty to provide compassionate nursing care to the patients in his or her care. Knowledge of appropriate handling and restraint of a variety of species is necessary to prevent injury to oneself and to the patient. It is important for the veterinary technician to be familiar with common animal diseases and conditions and preventative health schedules.

Safe methods of restraint and handling that utilize understanding of normal species behavior form the foundation of providing effective nursing care to animal patients. Nutritional needs, disease risk, and vaccination schedules are influenced by species, age of the animal, and the geographical locality.

Key Terms

Bordetella bronchiseptica
bovine respiratory syncytial virus (BRSV)
canine adenovirus type 1 (CAV-1)
canine adenovirus type 2 (CAV-2)
canine distemper virus (CDV)
canine parainfluenza virus (CPIV)

canine parvovirus (CPV)

Clostridium perfringens

EEE/WEE/VEE (Eastern, Western, and
Venezuelan equine encephalomyelitis)

equine infectious anemia (EIA)

equine influenza

equine rhinopneumonitis (EHV-1 and
EHV-4)

equine strangles

erysipelas

Escherichia coli

feline calicivirus

feline herpesvirus (feline viral
rhinotracheitis)

feline immunodeficiency virus (FIV)

feline infectious peritonitis (FIP)

feline leukemia virus (FeLV)

feline panleukopenia (feline distemper)

hardware disease (traumatic reticulo-
pericarditis/-peritonitis)

infectious bovine rhinotracheitis (IBR, or
bovine herpesvirus type 1)

kennel cough

leptospirosis

Mannheimia haemolytica (formerly *Pasteurella
haemolytica*)

milk-and-meat withdrawal time

parainfluenza type 3

Pasteurella multocida

Potomac horse fever (equine monocytic
ehrlichiosis)

rabies

Salmonella

scours

snuffles

tetanus antitoxin

tetanus toxoid

vent disease

West Nile virus (WNV)

Concepts and Skills

The following nine concepts are reviewed in this chapter:

- methods of restraint used for animals
- basic nursing and clinical procedures
- administration of medications
- catheters and catheterization
- clinical nutrition
- emergency care and procedures
- common diseases of animals
- pediatric medicine
- preventative health care

Methods of Restraint Used for Animals

The goal of the veterinary technician is to use the minimal amount of restraint necessary to perform the procedure safely. The objective of restraint is to keep the animal from injuring itself or the caregivers. Restraint techniques are broken down into those appropriate for large animals such as horses, cattle, sheep, and pigs, and those for small animals such as dogs, cats, birds, reptiles, and pocket pets.

Restraint of Large Animals

Horses

Horses should be approached in a quiet, calm manner. Address the horse by name and speak quietly to it as you approach it. Avoid approaching from or standing in the animal's blind spot directly behind it. The horse's halter should be secured while standing on the left, or near, side of the animal (the right is known as the offside), and a lead rope should also be attached to the halter. *Never* wrap the lead rope around your hand in case the animal is startled; instead, hold the excess lead folded within your hand.

A horse should be led from its stall prior to the physical examination. The handler should lead the horse from the left side and should always stand on the same side of the horse as the examiner. For additional control, a chain on the lead shank may be passed over the muzzle and attached to the halter. A chain twitch or humane twitch may be applied to the horse's upper lip to keep the animal still.

A nervous or aggressive horse can kick up to 6 to 8 feet directly backwards and may strike with its front legs as well. For maximum safety an aggressive or nervous horse can be placed in stocks. Always close the rear gate before attempting to tie the head of a horse in stocks.

A foal can be restrained by grasping it around the neck and under the tail simultaneously. Care must be taken not to alarm the mare and not to unintentionally move one's body between the mare and the foal.

Cattle

Dairy cattle in free stall barns are easily captured in head locks at the feed bunk or by simply standing behind their stall and blocking the exit. Cows in stanchion or tie-stall barns are already captured, but may require additional restraint for certain procedures. A halter or nose leads or tongs can be used to tie the cow's head to one side for jugular venipuncture.

Raising the cow's tail to an erect midline position (tail-jacking) can provide additional restraint for examination of the mammary glands or for intramuscular injections.

Beef cattle are generally captured by driving them into successively smaller enclosures until finally they are driven into an alleyway just wide enough for the animal to pass through without attempting to turn around. A mechanical chute at the exit point of an alleyway can be used to trap a beef animal for routine veterinary procedures.

Cattle are cast (pulled into recumbency) by placing a single long rope as a loop around the haltered animal's neck (or around the animal's neck but passing between the forelimbs), then placing a half-hitch around the girth and another around the flank. The animal can now be pulled to the ground by a person standing directly behind it and pulling on the rope. Care must be taken not to incorporate a bull's testicles or a cow's udder into the half hitch. Alternatively, cattle may be cast by marking half the length of a rope and placing it on the back of the animal's neck; the ends of the rope are now criss-crossed between the animal's forelegs, then both ends of the rope are brought up to the dorsum where they are criss-crossed again, and finally both ends of the rope are passed ventrally between the udder or testicles and leg. Both ends of the rope are pulled straight back to cast the animal.

Sheep

Sheep are easily driven into small enclosures as they tend to flock together when approached and will want to stay with the other animals. An individual animal is caught similarly to a foal, that is, by grasping it around the neck and around the rump simultaneously.

Sheep are set up on their rumps for routine clinical procedures. To accomplish this, the handler reaches between the forelimbs with one hand to tilt the animal backwards as the other hand reaches for the hindlimb of the opposite side and lifts the sheep's weight off of the leg. The animal is sitting upright and leaning against the legs of the handler.

For tail docking and castration of lambs, the lamb is held in dorsal recumbency with its hind legs grasped between the hock and fetlock, pulled forward and grasped with the forelegs to secure all four limbs.

Pigs

A hog snare can be used to capture and immobilize pigs in a small enclosure. The handler stands behind the animal, and a metal cable attached to a handle is placed around the pig's upper jaw behind the incisors. The pig will usually pull back against the snare and squeal loudly and continuously until the snare is removed. Ear protection is essential for the technician who will be working with swine.

Restraint of Small Animals

Dogs

Always make sure that doors, runs, and exercise yards are closed and secure before removing a dog from its ward (cage or run). A dog that has escaped may avoid capture with submissive behavior, or may become aggressive when cornered (fear biting). Use caution, speak softly, and reassuringly, and offer the back of the hand with one digit protruding to form a nose. Continue to watch the dog's eyes, ears, face, and body posture for clues about aggression. Small dogs can be distracted with a duster or similar long object that can be safely used to give the dog something to strike or attack.

Handling Aggressive Dogs

Small breeds may be handled with heavy leather gloves. Dogs can often be induced to bite at the fingers of the glove on one hand, while the other hand can grab the dog, and put on a lead rope with a slip knot. Before letting go, the other handler can then attempt to muzzle the dog. Sometimes a gauze muzzle works well; a commercial muzzle can be applied over the gauze strip if desired. Usually when a dog is muzzled, its behavior becomes more submissive. Never leave a muzzle on any longer than necessary. Dogs can asphyxiate in a muzzle if they vomit, their body temperatures will increase because they cannot pant as effectively, and geriatric patients and patients with certain medical conditions, especially heart or lung disease, can die if they are restrained too vigorously

An aggressive large dog is a major challenge but may be handled with a pole restraint or a cable snare called a *rabies pole*. Use two poles and two handlers for very large dogs.

Another method that is useful if the dog comes into the office on a leash involves trapping (known as *snubbing*) the dog close to a door with the door open a crack, thread the leash through to a handler on the other side. This handler will pull the leash through the cracked door until the dog's collar is pulled snug to the door. This restrains the dog's head to prevent biting when a dog cannot be muzzled. The veterinarian or technician can then grab the dog's hind leg and administer vaccinations or sedatives.

Cats

A cat that seeks to escape will seek out a hiding place. Covering the animal's head or putting a large towel in the cage can help capture a stressed cat. Heavy leather gloves or a large towel can also be used if a cat is responding to the handler with flattened ears, hissing, scratching, growling, and biting.

As was done with small dogs (above), a duster or similar long object that can be safely introduced to the cat's vicinity can be used to give the cat something to strike or attack. Nets, which may have a handle or a metal frame, are sometimes used to hold a fractious cat for IM or IV injection of a chemical restraining agent. The net method can be used for vaccines as well. A loop leash can be placed over the cat's head, then the scruff of the neck may be grasped to lift the cat out of a cage. Quickly stretch the cat by grasping the hind legs with the other hand. Extremely aggressive cats may be tranquilized in the carrier if the carrier has a wire mesh door or wire mesh sides. Extremely aggressive cats in ward cages may have to have a loop put around their neck and be pulled to the door of the cage to have a chemical restraint agent injected or squirted into the mouth.

Capture boxes (chambers) have ports so inhalation anesthetic agents can be piped in. These are used for the most difficult cats. In a pinch, placing a large plastic bag over the carrier can create a temporary capture chamber. Both of these methods have a disadvantage: a lot of anesthetic gases will be vented into the immediate environment, exposing personnel to the anesthetic.

Many cats will lie in a prone position on the exam table. They need only minimal restraint (mild neck scruff) that does not completely limit their movement. Some cats do better when they can clutch a towel for security. An aggressive cat may need to be stretched: one hand grasps it by the scruff of the neck and the forearm of the handler supports the cat's back as the other hand grasps its hind legs; the handler stretches the hind legs as the neck is held in extension. Some cats do better if they are left in the carrier for exams or treatments. Unless the carrier opens from the top or is a soft-sided carrier with zipper openings, this will require taking the carrier apart and putting it back together at the end of the appointment.

Birds

For smaller birds, hold the neck on either side of the skull with one hand and the legs with the other hand. Control the wings to avoid trauma by reaching over the back of the bird and holding the wings down to the body. Larger birds may be wrapped in a towel that holds the wings against the body. If possible, grasp the wings with one hand while holding the legs between the fingers of the other hand. *Do not* immobilize the sternum as birds lack a diaphragm and may suffocate. A restraint board can be used for radiographs.

Reptiles

Turtles and tortoises may have sharp beaks and claws that should be avoided. A towel may be placed over their heads to prevent their walking off the examination table. Gentle digital pressure or delivery forceps may be used to extend the head from the shell.

Examination of the snake is managed by immobilizing the head with your hand, tongs, plexiglass tubes or shields, or a snake hook. A snake may also be placed into a plastic box filled with inhalant gases to induce anesthesia and facilitate examination.

Care must be taken when handling small lizards to avoid the mouth and teeth. Lizards should never be grabbed by the tail as they may automatize (spontaneously separate) the tail from the body.

Ferrets

When picked up by the scruff of the neck, ferrets generally yawn and hang limply from the scruff. Many clinical procedures such as examination, ear cleaning, nail trimming, and injections may be attempted in this position. Ferrets love sweet tastes and may be distracted with Nutrical® or hairball remedies. Remember that certain states have made it illegal to keep a ferret as a domestic pet.

Rabbits

Rabbits are carried securely, supporting both the forequarters and hindquarters, with the head tucked into the crook of the handler's arm. To restrain a rabbit for examination, the handler should place the hands between the animal's front legs to control the forequarters and support the chest; as well, the hindquarters need to be controlled to prevent kicking and injury to the animal's back. A towel placed on the exam table adds security. Alternatively, a rabbit can be wrapped snugly in a towel (to make a kind of bunny burrito). Aggressive rabbits should be handled with heavy leather gloves as they can scratch. Never restrain, grab, or carry a rabbit by the ears. Always return a rabbit to the cage hind end first.

Rodents, Guinea Pigs, and Hamsters

Rats are picked up by grabbing them over the neck and shoulders. To provide additional restraint for procedures, hold the tail and hind limbs with the opposite hand. The tail base may be used to catch a rat in its cage temporarily, but you must be cautious as the tail skin can easily tear. Small rodents are captured by grabbing the tail close to the body and moving the animal to your forearm or hand. They can be held by the scruff of the neck for routine clinical procedures and injections. Alternatively, mice can be lifted by the tail as they are allowed to grasp onto a wire cage to restrain for subcutaneous injections.

Guinea pigs may whistle loudly when restrained. They feel comfortable in close quarters and often feel secure if held snugly. When removing a guinea pig from the cage, it is best to scoop him up with one hand and immediately support the rump with the free hand.

Hamsters are picked up by grasping its scruff with one hand and supporting its body with the other hand. Alternatively, the hamster may be picked up by cupping it in the hands, or by gripping over the back.

Basic Nursing and Clinical Procedures

All patients should be provided with a clean, comfortable environment. Fresh water and food should be available at all times, and adequate exercise needs to be provided, unless restricted for medical reasons. Dogs need to be given the opportunity to urinate or defecate outside or in a run at least twice daily. Litter boxes need to be changed at least daily, and smaller or disposable litter pans may need more frequent cleaning. Nonambulatory patients need to be checked and rolled from side to side frequently to prevent bedsores (known as *decubital sores*).

Anal sacs hold the secretions produced by the anal glands lining the walls of the sacs. Signs associated with impacted anal glands include scooting or dragging the perineum on the floor and excessive licking. Empty the anal glands by inserting a lubricated gloved forefinger into the rectum. Palpate the glands at the 4 o'clock and 8 o'clock position, and apply gentle pressure. The glands produce a foul-smelling discharge, and the animal may require bathing after expression of the sacs.

When animals are bathed, a protective lubricant ointment should be placed in the eyes and dry cotton placed in the ears until the end of the procedure. *Never* leave a tied animal unattended in the tub.

Administration of Medication

There are three ways to administer medication: enteral, topical, or by injection.

Enteral administration means that the medication is introduced into the digestive tract, either orally or rectally.

Oral administration is the most common route of administration of medication. For dogs, hiding a tablet or capsule in a piece of meat, cheese, or peanut butter usually works. For cats, pry open the mouth, place the tablet on the back of the tongue, quickly close the mouth and then stroke the cat's throat or blow in its nose to encourage the cat to swallow. For cattle and other livestock, oral medications may be administered in bolus form using a balling gun, as a paste, or mixed in with the ration or drinking water. Orogastric intubation is used to deliver medications such as mineral oil, barium, and charcoal. The tube is measured in advance from the nose to the level of the thirteenth rib and marked to indicate how far it should be passed. The tube should be lubricated and a speculum placed in the animal's mouth to keep it from biting and swallowing the tube. The tube should be bent to occlude it prior to removal to prevent aspiration of liquids.

The rectal mucosa can absorb certain medications such as diazepam and antiemetics. Enemas may be used to soften stool or to stimulate defecation; they may consist of warm soapy water, petrolatum, or glycerine. No phosphate enemas (such as Fleet®) should be given to cats or small dogs.

Topical Treatments

Topical treatments are administered either on the skin (dermal) or through the eyes (ophthalmic) or the ears (otic).

Dermal Treatments

Gloves should be worn when applying topical drugs including transdermal patches and insecticidal shampoos and dips. Alternatively, liquid and semiliquid preparations may be applied via cotton or wooden applicators.

Ophthalmic Treatments

The Schirmer tear test utilizes sterile, absorbent paper strips to measure the production of tears. Any samples for bacterial culture or cytology are collected *before* any drops, ointments, solutions, or medications of any kind are applied to the eye. Tonometry is used to measure intraocular pressure (IOP) with a Tono-Pen® or a Schiotz tonometer, and should be performed *after* a topical anesthetic has been applied, but *before* a mydriatic is applied. Funduscopic exam (examination of the retina) is performed with an ophthalmoscope after a mydriatic has been applied. Fluorescein staining is a test that utilizes a fluorescent dye to evaluate the integrity of the corneal surface. Liquid ophthalmic medications should be instilled onto the bulbar conjunctiva at the 12 o'clock position, taking care not to touch the tip of the applicator to the cornea; ointments should be applied in a thin ribbon along the palpebral conjunctiva, working laterally from the medial canthus.

Otic Treatments

Samples for culture or cytology should be collected before cleaning the ear. The integrity of the tympanic membrane should be confirmed via otoscopic exam prior to instilling medication or cleaners. The pinna is pulled dorsally and slightly caudally to open the vertical ear canal to facilitate examination and treatment.

Injections

Subcutaneous (SQ or SC) administration is the easiest, most frequently performed type of injection. The needle is inserted at a 45-degree angle. It is the most common route for vaccine administration, and is also frequently used for administering isotonic fluids at 10 to 30 mL/lb (ideally 50 to 100 mL per site). The absorption rate is slow because fat has a relatively poor blood supply. The subcutaneous route should not be chosen for fluids containing >2.5% dextrose or other substances that are potentially irritating when administered via this route.

Intravenous (IV) administration is the fastest route for a medication to reach high blood levels. Examples of drugs administered via the IV route include some anesthetic agents, chemotherapeutic agents, anticonvulsants, and CPR drugs. Cloudy or opaque drugs are not injected intravenously; an exception would be the intravenous anesthetic propofol. Caution must always be exercised when administering IV drugs. Perivascular (the tissues surrounding the blood vessel) injection can be painful and lead to tissue necrosis and sloughing. In addition, certain drugs can be potentially fatal if injected too quickly.

Intramuscular (IM) administration generally results in a faster absorption of drug than the SC route, and slower absorption than the IV route. The needle is inserted at a 90-degree angle, and aspiration should always be performed to confirm that the needle has not entered a blood vessel. The lumbar muscles (epaxial muscles) may be used for IM injections in cats, dogs, and sometimes horses; these muscles should be avoided in food animals to preserve the quality of the carcass at slaughter. The caudal hind leg muscles are commonly used in small animals and horses. Care must be taken to avoid the sciatic nerve. The hind leg muscles should also be avoided in food animals. The cervical muscles are the preferred sites for IM injection in livestock and horses; the injections are given within a triangular region between the head and the shoulder, located dorsal to the jugular vein and ventral to the transverse processes of the vertebrae. For cattle, the IM injection is given in the triceps muscle, and for horses in the pectoral muscles.

Intradermal (ID) administration is used for TB testing of livestock, allergy testing, and local anesthesia. The injection site will appear as a raised lump if done correctly

Intraosseous (IO) administration involves injection into the bone marrow cavity and is used in *small* patients (such as neonates) to rapidly administer medications, fluids, or blood when IV catheterization cannot be performed (for example, in circulatory collapse).

The locations chosen in small-animal patients are the proximal humerus, the femur at the level of the trochanteric fossa, and the wing of the ilium. A local anesthetic and aseptic site preparation must be employed.

Intraperitoneal (IP) administration places drugs directly into the abdominal cavity. The IP route is commonly used in lab animals for anesthetic agents or euthanasia solutions, and also may be used in neonates if IV or IO injection is unsuccessful. There is a risk of accidental puncture of abdominal organs, and care must be taken to avoid the spleen on the left side of the abdomen.

Epidural injection involves administering local anesthetic into the epidural space of the spinal canal (above the dura mater) at the lumbosacral or first interlumbar space. This method is used for pain associated with pelvic surgery and fractures.

Catheters and Catheterization

IV catheter types include butterfly, over-the-needle (OTN), and through-the-needle (TTN). Butterfly catheters have short, rigid needles and wings that may be taped into place. They are for injection or removal of small volumes of fluid, and are not for indwelling use in peripheral veins. OTN are the most common indwelling catheter; a needle (stylet) passes into the vein first, and the catheter is advanced over the needle. Indwelling jugular catheters are TTN catheters; a large needle is inserted first, and the catheter (smaller gauge) passes through the needle. The catheter site should be monitored frequently for redness, swelling, or discharge, and the catheter should be flushed frequently with heparinized saline. Injection caps and ports should be wiped with alcohol before any liquid is injected or withdrawn. Administration sets should be changed every 48 hours and the catheter should be removed after 72 hours and a new one placed in a different vein, unless it is a dedicated catheter used to administer total parenteral nutrition (TPN).

Fluid Administration Rates

Maintenance fluids are given at a rate of 40 to 60 ml/kg/24 hours (30 mL/lb/day). The dehydrated animal will require replacement fluids, which depend on the hydration status. Replacement fluids (fluid deficit) are calculated based on the following formula:

% dehydrated × body wt. (kg) × 1000 = volume of replacement fluid (in ml)

To estimate the degree of dehydration, assess skin turgor and degree of sunken eyes, capillary refill time (normal is <2 seconds), and laboratory criteria such as hemoconcentration on the hematocrit (Hct, or PCV) and/or a urine SG of >1.035 (dog) or >1.040 (cat).

The total daily fluid requirement for a dehydrated animal equals the sum of maintenance and replacement fluids. In addition, ongoing losses (vomiting, diarrhea, etc.) must be corrected for, and it is recommended that you double the estimated volume of the vomit or diarrhea produced (per day):

Total daily fluids = maintenance fluids + fluid deficit + ongoing losses

The rate of fluid administration during anesthesia or surgery is 10 ml/kg/hour. This rate may need to be adjusted in geriatric or ill patients.

Critical or shock fluids are administered to correct hypovolemia. For dogs, a volume of 20 to 40 ml/kg is administered for the first 15 minutes, then 70 to 90 ml/kg over a 1-hour period, then a shock maintenance rate of 10 to 12 ml/kg/hour is administered. For cats the shock rate is 10 to 20 ml/kg for 15 minutes, then 35 to 50 ml/kg over 1 hour, then shock maintenance of 5 to 6 ml/kg/hour. A general rule of thumb across species is that 90 ml/lb can be administered during the first hour, and approximately one quarter of this volume may be initially administered as a fluid bolus.

IV fluid infusion (administration) sets are generally calibrated to deliver 10 drops/ml, 15 drops/ml, or 60 drops/ml (microdrip set). To calculate the number of drops per minute that a patient should receive when a gravity drip method is used, we must know how much fluid is to be administered over what period of time and using which type of drip set:

$$\frac{\text{fluid volume to be infused (ml)}}{\text{number of hours desired}} \times \frac{1 \text{ hour}}{60 \text{ mins}} \times \frac{\# \text{ drops}}{\text{ml}} = \text{drops/min}$$

Alternatively, an IV infusion pump may be used to deliver a specified amount of fluid for a given time period. Patients on IV fluids should be weighed daily and monitored for signs of fluid overload: restlessness, increased respiratory rate, pitting edema, serous nasal discharge, and chemosis.

Clinical Nutrition

The maintenance or resting energy requirement (RER) in kilocalories is calculated according to the following formula:

$$\text{RER} = 70 \times (\text{Body Weight in kg})^{0.75}$$

Energy requirements are influenced by five factors: (1) life stage, (2) activity level, (3) environment, (4) reproductive status, and (5) health status. Young animals may require 2 to 3 times the adult RER. Active animals may need to have their RER multiplied by an activity factor of 1.2 to 1.6; this factor may be as high as 4 to 8 times the RER for certain working dogs in cold environments. During the last third of gestation, RER increases to up to 2 times normal, and during peak lactation, the energy requirement increases by a factor of 3 to 4 times the RER.

Nutrient requirements vary between species. Cats are obligate carnivores, and because of this have several unique increased nutritional requirements compared to dogs and other animals. Essential fatty acids for dogs are linolenic and alpha-linolenic; in ad-dition cats require a dietary source of arachidonic acid. Cats also require high levels of the amino acid taurine, which is only found in appreciable levels in meat. If they are fed taurine-deficient diets they are at risk for developing dilated cardiomyopathy and retinal atrophy. Dogs may synthesize vitamin A from beta-carotene, but cats require a dietary source of vitamin A. Additionally, cats require the B vitamin niacin at four times the level required in dogs because dogs are capable of synthesizing niacin from the amino acid tryptophan. Rumen microbes synthesize B vitamins and vitamin K, which the host ruminant can utilize to meet nutritional needs.

Diet may need to be adjusted to prevent a particular disease, slow the progression of a disease, or treat a specific disease. For patients with food allergies it is important to reduce antigen ingestion through a novel protein source, low allergen ingredients, limited ingredients, or low molecular weight proteins. For patients with cancer, longevity and quality of life can be improved by decreasing soluble carbohydrates to starve cancer cells, increasing fat to meet energy demands, and increasing arginine and omega-3 fatty acids to boost the immune system. The goal with constipation is to normalize GI motility by increasing dietary fiber to >10% and encouraging water intake. Diets for diabetes mellitus should even out the rate of glucose absorption. For dogs with diabetes, feed >10% fiber and decrease the amount of soluble carbohydrates; cats do well with high-protein, low-carbohydrate diets. Diets for heart failure should be sodium restricted. In liver disease states, the protein metabolism may need to be reduced, while maintaining liver glycogen with increasing digestible energy. With obesity, the goal is to maintain intake of all nutrients except energy by decreasing energy digestibility, and replacing digestible calories with indigestible fiber. For renal failure, diets should be designed to reduce signs of uremia, by decreasing the protein and/or feeding high biological value protein. Cats, dogs, and ruminants with a history of uroliths or crystalluria require diets that alter the urine components and urine pH.

Enteral feeding is the preferred method of delivering nutrients whenever possible. Animals can be encouraged to eat by offering a more palatable food, placing a small amount of food on their paw, or by hand feeding. Tube feeding can be accomplished via nasoesophageal or nasogastric (NG), esophagostomy, pharyngostomy, gastrostomy (G-tube), or jejunostomy (J-tube) tubes. When a feeding tube has been surgically placed, the site should be kept clean and covered with a bandage. Commercial liquid diets can be passed through smaller diameter NG tubes, whereas diets such as Hill's a/d® for small-animal patients, or pelleted diets for herbivores, may be blenderized and administered via larger-diameter tubes. Feeding tubes should be flushed after use, and clogs may be broken up with carbonated soft drinks such as cola.

TPN is a sterile liquid nutrient diet that is given IV through a fresh, aseptically placed, dedicated jugular catheter. TPN can lead to sepsis and thrombosis and is only used when other feeding options are not possible.

Emergency Care and Procedures

Triage is the process of sorting out patients according to the severity of their injury or illness. It is broken down into the primary survey and secondary survey. The primary survey consists of the ABCDEs of triage (airway, breathing, circulation, dysfunction, examination). The airway is checked for patency, and the patient is checked for signs of inadequate breathing or respiratory distress. The patient is checked for a heartbeat and pulse. Level of consciousness is evaluated, and papillary light reflex may need to be assessed. Finally an examination for vital signs and baseline data is performed. The secondary survey consists of performing a complete physical, and collecting a patient history, and performing needed laboratory tests.

If respiratory and/or circulatory arrest has occurred, then cardiovascular/cerebrovascular pulmonary resuscitation (CPR/CCPR) is initiated if desired by the client. Basic life support consists of the ABCs of airway, breathing, and circulation. An endotracheal tube is placed, and connected to a source of 100% oxygen. Positive pressure ventilation is supplied via an Ambu bag or an automatic ventilator, or by utilizing the rebreathing bag on a gas anesthetic machine. External cardiac compressions are initiated with the patient in lateral or dorsal recumbency at a rate of 80 to 120 compressions/minute. If one person is performing CPR, 15 compressions are followed by 2 ventilations. With two-person CPR, approximately 20 ventilations per minute (or as fast as the Ambu bag or rebreathing bag can refill) are administered while chest compressions are given continuously. Counterpressure may be applied to the abdominal cavity, alternating with chest compressions to improve blood flow cranially. Internal cardiac massage is indicated when external efforts have not established circulation within 5 minutes.

Advanced life support measures include drugs and electrical defibrillation. IV fluids are administered at shock fluid rates. Some drugs such as atropine, epinephrine, and lidocaine can be administered intratracheally via the ET (endotracheal) tube if given at 2 times the dose. Doxapram and dobutamine may be administered as respiratory and myocardial stimulants respectively. It is advisable for every veterinary hospital and clinic to have a crash cart of emergency drugs and supplies that is stocked and always ready for use. Specific hospital drug protocols for CPR should be posted and readily visible as well.

Common Diseases of Animals

Leptospirosis is a disease caused by the spirochete bacterium *Leptospira interrogans*. There are over 200 distinct subtypes of this bacterium, affecting a variety of species including cattle, horses, pigs, sheep, goats, dogs (rarely cats), and wildlife. The bacterium is very contagious and potentially zoonotic, and PPE must be worn when handling or cleaning leptospirosis suspects. Leptospires is transmitted via the urine of infected animals or by contact with objects that have been contaminated with the urine of infected animals. The disease affects the liver and kidneys, and other organs, although affected animals may be asymptomatic. The clinical presentation of symptoms includes fever, hepatic disease with icterus (jaundice), renal failure, vomiting/diarrhea, and hemoglobinuria. If death results, it is usually from vascular damage and renal failure, but may be from DIC. In large animals, leptospirosis causes infertility, abortion in the middle or last third of gestation, and is also a causative agent of equine recurrent uveitis (moon blindness).

Rabies is an acute viral encephalomyelitis caused by a lyssavirus of the Rhabdoviridae family and is capable of affecting all species of mammals. The affected animal sheds rabies virus in the saliva. Rabies is spread primarily via bite wounds, although it is also possible for rabies to be transmitted via contact of saliva in open wounds or even via intact mucous membranes. The incubation period from time of exposure until development of clinical signs is prolonged (up to 6 months) and variable; however, the majority of cases develop 21 to 80 days post-exposure.

The virus travels via peripheral nerves from the point of inoculation to the spinal cord and the brain where it replicates and is shed. Then it travels, again via peripheral nerves, to the salivary glands, where it is shed in the saliva. Rabies is considered 100% fatal, and death results within a few days of the onset of clinical symptoms. Rabies produces neurologic signs including acute behavioral changes and unexplained progressive paralysis. Other symptoms may include anorexia, signs of apprehension or nervousness, irritability and hyperexcitability, ataxia, dysphagia, changes in voice, circling, seizures, aggressiveness, coma, and anorexia. Wild animals may lose their fear of humans, and nocturnal animals may wander during the daytime. Laboratory confirmation of a diagnosis of rabies is made via testing of brain tissue. The suspect animal is euthanized and the refrigerated (not frozen) head or brain tissue is submitted for testing.

Other common diseases can be readily grouped by the size of the animal they affect.

Large Animals

Cattle

Lactating cows can experience a variety of periparturient problems. Dystocia may be caused by malpositioning of the fetus or by maternal factors such as uterine torsion, uterine inertia, and hypocalcemia. Hypocalcemia, or milk fever, presents as a down cow or an extremely weak animal; care must be taken when administering IV calcium, as too rapid administration may cause cardiac arrhythmia and arrest. A reusable rubber IV simplex with an attached 2-inch 12-gauge or 14-gauge needle is normally used for IV administration in adult cattle. Toxic mastitis can also be life-threatening and results in a down cow that will require treatment with intravenous fluids, anti-inflammatories, and antibiotics. Retained placenta, metritis (uterine infection), and uterine prolapse (*cast her withers*) are also frequently encountered periparturient problems.

High producing animals may develop ketosis from utilizing body stores of fat to meet increased metabolic needs. Lactating dairy cattle are predisposed to forming a displaced abomasum, which may twist if it occurs on the right side. Hardware disease (traumatic reticuloperitonitis) results from a sharp, usually metallic object penetrating through the cow's reticulum and/or the diaphragm and pericardium. It is an intensely painful condition that may require surgery to correct. It is critical to observe **milk-and-meat withdrawal times** when medications are administered to cattle.

Bovine respiratory disease complex (BRD), or shipping fever, is one of the most economically important disease conditions affecting dairy and feedlot cattle. BRD refers to a group of diseases typically affecting young cattle and characterized by nonspecific signs such as coughing, nasal discharge, and auscultable evidence of pneumonia. Viruses associated with respiratory tract disease in ruminants include IBR, PI-3, BRSV, and BVD. **Infectious bovine rhinotracheitis** (IBR) or bovine herpesvirus type 1, causes mild to severe disease.

In feedlot cattle, respiratory disease is the most common presentation of IBR, whereas in breeding cattle IBR can also produce abortions, genital infections, infectious pustular vulvovaginitis (IPVV), and balanoposthitis in bulls. Bovine parainfluenza-3 Virus (PI-3) is capable of causing disease but usually associated with mild to subclinical infections. BVD (bovine viral diarrhea) virus generally produces mild symptoms of respiratory disease and diarrhea, but can result in abortion and congenital defects if a cow is infected during gestation. **Bovine respiratory syncytial virus** (BRSV) is a major agent in initiating BRD, with symptoms of clinical disease resulting from stress and concurrent bacterial infection of the respiratory tract. Bacteria associated with bronchopneumonia in ruminants include *Mannheimia haemolytica* (formerly *P. hae-molytica*), *Pasteurella multocida*, *Haemophilus somnus*, and *Mycoplasma bovis*.

Horses

A common noninfectious disease of horses is chronic obstructive pulmonary disease (COPD, or heaves). COPD is usually seen in horses and ponies >6 years of age, but can occur in younger horses as well. The most common etiology is an allergic and inflammatory response to barn and hay dust (i.e., COPD is a hypersensitivity). COPD is best treated by management changes to reduce exposure to antigen; additional medications such as bronchodilators, antihistamines, and anti-inflammatory drugs may be needed as well.

Another common noninfectious disease of horses is colic, more accurately described as gastrointestinal pain rather than a specific disease. Signs of colic include stamping feet, kicking at the abdomen, lying down, rolling, sweating, and grinding of teeth. Common causes include gas accumulation in the intestines, obstruction, gastric ulcers, colitis/enteritis, colonic volvulus (twisted colon), foreign bodies, and parasites. Treatment of colic ranges from conservative measures (walking, injectable analgesia such as flunixin meglumine, nasogastric intubation with mineral oil, and/or docusate sodium) to surgical correction (for torsions and impactions).

Horses are susceptible to a variety of mosquito- and arthropod-borne causes of equine encephalomyelitis including **Eastern, Western, and Venezuelan equine encephalomyelitis** (EEE/WEE/VEE). Encephalomyelitis is characterized by disturbed consciousness, motor irritation, and commonly high mortality rates.

All of these viruses are potentially zoonotic, although typically the affected horse harbors low levels of virus in the bloodstream. EEE is the most pathogenic and is seen in the eastern United States and Canada. WEE occurs in the western United States and Canada. VEE is seen in South America and Mexico, and horses in border states are vaccinated to provide a barrier to entry of this disease into the United States. **West Nile virus** (WNV) was previously a foreign animal disease, but has been endemic in the United States since 1999. Symptoms include weakness and muscle tremors, with high mortality seen in horses (30% to 40%). Vaccines are available for all of the aforementioned causes of encephalomyelitis.

Common causes of equine respiratory disease include equine rhinopneumonitis, equine influenza virus, and *Streptococcus equi*. **Equine rhinopneumonitis** is caused by a herpesvirus (types EHV-1 and EHV-4), and in addition to respiratory disease, it may result in abortion in pregnant mares. **Equine influenza** virus usually causes mild flu-like symptoms of fever, cough, and depression, and has an increased incidence in young animals (1 to 3 years). *Streptococcus equi* (strangles) is a very contagious respiratory disease characterized by abscessation of the submandibular and retropharyngeal lymph nodes. An immune-mediated disease known as purpura hemorrhagica is a possible severe adverse effect of strangles infection or vaccination.

Potomac horse fever (equine monocytic Ehrlichiosis) is a rickettsial disease caused by *Ehrlichia risticii*. Mosquitoes and ticks are the suspected insect vectors of this diarrheal disease, which may result in death. It is unknown whether the vaccine reduces incidence of disease.

Tetanus (lockjaw) is caused by the organism *Clostridium tetani*, a gram-positive rod found in the soil and in the gastrointestinal tract of normal animals. *C. tetani* is contracted via deep puncture wounds or incisions, and may occur in small ruminants at the time of tail docking (lambs), dehorning, or castration. *C. tetani* produces a potent neurotoxin in necrotic tissue to which all mammals are susceptible, although horses are the most susceptible animal, secondary only to humans.

Tetanus is characterized by spasmodic, tonic contractions of voluntary muscles triggered by stimulation such as noise. Typical symptoms in horses consist of erect ears, stiff, extended tail, prolapsed third eyelid, dilated nares, extension of the head and neck, a sawhorse stance caused by stiff leg muscles, and difficulty walking, turning, and backing. Sheep, goats, and pigs may fall to the ground when startled in opisthotonos (stargazing) posture. Mortality is up to 80%. Prevention and control are via immunization with tetanus toxoid and/or tetanus antitoxin. **Tetanus toxoid** produces active immunity or increased antibody levels against *C. tetani*. **Tetanus antitoxin** provides passive protection by neutralizing unbound toxin; this effect lasts up to two weeks.

Small Animals

Dogs

Canine distemper virus (CDV) is a contagious, incurable, often fatal, multisystemic viral disease that affects the respiratory, gastrointestinal, and central nervous system. The initial symptom is fever (103°F to 106°F), and dogs may subsequently experience eye and nose discharge, depression, and anorexia. After the fever, symptoms vary considerably, depending on the strain of the virus and the dog's immunity, but may include conjunctivitis, rhinitis, diarrhea and vomiting, fever, pneumonia, secondary bacterial infections, neurological symptoms, and death (50% mortality). Puppies may develop enamel hypoplasia if infected prior to the eruption of permanent teeth, and hyperkeratosis of the footpads and nose (hardpad disease) may be seen. The disease is spread via aerosol droplet secretions, and young, unvaccinated animals are the most susceptible to CDV.

Many different agents contribute to the disease process of infectious tracheobronchitis (**kennel cough**). The most common viral causes are **parainfluenza type 3** and **canine adenovirus type 2** (CAV-2), and the most common bacterial cause is *Bordetella bronchiseptica*. CAV-2 commonly exhibits comorbidity with B. bronchiseptica in cases of kennel cough. Usually the dog has a history of contact with other dogs in the past 2 to 10 days. Symptoms include a dry hacking cough sometimes followed by a retching, honking sound, and watery nasal discharge may also be present.

In mild cases, the dog continues to eat and be alert and active. With severe cases the symptoms may progress and include lethargy, fever, anorexia, pneumonia, and in very severe cases, even death. The majority of severe cases of CAV-2 occur in immunocompromised animals or in young unvaccinated puppies. **Canine parainfluenza virus** (CPIV), another virus that may cause kennel cough, is commonly comorbid with *B. bronchiseptica*. Parainfluenza causes mild to severe respiratory symptoms of coughing and gagging, wheezing, and sneezing, and is easily transmissible through contact with the secretions of infected dogs. Treatment consists of supportive care based upon symptoms, and the patient is preferably treated at home unless critically ill, as the virus is highly contagious. Although the disease is rarely fatal, it can be, especially in young puppies.

Canine hepatitis is a disease of the liver and other body organs caused by **canine adenovirus type 1** (CAV-1). The disease is spread by body fluids including nasal discharge and urine. Symptoms include coughing and occasionally pneumonia. The cornea may appear cloudy or bluish (hepatitis blue eye), and as the liver and kidneys fail, one may notice seizures, increased thirst, vomiting, and/or diarrhea. CAV-1 vaccination is no longer recommended because the CAV-2 vaccine protects against both strains, and there is significant risk of vaccine-induced blue eye.

Canine parvovirus (CPV) is a potentially fatal, extremely contagious virus that commonly occurs in shelters or anywhere there are high volumes of unvaccinated puppies. Symptoms include vomiting and severe diarrhea, depression, lack of appetite, and leucopenia. Affected canines often succumb to dehydration, and untreated pups can die within hours. The disease is caused by a mutation of the virus that causes feline distemper. Parvovirus is transmitted through the fecal matter of infected dogs. Key isolation and cleaning procedures are necessary within the clinic to prevent transmission to other patients. Canine coronavirus affects the intestinal tract of dogs and also causes diarrhea. Coronavirus rarely causes clinical disease, and if the disease occurs it is usually mild and self-limiting.

Lyme disease, or borreliosis, caused by the spirochete bacterium *Borrelia burgdorferi*, is a relatively new disease, first identified in the town of Lyme, Connecticut, in the 1970s. Disease results from exposure to bacteria that are introduced to the body via an *Ixodes* tick bite. Lyme disease cannot be spread directly between infected patients, but rather requires intermediate hosts (deer, ticks). Borreliosis produces a wide range of symptoms such as shifting-leg lameness, swollen joints, fever, lethargy, lymphadenopathy, and anorexia. Blood tests can identify patient infection, and infected patients are treated with long courses of antibiotics. Other tick-borne diseases that produce similar symptoms to Lyme disease and are likewise treated with antibiotics include Rocky Mountain spotted fever, carried by *Dermacentor* ticks, and canine Ehrlichiosis, which is transmitted via dog ticks.

Cats

The feline upper-respiratory infection complex is a group of viral and bacterial infections that cause sneezing and discharge from the eyes and nose. Disease is spread via aerosol droplets and fomites, and is highly contagious. Cats often have two or more of these upper respiratory infections at the same time, and feline viral rhinotracheitis and calicivirus are the most common viral causes of clinical disease.

Feline viral rhinotracheitis (**feline herpesvirus type 1**, or FHV-1) produces the hallmark sign of sneezing that worsens over 3 to 5 days. Other clinical symptoms may include ulcerative stomatitis or ulcerative keratitis (corneal ulcer), fever (≤105°F), conjunctivitis, anorexia, and nasal and ocular discharge. The mortality rate is low, except for young kittens and aged cats. As with other herpesviruses, infection is chronic, and clinical signs may reappear with stress. Suspected infected cats should be kept in isolation from other cats.

Feline calicivirus is characterized by upper respiratory symptoms, pneumonia, oral ulceration (sores in the mouth), and occasionally arthritis. Normally, calicivirus produces fairly mild flu-like condition and rarely causes serious complications, but novel strains may have unusually high morbidity and mortality. Feline chlamydiosis (also known as feline pneumonitis) is caused by the bacterium *Chlamydophila felis* (formerly *Chlamydia felis*), and produces relatively mild, chronic upper-respiratory disease.

Symptoms include conjunctivitis, nasal discharge, sneezing, and pneumonia. Left untreated, the infection tends to become chronic, lasting weeks or months. Feline *Bordetella* is caused by the same bacterium that may produce kennel cough in dogs. Clinical signs include sneezing, dry cough, nasal discharge, fever, increased lung sounds, swelling of submandibular lymph nodes. In some cases, the animal may be asymptomatic.

Feline panleukopenia (feline distemper) is caused by a parvovirus and is a highly contagious disease that is common wherever cats exist. Transmission is via direct contact with the secretions of the infected cat via aerosol droplets or fomites. Isolation practices and disinfection are crucial to preventing spread of the disease within the clinic; the virus is stable outside of the body for a year. Feline distemper can present with a wide variety of symptoms, ranging from mild to severe, and including depression, anorexia, fever, panleukopenia (greatly reduced numbers of all types of white blood cells), and vomiting leading to dehydration. Without quick identification and supportive care, feline distemper can result in death.

Feline leukemia virus (FeLV) is a devastating, fatal virus that affects the immune system, leaving the cat vulnerable to all infections. Transmission occurs through direct contact with infected saliva from bite wounds, saliva left on food or water bowls, and typically an infected queen (as female cats with litters are known) will transmit the virus to her kittens via grooming activity. Symptoms include fever, frequent infections, weight loss, depression, decreased appetite, swollen lymph nodes, and sometimes leukemia. The disease is incurable, and can only be treated with supportive care. All new cats and kittens should be blood tested for feline leukemia prior to introducing them to other cats in a household. The disease may be prevented in at-risk cats by vaccination.

Feline immunodeficiency virus (FIV) is another destructive and fatal virus for which there is no cure. FIV is spread primarily via bite wounds and fighting. The infected cat may live a relatively normal life for a period of time, but eventually the virus affects the immune system, and the infected cat becomes unable to fight off infections and illnesses. Common symptoms include fever, recurring infections and illnesses, weakness, depression, weight loss, and lack of appetite. Preventing contact with potentially affected cats is the best method for avoiding the virus.

Feline infectious peritonitis (FIP) is another serious, destructive virus affecting cats, It is commonly found in high-population areas such as shelters, hoarders, and large stray populations. It is caused by a coronavirus, which is stable outside of the body, and disinfection is important to minimize spread. Transmission is primarily fecal-oral and occurs via contact with the infected cat's secretions: saliva, feces, dirty litter box, water bowl, and so on. Infected asymptomatic queens usually infect their kittens. Initial symptoms include upper respiratory symptoms, depression, weight loss, and lack of appetite. Weeks to months later, the virus may produce a lethal form of the disease. Two types of the lethal disease are recognized, the wet or effusive form, and the dry or non-effusive form. Wet type FIP infected cats typically have large pot-bellied abdomens filled with fluid and/or pleural effusion that eventually causes respiratory distress. Dry type FIP infected cats can exhibit a variety of clinical signs depending on where immune-mediated granulomas develop.

Ferrets

Most ferrets have been neutered and descented (that is, their anal sacs have been removed) prior to adoption as indicated by their ear tattoos. Females that have not been spayed can experience prolonged estrus which results in a swollen vulva, hair loss, and potential aplastic anemia (lack of production of all types of blood cells in the bone marrow) due to high estrogen levels. Ferrets are commonly infected with ear mites and fleas, and may be treated with topical products such as imidocloprid for fleas, selamectin for fleas and mites, and otic products containing ivermectin.

Unfortunately, ferrets exhibit an extraordinarily high level of neoplasia, with most ferrets developing at least one of three common types of cancer in adulthood: lymphoma, adrenocortical adenocarcinoma, and insulinoma. Adrenocortical disease should be suspected in any neutered ferret exhibiting signs of hair loss or a swollen vulva. These conditions may be managed with chemotherapy, surgery, or a combination of chemotherapeutic agents and surgery.

Respiratory viruses affecting ferrets include influenza and canine distemper. Influenza is a reverse zoonosis, that is, a ferret may become ill from contact with sick humans in the household. Canine distemper has a 100% mortality rate in ferrets, but can be prevented with ferret-specific vaccines. A common ferret GI problem is gastrointestinal foreign body, and owners should be cautioned about allowing ferrets to roam about the house without supervision. Gastric ulcers caused by the *Helicobacter* bacterium are another common ferret GI problem that can be treated with oral medications.

Avian and Exotic Animals

A common disease of pet birds is ornithosis, caused by the bacterium *Chlamydia psittaci*. The disease is transmitted via inhalation of the bacteria, and may cause a potentially fatal zoonotic pneumonia (psittacosis) in humans. Affected birds may be asymptomatic or may have signs of air sacculitis, nasal and ocular discharges, or nonspecific signs such as weight loss, anorexia, ruffled feathers, weakness, or lethargy.

Poultry commonly harbor **Salmonella** species, which are passed via the fecal-oral route and can cause severe diarrhea in humans. Care should always be taken when handling chickens, turkey, and ducks to exercise hygiene and utilize PPE. Poultry also may develop respiratory disease from the avian influenza (bird flu) virus, another zoonotic disease. Suspect animals should be quarantined and/or euthanized to minimize spread to commercial flocks and humans.

More than 90% of reptiles harbor *Salmonella* bacteria, and clients must be counseled with regard to the zoonotic potential. Good hygiene and use of PPE are a must. A pet reptile should never be placed in the family bathtub while the aquarium is being cleaned as this is one of the common ways that humans are exposed to *Salmonella*.

Laboratory Animals

Laboratory animals include rabbits, rodents, mice, hamsters, gerbils, and guinea pigs.

Rabbits

Rabbits should be fed a high-fiber timothy hay–based ration for healthy digestive tract function, to prevent trichobezoars (hairballs), and to help prevent overgrowth of incisors. Rabbits produce both day feces, a firm pelleted fecal ball, and night feces, a wet, soft feces, which the rabbit ingests to undergo further digestion to maximize the nutritional value of the feed. A sick rabbit might have night feces that has not been reingested visible in its cage or enclosure. Malocclusion and overgrowth of incisors and/or molars are common problems in the rabbit, with genetics playing an important role. Malocclusion and overgrowth can lead to weight loss and anorexia, and routine dental care is important for affected animals.

A major disease of rabbits is **snuffles**, caused by the bacterium *Pasteurella multocida*. *P. multocida* can produce a range of respiratory, neurologic, and dermal signs including nasal discharge, torticollis (wry neck), caseous skin abscesses, conjunctivitis, ocular discharge, and dyspnea. The disease is not readily eliminated by antibiotics; however, intermittent use of antibiotics such as enrofloxacin may be employed to reduce the severity of clinical signs. Caution must always be used when administering antibiotics to rabbits, as diarrhea may be induced. Infectious and parasitic causes of diarrhea in rabbits include coccidiosis and clostridial bacteria.

Rabbits are prone to skin conditions associated with ear mites, fur mites, lice, and fleas, and may be treated with imidocloprid, fipronil, or ivermectin, depending on the condition. In addition, fight wounds are common as rabbits can be surprisingly aggressive toward other rabbits; routine spaying and castration may reduce the incidence. Rabbit syphilis (**vent disease**) is caused by the spirochete bacterium *Treponema cuniculi*. Vent disease causes infertility, and is treated with penicillin and probiotics to prevent diarrhea.

Rodents

Rats are prone to developing mammary tumors, which may be benign or malignant and are routinely removed surgically. Upper respiratory infection (URI) with signs of nasal discharge and dyspnea is common in rats, often due to infection with Mycoplasma bacteria. Porphyrins or red pigments produced by the harderian glands may color ocular and nasal discharge and can be confused with blood. Rats with paraplegia may have spinal lymphoma causing compression of the spinal cord.

Mice

Mice are territorial, and fight wounds tend to be seen on the rumps of group-housed males. Mammary tumors are common and tend to be malignant. Ulcerative dermatitis is an intensely pruritic skin condition caused by mites.

Hamsters

Hair loss in hamsters may be caused by the *Demodex* mite. Hamsters tend to be aggressive toward other hamsters, and females may cannibalize their litters if disturbed by humans or other hamsters. *Wet tail* is a nonspecific term for diarrhea (enteritis) and can be fatal in the case of antibiotic-induced enteritis. Fluid distension of the abdomen may be seen associated with ovarian tumors and heart failure.

Gerbils

Gerbils are prone to developing a staphylococcal bacterial dermatitis around the nose due to their burrowing behavior. Some lines of gerbils are also prone to epilepsy, which may be treated with a phenobarbital elixir.

Guinea Pigs

Cavies (guinea pigs) require vitamin C in their diets or else they develop symptoms associated with scurvy (vitamin C deficiency). Milled foods should be fed within 90 days of production; otherwise the guinea pig should be supplemented with a source of vitamin C such as tablets, oranges, or powdered Tang in the drinking water. Strangles (cervical lymphadenitis) is a condition characterized by submandibular abscesses and is caused by inoculation with *Streptococcus zooepidemicus* following trauma to the oral cavity. Treatment of strangles consists of sedation, lancing

and flushing the abscesses, and antibiotics. Care should be taken when administering antibiotics to cavies, as they are susceptible to clostridial overgrowth. Mange mites and fleas are common skin problems that can be treated with ivermectin and imidocloprid respectively. Dystocia requiring C-section is likely to occur if the first breeding has not occurred prior to 6 to 8 months of age, because the pelvic symphysis will fuse to a narrow position.

Pediatric Medicine

Young animals such as calves, foals, puppies, and kittens need special attention.

Calves

Immediately after the birth of a calf, the navel is dipped into an antiseptic such as Betadine® solution, and within 12 hours, the calf should receive a minimum of 2 quarts of colostrum. The calf may also receive an injection of vitamin E and selenium to prevent white muscle disease. The cow is typically allowed to lick the placenta and amniotic fluid off the calf, and then the calf may be allowed to nurse from the cow (beef animals), or the calf is removed from the cow (dairy animals) and bottle-fed the colostrum to ensure adequate passive transfer of maternal antibodies. Between one week and 3 weeks old, routine dehorning is performed, permanent identification (ear tag) may be applied to the ear, and in the case of dairy animals, any supernumerary teats may be removed by the veterinarian, tails are sometimes docked for cleanliness, and any bull calves that are still on the farm may be castrated.

A common health problem of calves that can be a source of high mortality is diarrhea (**scours**). Common causes of scours in calves less than 3 weeks old include *E. coli*, rotavirus, and coronavirus, all of which can be prevented or reduced in severity by vaccinating the dam during the dry period and ensuring adequate intake of colostrum or commercial oral monoclonal antibodies at birth. Treatment of scours includes frequent small feedings alternating milk replacer and electrolytes, and IV fluids in severe cases. The coccidian *Cryptosporidium parvum* and *Salmonella* are potentially zoonotic causes of diarrhea that typically strike slightly older calves. There is no effective treatment for cryptosporidium, but coccidia can be prevented with feed supplements or treated with anticoccidial drugs.

Foals

Neonates should have the navel dipped in an antiseptic such as Betadine® shortly after birth. An enema is given to assist in the passing of the first stool, known as *meconium*. A blood sample is taken for an immunoglobulin test at 12 to 24 hours to evaluate for failure of passive transfer. Passive transfer refers to the passage of protective immunoglobulin proteins from the mare into the colostrum, or mare's first milk, which is ingested by the foal. Passive transfer is a method of providing natural immunity to diseases that the foal has never been exposed to. A foal that has received no or inadequate colostrum will be at greatly increased risk for developing disease in the neonatal period. No vaccines are indicated for the neonatal foal if the mare was vaccinated prepartum, the mare received a vitamin E and selenium injection perpartum, and there has been no failure of passive transfer.

Otherwise, the foal should be given a dose of tetanus toxoid, 1,500 U of tetanus antitoxin (not in the same syringe as the tetanus toxoid, and not in the same injection site!), and a vitamin E and selenium injection.

Small Animals: Puppies and Kittens

Resuscitation may be required following dystocia or C-section. The umbilical cord is ligated by clamping, suturing, or tying off. The airway is cleared of amniotic fluid, placental membranes, and meconium by vigorously swinging the neonate in a back and forth motion between the handler's legs while the spine and body are carefully supported in a towel. Stimulate the neonate to breathe by rubbing vigorously with a towel; if there is apnea, administer a drug such as Dopram (doxapram) injected sublingually. In addition, a 25-gauge needle may be placed to stimulate at an acupuncture point located at the midline of the point where the nose meets the upper lip as an aid to stimulate breathing. Just as in calves and foals, colostrum is essential in the first 24 to 48 hours to provide the neonate with passive immunity to disease. Check the neonate for the presence of a cleft palate, which may be evidenced by difficulty nursing or milk passing through the nares. The umbilical cord falls off at 2 to 3 days, and the umbilicus is checked for hernia and/or infection. Eyes open at 5 to 14 days, and ear canals open at 6 to 14 days.

The typical neonatal puppy and kitten has a body temperature of 95.9°F–97.9°F and a heart rate of 180 to 250 beats per minute. Neonatal puppies are poikilothermic (the body temperature varies with the ambient temperature), and the whelping box should be maintained between 86° and 95°F, gradually reducing ambient temperature to 75°F over the next 3 weeks. Because body fat stores are only 1% to 2% of body weight at birth, the neonate is at increased risk for hypoglycemia, hypothermia, and starvation. Hypothermia leads to inadequate nursing, which further complicates hypoglycemia. Puppies and kittens should be weighed *daily*. Healthy neonates should gain between 10% and 20% of their body weight daily during the first two weeks of life. The birth weight should double in 12 days. Supplemental feedings with milk replacer may be required

Signs of distress in the neonate include crying (or lack of crying), restlessness, failure to gain weight, and failure to thrive, and may be caused by factors such as crowding, lack of maternal milk, and cleft palate. Management of severely ill neonates includes external warming, parenteral fluid (which may require intraosseous catheterization), glucose supplementation to prevent or treat hypoglycemia, and good nutrition. In addition, the neonate may require oxygen or antibiotics, the doses of which are reduced by 30 to 50% if the patient is less than 5 weeks old, as liver enzymes will not be fully functional.

Hand-rearing orphan puppies or kittens can be accomplished by tube feeding or bottle feeding. Tube feeding (orogastric intubation) is safer (less risk of aspiration) and is faster. Commercial milk replacement formulas are available for puppies and kittens, and should be delivered to meet a daily energy requirement of 25 kcal/100g body weight. The total daily requirement is divided into four feedings. Food in gruel form is introduced at 3 to 4 weeks of age. Puppies and kittens under 2 weeks of age often do not urinate or defecate spontaneously. A cotton ball or paper towel is used to gently rub the abdomen and perineum to stimulate urination and defecation several times daily.

Preventative Health Care

Preventative medicine involves ways to prevent diseases rather than simply treating the symptoms of illness. Our discussion is divided into large and small animals.

Large Animals

Vaccination schedules for cattle vary depending on history of herd problems and potential exposure to disease. A 3-month-old heifer may receive a rabies vaccine and a clostridium 7-way vaccine (to prevent various diseases), and vaccination against the bovine respiratory disease complex (BRSV, PI-3, *Pasteurella*).

At 4 to 8 months old, heifers are vaccinated for the bovine respiratory diseases IBR, BVD, PI3, and BRSV. This vaccination is repeated in 3 to 4 weeks and then boosted annually; heifers may be vaccinated for brucellosis as well. Brucellosis vaccination can only be given by a USDA-accredited veterinarian. Vaccinated animals are identified with a tattoo on the right ear; the tattoo consists of the letter *R* followed by a V-shaped vaccine shield and a number. The R indicates that the recombinant vaccine was used, the V indicates

that the animal was vaccinated, and the number represents the last digit of the year in which the vaccine was given. Vaccinated animals are identified with an orange ear tag in the right ear, the first 2 digits of which identify the state in which it was given. Brucellosis vaccine cannot be given at less than 4 months old due to maternal antibody interference. If it is given after 12 months old, it will interfere with testing for routine surveillance and sale purposes (the animal may be a false positive). Brucellosis causes contagious abortion in cattle, also called Bang's disease, but it has been eliminated from most of the United States. Brucellosis is zoonotic and causes undulant fever, a chronic recurring disease in humans.

Lactating cows should be vaccinated for leptospirosis, IBR, and BVD, all of which can cause abortion in pregnant animals. Modified live virus vaccines of BVD should not be administered to pregnant cows as they can produce calves that are persistently infected with the virus.

Ideally a dairy cow will be in lactation for 10 months of the year and then be dried off 60 days prior to her due date. A dry cow antibiotic treatment is infused into each teat to prevent mastitis. *E. coli*, rotavirus, and coronavirus multivalent vaccines are recommended to prevent calf scours, and are administered one month before the due date; first calf heifers should initially receive a series of 2 vaccines given 3 weeks apart and then revaccinated annually, along with a vitamin E and selenium injection to help prevent retained placenta after calving.

Vaccination and testing requirements for cattle prior to sale depends on the state of origin and the destination state. The usual requirements are TB dermal testing (which must be performed by an accredited veterinarian), brucellosis blood testing, and an interstate health certificate. Blood testing for bluetongue or other additional tests may also be required prior to sale. A shipping fever vaccine (vaccine(s) containing BRSV, PI3, IBR, BVD and *Pasteurella*, +/– *Hemophilus*) is recommended before the animals leave the farm.

Small ruminants are routinely vaccinated for enterotoxemia (overeating disease) caused by **Clostridium perfringens** types C and D. In addition, sheep and goats should have limited access to lush pasture and grain to help prevent enterotoxemia. Lambs and kids should receive 2 doses administered 2 weeks apart starting at 6 to 8 weeks of age in their first year, and then boosted annually. The dam is vaccinated 4 to 6 weeks prior to delivery. Kids and lambs are given antitoxin at birth for passive immunity. The bacterium that caused tetanus (*Clostridium tetani*) exists in soil, and enters wounds associated with tail docking and castration. Tetanus toxoid is usually included with *Cl. perfringens* in the C, D, and T vaccine. Some brands of rabies vaccine are labeled for use in sheep, but use in goats is extra-label. Animals receiving rabies vaccinations must be at least 3 months old, and rabies is boosted annually in livestock.

Orf (also known as *contagious ecthyma* or *sore mouth*) is a common zoonotic viral disease of small ruminants that causes crusting pox-type lesions on the nose and muzzle. A vaccine is available but is only used if there is a serious problem with orf on the farm as the vaccine is live and can produce zoonotic lesions in the person administering it. The feet of small ruminants should be checked regularly for overgrowth and for the presence of contagious foot rot, a disease for which a vaccine is available. Deworming should be performed regularly as well. The biggest nutritional problem in pet sheep and goats is overnutrition, and the client may need to be counseled on ways to prevent urolith formation.

Core vaccinations for all horses are tetanus, EEE/WEE, WNV, and rabies. The vaccination schedule for foals includes tetanus vaccination at 2, 4, and 6 months of age; EEE, WEE, and/or VEE at 3, 5, and 7 months of age (or administered concurrently with tetanus); rabies at 3 months of age, then boosted annually; WNV at 4, 6, and 8 months of age. In addition it is recommended that foals receive vaccinations for EHV at 4, 6, and 10 months of age and equine influenza at 3 and 5 months of age, since young animals are most susceptible. Once the primary vaccination series is completed, adult animals should receive boosters of the core vaccines annually.

In addition, because of high species susceptibility, any horse with a puncture wound, laceration, or other injury should receive a tetanus booster if it has not received one in the past month. Mares should be vaccinated 6 weeks before foaling. Tetanus antitoxin provides passive protection (neutralizes unbound toxin) and lasts up to 2 weeks. A horse with a wound and no history of vaccination should receive 1,500–3,000 IU or more of tetanus antitoxin; in addition, it is vaccinated with tetanus toxoid (not in the same syringe and not at the same injection site!), and the toxoid is repeated in 30 days.

Pregnant mares should be vaccinated with equine rhinopneumonitis (EHV-1 and EHV-4) at 5, 7, and 9 months gestation to prevent abortion. In addition, the mare should receive boosters for tetanus and other core vaccines 6 weeks prior to foaling.

Noncore vaccines for horses include equine influenza virus, strangles, and Potomac horse fever. There is an increased incidence of equine influenza in young (1 to 3 years) animals, and they should be revaccinated every 2 to 3 months if at increased risk of exposure (for example, show animals) in addition to receiving equine rhinopneumonitis vaccine every 3 to 4 months. Due to the high incidence of abscesses and other postvaccination reactions (IM injection), strangles (*Streptococcus equi*) vaccination is not routine unless the disease is a problem on the farm. Newer intranasal vaccines may reduce the incidence of abscesses. Potomac horse fever vaccine is available, but it is controversial as it is not known whether the vaccine actually reduces the incidence of disease.

Horses that will be traveling or attending shows or sales must have a screening blood test called the Coggins test for **equine infectious anemia** (EIA). This disease is spread by biting insects or blood-contaminated needles or instruments; once infected, the animal remains infected for life. To prevent the spread of the disease, a horse that tests positive is branded and then either quarantined or euthanized, depending on the testing and control measures followed in the locality.

Preventative health programs for pigs vary depending on the purpose of the animals and the history of disease on the premises. For a situation where 1 or 2 Vietnamese pot-bellied pigs are kept as pets, the minimum vaccines would consist of erysipelas, leptospirosis, and rabies. Erysipelas (*Erysipelothrix rhusiopathiae*) causes chronic arthritis, joint disease, heart disease, diamond-back skin disease, and death, and produces a zoonotic skin rash (erysipeloid) in humans. Pigs should be vaccinated annually for erysipelas. A 5-way vaccine for leptospirosis should be given annually to pigs; leptospirosis is a cause of abortion in pregnant sows and is potentially zoonotic. Although pigs are relatively resistant to rabies virus, pet pigs should still receive a rabies booster annually due to the seriousness of this disease.

Production animals receive routine twice-yearly vaccinations for leptospirosis, porcine parvovirus, and erysipelas. Gilts and sows are given prefarrow vaccines for *E. coli* diarrhea and atrophic rhinitis (*Pasteurella multocida* and *Bordetella bronchiseptica*). Atrophic rhinitis causes distortion of the nasal passages; baby pigs should receive an atrophic rhinitis vaccine once or twice before weaning. Other vaccines may be given to production pigs if the particular diseases have been a herd problem, but this requires a cost–benefit analysis as prevention costs can sometimes outweigh treatment costs and costs associated with lost production. Examples of noncore vaccines include PRRS (porcine reproductive and respiratory syndrome), pseudorabies, *Clostridium perfringens*, *Mycoplasma*, *Haemophilus*, rotavirus, and swine influenza.

Deworming pigs for intestinal parasites may be accomplished with 2 doses of 1% ivermectin given 2 weeks apart at a dosage of 1 mL per 75 lbs. Observe meat-withdrawal times in production animals.

Small Animals

All puppies should be vaccinated with a multivalent distemper vaccine such as DA2PP, which contains canine distemper virus, canine adenovirus type 2, canine parainfluenza virus, and canine parvovirus. Schedules will vary with location and veterinarian preference; however, a minimum of 3 doses of DA2PP should be given 3 to 4 weeks apart with the final dose given between 14 and 16 weeks of age.

The first dose is given at the first puppy visit (*typically* at 6 to 8 weeks of age). At this time a physical should be performed to check for the presence or absence of congenital defects such as heart murmur, cleft palate, open fontanel, umbilical hernia, inguinal hernia, and undescended testicles. In addition, a fecal examination should be performed to check for the presence of parasites, heartworm preventative is dispensed, and a routine deworming treatment is given regardless of whether ova are seen on fecal examination (>95% of puppies harbor intestinal parasites).

During the second puppy visit (9 to 11 weeks of age), a second dose of DA2PP is administered, fecal examination and deworming are repeated, a heartworm preventative is dispensed, and rabies vaccination may be performed if the puppy is at least 3 months old. Noncore vaccines for *Bordetella* and Lyme disease may be started if the puppy will be at risk for exposure to kennel cough (such as boarding or obedience class) or in an endemic area for Lyme disease.

At the final puppy visit (approximately 16 weeks of age), DA2PP is repeated, and/or kennel cough, a second Lyme vaccination, and rabies if it was not given previously. Fecal exam, deworming, and heartworm prevention are repeated. Leptospirosis vaccines may be recommended for dogs that will have access to water or other areas potentially contaminated by infected wildlife, but there are increased chances of vaccine reactions associated with leptospirosis (including anaphylaxis) compared to other vaccines, particularly in puppies less than 12 weeks old and in smaller dogs. Leptospirosis may be incorporated into a DA2PP-L vaccine and initially should be administered as a series of 2 vaccines given 3 weeks apart. A fourth DA2PP is sometimes recommended at 20 weeks of age for dogs that seem to be at increased risk for parvovirus infection, such as dobermans and rottweilers. Client education at routine puppy visits should include discussion of spay, neuter, dewclaw removal, and breed-specific health problems.

Adult dogs should receive an annual DA2PP booster (and/or leptospirosis) or titer. If the hospital is using a DA2PP vaccine that is labeled as a 3-year vaccine, a booster is given at 1 year of age and then every 3 years, but leptospirosis, if given, still needs to be boosted annually. A rabies booster is given 1 year following initial vaccine, then every 3 years subsequently in most localities. (Note: Annual rabies vaccination are required in some states.) The Lyme vaccine, if given, is boosted annually. *Bordetella* vaccines for kennel cough tend to provide short-term immunity and need to be boosted every 6 to 12 months. Adult dogs should have an annual or biennial blood test for the presence of heartworm disease, depending on owner compliance with administration of preventative.

Kittens should present for the first office visit at 8 to 10 weeks of age. As with puppies, the kitten is examined for signs of congenital defects, and routine fecal examinations and deworming are performed at every visit. All new kittens should be blood-tested for FeLV and FIV. A positive ELISA test for FIV needs to be repeated at 6 months of age to distinguish the presence of maternal antibody from actual infection. The core vaccines for kittens are FVRCP and rabies. *All* kittens should receive 3 doses of the feline distemper or FVRCP vaccine (feline viral rhinotracheitis, calicivirus, and panleukopenia), with the final dose given at 16 to 18 weeks. Vaccinate against FeLV if the kitten's environment puts it at risk. During the second visit, at 12 to 14 weeks of age, a second FVRCP combination, and/or a second leukemia vaccine, and first rabies vaccine (boosted in one year) are given. For the third visit (16 to 18 weeks) a final FVRCP combination vaccination is given. Noncore vaccines for kittens include chlamydia (*Chlamydophila*), FIV, FIP, and *Bordetella*. The feline chlamydia vaccine, like other URI vaccines, is not 100% effective. It is administered subcutaneously as 2 doses, given 3 to 4 weeks apart and then boosted annually. It may be incorporated into the FVRCP-C vaccine; however, vaccination is generally reserved as part of a control regimen for cats in multiple-cat environments in which infections associated with clinical disease have been confirmed. Feline infectious peritonitis (FIP) is not generally recommended and the vaccine is somewhat controversial. FIP vaccination is sometimes recommended only for cats at high risk; however the AAFP (American Association of Feline Practitioners) does not recommend for *any* cat due to complications. Feline *Bordetella* vaccination may be used in kittens as young as 4 weeks of age. The vaccine is not routinely recommended except in high-risk environments.

Adult cats should receive an FVRCP booster at 1 year of age, followed by a booster once every 3 years, although some brands of vaccine may need to be given annually. A rabies booster is given 1 year following the primary vaccine and then is boosted annually or triennially depending on the product used and local laws. If they are used, FeLV, FIV, FIP, *Bordetella*, and chlamydia vaccines would be boosted annually.

The core vaccines administered to ferrets are canine distemper virus and rabies. For the primary series of canine distemper vaccinations, kits should receive a series of 3 vaccines administered 3 to 4 weeks apart; adults receive a series of 2 distemper vaccines if it is their primary series. A ferret-specific canine distemper vaccination must be administered, and is boosted annually. MLV (modified live virus) multivalent canine distemper vaccines such as the DA2PP vaccine administered to canine patients may produce clinical disease in ferrets and should be avoided. Ferrets should also receive their first rabies vaccine at 3 months old, with subsequent annual boosters. Although a brand of rabies vaccine may be labeled for use in ferrets, a ferret may still be considered as unvaccinated wildlife in the event of a human bite incident, and in some states (such as New York, California, Oregon, and Washington) it is still illegal to have a pet ferret.

Practice Questions

1. A horse should be approached in which of the following ways?
   a. from the right, or off, side
   b. from the left, or near, side
   c. from directly behind the horse since it will not see you approaching and have time to escape.
   d. while loudly shouting or making loud noises so the horse knows that you are approaching

2. Retinal atrophy and dilated cardiomyopathy are linked to deficiency of which amino acid in the feline?
   a. arginine
   b. histidine
   c. taurine
   d. tryptophan

3. Dogs can synthesize this vitamin from beta-carotene, but cats require it in their diet.
   a. vitamin A
   b. vitamin B complex
   c. vitamin C
   d. vitamin D

4. Cats require this nutrient at four times the level needed in the canine diet because dogs can synthesize it from tryptophan.
   a. vitamin A
   b. niacin
   c. taurine
   d. arachidonic acid

5. By what factor does a bitch's energy requirements increase during peak lactation?
   a. 0
   b. 1 to 2 times
   c. 3 to 4 times
   d. 5 to 8 times

6. Goats should have limited access to grain and lush pasture or else they are likely to develop which of the following?
   a. *Clostridium tetani*
   b. *Clostridium perfringens* C and D
   c. ketosis
   d. sweet tooth

7. Scours, a term commonly used in livestock, is also known as what?
   a. diarrhea
   b. cleaning the coat
   c. combing the coat with a metal brush
   d. vitamin C deficiency

8. Canine adenovirus type 1 causes which disease?
   a. hepatitis
   b. infectious tracheobronchitis
   c. measles
   d. parainfluenza

9. Abdominal distention secondary to buildup of peritoneal fluid is a symptom of which of the following?
   a. FeLV
   b. FIP
   c. FIV
   d. giardia

10. How old must a puppy or kitten be to receive its first rabies vaccine?
  a. 8 weeks or 56 days
  b. 12 weeks or 84 days
  c. 13 weeks or 91 days
  d. 6 months or 182 days

11. Which of the following vaccines should be given to indoor-only cats?
  a. chlamydia
  b. FeLV
  c. FIV
  d. rabies

12. Which of the following canine diseases is zoonotic?
  a. distemper
  b. parvovirus
  c. parainfluenza
  d. leptospirosis

13. Which of the following vaccines should be given to brood mares during the fifth, seventh, and ninth months of gestation to prevent abortion?
  a. EEE/WEE
  b. EHV-1
  c. rabies
  d. tetanus

14. Which of the following causes of calf diarrhea is NOT potentially zoonotic?
  a. *Coronavirus*
  b. *Cryptosporidium parvum*
  c. *E. coli*
  d. *Salmonella*

15. Which vaccine is typically given to cattle between 4 and 12 months by a USDA-accredited veterinarian?
  a. BRSV
  b. brucellosis
  c. rabies
  d. BVD

16. *Milk fever* is the lay term for
  a. hypercalcemia
  b. hypocalcemia
  c. hypokalemia
  d. hypermagnesemia

17. When farmers say that a cow has *cast her withers*, they are referring to what?
  a. an injured teat
  b. metritis
  c. a retained placenta
  d. a uterine prolapse

18. Core vaccinations for potbellied pigs kept as pets include all of the following *except*
  a. erysipelas
  b. leptospirosis
  c. pseudorabies
  d. rabies

19. Which of the following zoonoses is invariably fatal once the animal or the human has begun to show clinical signs?
  a. rabies
  b. tularemia
  c. plague
  d. anthrax

20. What percentage of pet reptiles harbor *Salmonella*?
  a. 0–25%
  b. 25–50%
  c. 50–75%
  d. >90%

21. What is the common term for the disease caused by the bacterium *Pasteurella multocida* in rabbits?
   a. snuffles
   b. sore hocks
   c. piles
   d. heaves

22. Which of the following vaccines would provide a horse or a foal with *immediate* protection against tetanus?
   a. MLV tetanus
   b. killed tetanus
   c. tetanus toxoid
   d. tetanus antitoxin

23. Which of the following routes of drug administration provides the quickest systemic absorption?
   a. SQ
   b. IM
   c. IV
   d. topical

24. What catheterization site is likely to be used in neonates and very small patients but NOT likely to be used in adults?
   a. jugular vein
   b. intraosseous
   c. cephalic vein
   d. femoral artery

25. Which of the following procedures is used to measure IOP?
   a. Schirmer tear test
   b. fluorescein staining
   c. ophthalmoscopic exam
   d. Schiotz tonometry/Tono-Pen®

26. An esophagostomy tube is placed when an animal is
   a. having difficulty breathing.
   b. anemic.
   c. having urinary problems.
   d. anorexic.

27. At approximately what rate should crystalloid fluids be administered to a dog in shock?
   a. 90 ml/lb/hr
   b. 50 ml/lb/hr
   c. 30 ml/lb/hr
   d. 20 ml/lb/hr

28. How soon should a puppy's birth weight double?
   a. by 5 days
   b. by 7 days
   c. by 12 days
   d. by 21 days

29. All of the following drugs can be administered via endotracheal tube in an emergency situation *except*
   a. atropine.
   b. dobutamine.
   c. epinephrine.
   d. lidocaine.

30. What is the correct ratio of chest compression to ventilations for one-person CPR?
   a. 1 compression:1 ventilation
   b. 2 compressions:1 ventilation
   c. 1 compression:1 ventilation:1 abdominal compression between ventilations
   d. 15 compressions:2 ventilations

31. What is the location of an acupuncture point that can be used to stimulate breathing with a 25-G needle?
    a. at the sternal notch
    b. midline on the dorsal aspect of the nose or the muzzle
    c. between the third and fourth digits of either front paw
    d. midline at the point where the nose meets the upper lip

32. Which of the following lab animals should be bred before 6 months of age to avoid serious risk of dystocia requiring C-section?
    a. gerbils
    b. hamsters
    c. guinea pigs
    d. rabbits

33. Insulinoma is a common tumor of
    a. cats.
    b. dogs.
    c. ferrets.
    d. hamsters.

34. Controlling food allergies in small animals may involve all of the following dietary changes *except*
    a. a novel protein source.
    b. a limited-ingredient diet.
    c. an enzyme hydrolysis to produce low molecular weight proteins.
    d. replacing rice with corn and wheat grains.

35. In addition to affecting dogs, canine distemper virus is an important cause of disease in
    a. hamsters.
    b. ferrets.
    c. cats.
    d. humans.

36. A mixed-breed dog has had a relatively severe, dry cough for the past 10 days. The cough began 4 to 5 days after the animal was housed at a kennel. What is the most likely cause of this dog's disease?
    a. herpesvirus
    b. *Streptococcus pneumonia*
    c. *Klebsiella pneumonia*
    d. *Bordetella bronchiseptica*

37. At what age should most kittens first be presented for initial immunization?
    a. 4 to 6 weeks
    b. 8 to 10 weeks
    c. 12 to 14 weeks
    d. 16 to 20 weeks

38. Lambs are routinely restrained for castration and tail docking by
    a. holding them in dorsal recumbency with the hind legs restrained.
    b. holding them still with a rabies pole.
    c. placing a cable snare around the upper jaw.
    d. distracting them with molasses.

39. All of the following diseases are caused by a single virus *except*
    a. feline infectious peritonitis.
    b. canine distemper.
    c. kennel cough.
    d. rabies.

40. At what age should most puppies first be presented for initial immunization?
    a. 4 to 6 weeks
    b. 6 to 8 weeks
    c. 12 to 14 weeks
    d. 16 to 20 weeks

41. What are the diet recommendations for canine diabetics?
a. foods that are high in fat for weight gain
b. foods that are high in sugar for energy
c. foods that are high in fiber for slow, consistent release of nutrients
d. foods that are high in moisture for compensatory hydration

42. Which of the following is the causative organism of Lyme disease?
a. *Borrelia burgdorferi*
b. *Ixodes dammini*
c. white-footed mice
d. *Dermacentor variabilis*

43. How are Eastern, Western, and Venezuelan equine encephalomyelitis (EEE, WEE, and VEE) transmitted to horses?
a. by ticks
b. by mosquitoes
c. by aerosolization
d. by ingestion of moldy feed

44. Young horses and performance horses (engaged in racing, showing, or off-site training) are at high risk of contracting _____ and should be vaccinated every 3 to 4 months for these diseases.
a. equine viral arteritis and Potomac horse fever
b. botulism and strangles
c. influenza and rhinopneumonitis
d. both **a** and **c**

45. What is the most important aspect of treatment for horses diagnosed with chronic obstructive pulmonary disease (COPD)?
a. regular vaccination
b. removal of the offending allergens (usually hay or straw) from the horse's environment
c. lifelong corticosteroid administration
d. lifelong antibiotic administration

46. What should a previously nonvaccinated mature horse that receives a traumatic puncture wound in the sole be given?
a. tetanus antitoxin only
b. tetanus toxoid only
c. both tetanus antitoxin and toxoid
d. neither tetanus antitoxin or toxoid; only local wound therapy is required

47. Which ailment is commonly known as Bang's disease?
a. botulism
b. tetanus
c. enterotoxemia
d. brucellosis

48. What are the most common viral agents involved in feline respiratory disease complex for which a vaccine exists?
a. papovirus and reovirus
b. herpesvirus and calicivirus
c. *Chlamydia* and *Mycoplasma*
d. calicivirus and myxovirus

49. It is imperative to a calf's survival to receive colostrum how soon after birth?
a. 12 to 24 hours
b. 3 days
c. 7 days
d. Calves do not require colostrum.

50. What is the ideal vaccination schedule for a 7-week old cocker spaniel puppy?
a. distemper at 12, 16, and 20 weeks, with rabies at 12+ weeks
b. Distemper at 8, 12, and 16 weeks, with rabies at 8 weeks
c. distemper at 8, 12, and 16 weeks, with rabies at >12 weeks
d. distemper at 8, 12, and 16 weeks, with rabies at 1 year of age

Answers and Explanations

1. b. A horse should be approached from the left, or near, side because this is the side from which it is used to being approached. A horse should never be approached directly from the rear as this may startle it and lead to human injury. For the same reason, one should avoid making loud noises when approaching a horse.

2. c. Retinal atrophy and dilated cardiomyopathy are linked to deficiency of taurine. Arginine, histidine, and tryptophan are also amino acids, but deficiencies do not produce feline dilated cardiomyopathy.

3. a. Dogs can synthesize vitamin A from beta-carotene, but cats require it in their diet. Both cats and dogs require exogenous sources of vitamin B complex, vitamin C, and vitamin D, but these are not precursors to vitamin A.

4. b. Cats require niacin at 4 times the level needed in the canine diet because dogs can synthesize niacin from tryptophan. Dogs can synthesize vitamin A from beta-carotene, but not from tryptophan. Taurine is an essential amino acid for the feline, but it is not synthesized from tryoptophan. Arachidonic acid is an essential fatty acid in the feline diet, but it is not synthesized from tryptophan.

5. c. A bitch's energy requirements increase by a factor of 3- to 4-fold during peak lactation. Her energy requirements increase by a factor of approximately 1.5 to 2 during the last third of gestation. Five- to 8-fold increases in energy requirements are seen in working sled dogs.

6. b. Goats should have limited access to grain and lush pasture or else they are likely to develop *Clostridium perfringens* C & D (overeating disease). *Clostridium tetani* is the causative agent of tetanus, which is caused by puncture and wound infections. Ketosis may develop when an animal's nutritional energy requirements are not being adequately met and it begins to use its body stores of fat for energy.

7. a. Scours, a term commonly used in livestock, is also known as diarrhea. Vitamin C deficiency produces scurvy.

8. a. Canine adenovirus type 1 causes hepatitis. CAV-2 may be a causative agent of infectious tracheobronchitis. Measles vaccine provides cross-immunity to CAV-1, but measles is not caused by CAV-1. Parainfluenza is another causative virus of tracheobronchitis.

9. b. Abdominal distention secondary to buildup of peritoneal fluid is a symptom of FIP. FeLV and FIV produce nonspecific symptoms associated with immunodeficiency. Giardia produces diarrheal disease.

10. c. Be careful: although the package insert usually states that the rabies vaccine may be used in animals 12 weeks or older, the eligible age for rabies vaccination is defined as three months = 91 days = 13 weeks. Eight- and 12-week-old kittens and puppies are ineligible for vaccination. There is no reason to postpone vaccination until the animal is 6 months old provided the animal has not been quarantined following a human bite incident.

11. d. Even though indoor-only cats are at decreased risk for rabies, due to the serious and fatal nature of the disease and the serious consequences when an unvaccinated pet bites a human, all pets should be vaccinated against rabies. Chlamydia is a noncore vaccine. FeLV and FIV vaccines are not necessary for cats that have no access to the outdoors and no contact with other cats.

12. d. Leptospirosis can cause severe liver and kidney dysfunction in humans. Canine parvovirus is a different species than human parvovirus; likewise human influenza is not caused by canine parainfluenza.

13. b. The EHV-1 vaccine should be given to brood mares during the fifth, seventh, and ninth months of gestation to prevent abortion. Pregnant mares should also be kept up to date on EEE/WEE, rabies, and tetanus for passive transfer of immunity to the foal.

14. a. *Coronavirus* is not potentially zoonotic. *Cryptosporidium parvum* can cause severe disease in immunocompromised humans. *E. coli* and *Salmonella* can cause diarrhea in previously healthy individuals.

15. b. Brucellosis vaccine is given to cattle by a USDA-accredited veterinarian. Rabies vaccine can be administered to cattle by any veterinarian licensed to practice in that particular state. BRSV and BVD vaccines may be given by the livestock producer.

16. b. *Milk fever* is the lay term for hypocalcemia, or low blood calcium. Hypercalcemia refers to *increased* blood calcium. Hypokalemia refers to low blood potassium, whereas hypermagnesium refers to high blood magnesium.

17. d. When a farmer says that a cow has *cast her withers*, he is referring to a prolapsed uterus. Metritis refers to a uterine infection. A farmer refers to a retained placenta as a cow that needs cleaning.

18. c. Pseudorabies is not a core vaccination for potbellied pigs kept as pets. Although pigs are fairly resistant to rabies, they should still be vaccinated due to the serious nature of the disease. Also, leptospirosis and erysipelas are potentially zoonotic, and any animal with access to the outdoors should be vaccinated for these.

19. a. Rabies is invariably fatal once the animal or human has begun to show clinical signs. Rabbits are the reservoir species for tularemia which produces skin lesions in humans and is treated with antibiotics. Desert rodents are the reservoir species for *Yersonia pestis* (plague) in the United States, but the disease has a good prognosis when treated with antibiotics. Most cases of anthrax in humans involve cutaneous exposure producing skin lesions and respond well to antibiotics; the inhalation form of anthrax carries a more guarded prognosis.

20. d. The percentage of pet reptiles that harbor *Salmonella* is >90%.

21. a. The common term for the disease caused by the bacteria *Pasteurella multocida* in rabbits is snuffles. Sore hocks is a lay term for a bacterial skin disease of the plantar surfaces of rabbit hind feet. Piles is a lay term for rectal prolapse in swine. Heaves is a lay term for COPD in horses.

22. d. Tetanus antitoxin provides a horse or foal with *immediate* (passive) protection against tetanus because it contains an actual antibody against the toxin. Tetanus toxoid induces active immunity against the toxin that produces tetanus, but it requires time for the animal to mount an immune response. Tetanus is caused by a bacterium, therefore choice **a** (modified-live virus vaccine) must be incorrect. Choice **b** is incorrect because it is not the presence of bacteria that produces disease, but rather the toxin produced by the bacteria.

23. c. The IV route of drug administration generally provides the quickest systemic absorption, followed by (in order of decreasing absorption) IM, SQ (SC), and topical routes.

24. b. Intraosseous catheters are more likely to be used in neonates and very small patients than in adults. The veins of neonates may be too small to accommodate even the smallest of IV catheters, or it may be technically too difficult to catheterize a small patient.

25. d. Schiotz tonometry or a Tono-Pen® are used to measure IOP (intraocular pressure). The Schirmer tear test measures tear production. Fluorescein staining evaluates corneal integrity. Ophthalmoscopic exam involves visual exam of the internal eye structures including the fundus.

26. d. An esophagostomy tube is a type of feeding tube that may be placed in the esophagus when an animal is anorexic. A tracheotomy tube or an endotracheal tube may be used if an animal is having difficulty breathing.

27. a. The *approximate* rate at which crystalloid fluids should be administered to a dog in shock is 90 ml/lb/hr. The more precise formula is 20 to 40 ml/kg administered for the first 15 minutes, then 70 to 90 ml/kg over a 1-hour period.

28. c. A puppy's birth weight should double by 12 days. Eyes open at 5 to 14 days, and gruel may be introduced at 3 to 4 weeks of age.

29. b. Dobutamine cannot be administered via endotracheal tube in an emergency situation. Atropine, epinephrine, and lidocaine may be administered via endotracheal tube, but at double the IV dose.

30. d. For one-person CPR, the correct ratio of chest compressions to ventilations is 15 compressions:2 ventilations. For two-person CPR, ventilations should be given as quickly as the Ambu® bag or rebreathing bag can refill. For three-person CPR, the goal is 1 chest compression:1 ventilation: 1 abdominal compression between ventilations.

31. d. An acupuncture point that can be used to stimulate breathing with a 25-G needle is located midline at the point where the nose meets the upper lip.

32. c. Guinea pigs should be bred before 6 months of age. Otherwise the pubic symphysis may fuse and not be able to widen to accommodate passage of the fetus. This phenomenon is not seen in gerbils, hamsters, or rabbits.

33. c. Insulinoma is a common tumor of ferrets. Insulinoma can occur in other species, but not with the frequency seen in ferrets.

34. d. Controlling food allergies in small animals does not involve replacing rice with corn and wheat grains. Corn and wheat are potential allergens to many animals. Novel protein sources, limited-ingredient diets, and enzyme hydrolysis to produce low molecular weight proteins are all ways to attempt to bypass the animal immune response to allergens.

35. b. In addition to affecting dogs, canine distemper virus is an important cause of disease in ferrets, and in fact is 100% fatal in this species. The virus that causes feline distemper is unrelated to canine distemper virus; feline distemper virus is actually more closely related to the canine parvovirus. Canine distemper is not zoonotic.

36. d. A dog that has severe, dry cough that began four to five days after the animal was housed in a kennel is most likely infected with *Bordatella bronchiseptica*, the most common bacterial cause of kennel cough. A herpesvirus causes rhinotracheitis in cats and bovines, but not in dogs. *Streptococcus* and *Klebsiella pneumonia* are not as common.

37. b. Most kittens should first be presented for initial immunization at 8 to 10 weeks old. At 4 to 7 weeks they would be expected still to have maternal antibody interference with vaccination. By 12 to 14 weeks, maternal antibodies have generally disappeared, and a kitten that has not yet been vaccinated is already at risk for disease.

38. a. Lambs are routinely restrained for castration and tail docking by holding them in dorsal recumbency with the hind legs restrained. Large, aggressive dogs may be restrained with a rabies pole. Hogs are restrained by placing a cable snare around the upper jaw. Distracting them with food would not provide adequate restraint.

39. c. Kennel cough is a disease complex caused by a variety of bacteria and viruses, and in most cases involves concurrent infection of *Bordetella* with either CAV-2 or parainfluenza.

40. b. Puppies should first be presented for initial immunization at 6 to 8 weeks old. At 4 to 6 weeks they would be expected still to have maternal antibody interference with vaccination. By 12 to 14 weeks, maternal antibodies have generally disappeared, and a puppy that has not yet been vaccinated is already at risk for disease.

41. c. Diet recommendations for canine diabetics are foods that are high in fiber for slow, consistent release of nutrients. High-moisture foods tend to be low-fiber diets. Foods that are high in fat would be contraindicated as they would predispose to weight gain, and obesity is a contributing factor to development of diabetes. Because diabetes is a derangement of the body's ability to utilize glucose, high-sugar foods are contraindicated.

42. a. The causative agent of Lyme disease is *Borrelia burgdorferi*. *Ixodes* is the deer tick, which is the insect vector of Lyme. The white-footed mouse is an intermediate host. The dog tick *Dermacentor variabilis* is not involved in the transmission of Lyme.

43. b. Eastern, Western, and Venezuelan Equine Encephalomyelitis (EEE, WEE, and VEE) are transmitted to horses by mosquitoes. Ticks play a role in the transmission of Lyme disease. EEE/WEE/VEE are not transmitted by aerosolization or by feed.

44. c. Young horses and performance horses (engaged in racing, showing, or off-site training) are at high risk of contracting influenza and rhinopneumonitis and should be vaccinated every 3 to 4 months for these diseases. Horses are not routinely vaccinated for equine viral arteritis. Potomac horse fever is transmitted by insect vectors and occurs sporadically. Botulism and strangles vaccines are only used in some cases where these diseases have been a problem on the farm.

45. b. Owners of horses diagnosed with COPD need to be counseled that the most important aspect of treatment is removal of the offending allergens (usually hay or straw) from the horse's environment. COPD cannot be prevented by vaccination. Although animals may require treatment with corticosteroids, bronchodilators, and/or antibiotics, these treatments are generally seasonal rather than continuous or lifelong.

46. c. A previously nonvaccinated mature horse that receives a traumatic puncture wound in the sole of the hoof should be given both tetanus antitoxin and toxoid. The antitoxin provides immediate passive immunity, whereas the toxoid induces active long-acting immunity. Because horses are a species very prone to developing tetanus, local wound therapy is not adequate in an unvaccinated animal.

47. d. Brucellosis in cattle is commonly known as Bang's disease. Enterotoxemia is known by the lay term *overeating disease*, tetanus is known as *lockjaw*. Botulism generally does not have a lay term associated with it, although in waterfowl is sometimes referred to as *limber neck*.

48. b. The most common viral agents involved in feline respiratory disease complex for which a vaccine exists are herpesvirus (FHV-1 or feline viral rhinotracheitis) and calicivirus. *Chlamydia* and *Mycoplasma* are bacterial diseases. Other viral causes of feline respiratory disease are not as common as FHV-1 and calicivirus, and currently no vaccines exist for them.

49. a. It is imperative to a calf's survival to receive colostrum within the first 12 to 24 hours of life, and preferably as soon as possible. Colostrum contains antibodies that provide the calf with passive immunity to disease. There is only a limited time window when antibodies can be absorbed directly from the abomasum into the bloodstream, and by 48 hours the window has generally closed.

50. c. The vaccination schedule for a new puppy includes a series of at least 3 canine distemper vaccinations given at approximately 8, 12, and 16 weeks of age, and a rabies vaccine when the puppy is at least 3 months old. Rabies should not be given to an animal that is only 8 weeks old, nor should it be delayed until the animal is a year old. Distemper vaccination should not be initiated as late as 12 weeks because maternal antibody will have declined weeks prior to this.

10 ▶ DIAGNOSTIC IMAGING

CHAPTER OVERVIEW

Diagnostic imaging is an essential part of any modern veterinary practice. This chapter discusses the theory and practice of diagnostic imaging from radiography to ultrasound and other forms of imaging technology such as magnetic resonance imaging (MRI) and computerized axial tomography (CAT or CT). The most commonly used imaging technique is radiography. Radiographs are images produced on film exposed to x-rays and then developed into a negative image. These allow the veterinarian to see internal structures of different densities.

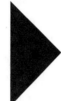

The veterinary technician is trained to obtain clean, clear, diagnostic radiographs to aid the veterinarian in examining and diagnosing patients. X-radiation is used to produce radiographs (x-ray films), which can be damaging to living tissue. That is why proper protection techniques for both the operator and the patient are essential.

Key Terms

acoustic shadowing
ALARA
alpha particles
anode

beta particles
cathode
collimating
computed radiography
computerized axial tomography (CAT)
contrast
direct digital radiography
direct radiation
dosimetry badge
film fog
gamma rays
grid
grid ratio
heel effect
hyperechoic
isoechoic
kilovolts peak (kVp)
milliampere seconds (mAs)
maximum permissible dose (MPD)
nuclear magnetic resonance imaging (NMRI)
Orthopedic Foundation of America (OFA)
PennHIP
Potter-Bucky tray (Bucky)
primary beam
protons
radiodense
radiolucent
reverberation
scatter radiation
transducer

Concepts and Skills

Diagnostic imaging plays a crucial role in veterinary medicine. This field has been broken down into three subject areas:

- radiography
- ultrasound
- other imaging techniques

Radiography

Radiographic imaging is one of the most important diagnostic tools in veterinary medicine. It allows the veterinarian virtually to see the structures inside the animal. Radiographs are very similar to regular photographic images. Light is used to make an image on a photographic plate, which is then processed to make a permanent image. The light used in photographic imaging is in the visual spectrum, while the light for a radiographic image is in the x-ray wavelength, which is higher frequency (above the ultraviolet wavelength).

History

In order to understand the production of x-rays, a basic understanding of atomic theory is necessary. Historically, the atom was thought to be an indestructible particle of matter. Marie Curie discovered that certain atoms could be broken down into smaller particles called *electrons*, and pure energy, or **gamma rays**. Marie Curie eventually died of radiation poisoning, because gamma rays can cause somatic damage. It was later discovered that nonradioactive atoms could also be broken down into smaller particles by the use of electrical charge in a vacuum environment. Depending on the charge difference (negative and positive), light of different wavelengths would be emitted. Wilhelm Roentgen discovered that some of these wavelengths, called x-rays, could be used to penetrate flesh and create an image either on a fluorescent plate or on film. These x-rays did not result in somatic damage as severe as gamma rays, but still caused very high rates of cancer and radiation burns with repeated use.

Theory of X-Ray Production

In order for radiographic imaging to work, x-rays need to be considered as both light (electromagnetic radiation, which has a wavelength) and as particles. The particles of light are called *photons*. X-rays are produced by the bombardment of a metal (usually tungsten) by a beam of electrons. This produces energy in the form of light (x-rays) and heat.

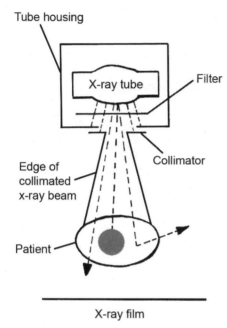

Figure 10.1 *x-Ray Film*

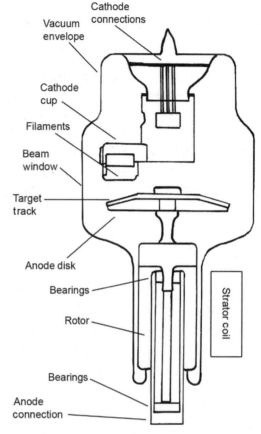

Figure 10.2 *Rotating Anode*

Electromagnetic Radiation

An x-ray machine is basically a magnetic tube. The part of the magnet that produces the electrons is called the **cathode**, the part that produces the x-rays (usually tungsten) is called the **anode**. The part of the anode that the electrons hit is called the *target*. The electrons are drawn across the gap in the tube to the target by a strong magnetic field. The speed of the electrons (penetration) is adjusted by the kVp, or **kilovoltage peak**. The number of electrons is adjusted by the mA or milliamperage. The amount of time the electrons bombard the target is measured in seconds (s). The mA and seconds are adjusted together on many machines. The multiplication of the mA by the number of seconds is termed the *mAs* or **milliampere seconds**. (See Figure 10.1.)

Most of the energy produced from the tungsten anode is heat, so a method for cooling must be provided. Two types of anodes exist: rotating anodes and stationary anodes. Rotating anodes allow the heat to dissipate because the same area is not being bombarded all the time. (See Figure 10.2.) The other way to dissipate heat is to decrease the time that the anode

is being bombarded by the electrons. For this reason, stationary anodes require higher mAs because they have to have shorter exposure times. (See Figure 10.3.)

Electrons do not selectively hit particular particles, so the heavy glass x-ray tube is kept in a vacuum to decrease the incidence of sparking from floating particles. When this occurs, it can blow the tube, similar to a light bulb burning out. The two parts of the tube are surrounded by an oil bath to help further with heat dissipation. In addition, the tube is encased by metal to protect the surrounding environment from x-radiation, because x-rays may travel in any direction in a straight line from the point of production. This means that the percentage of x-rays produced that go in the desired direction is very small.

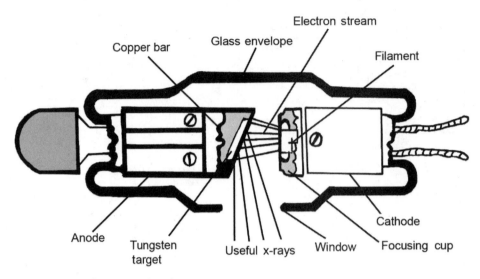

Figure 10.3 *Stationary Anode*

Electricity from a wall plug is produced as a cyclical wave. Electrons are only produced by the cathode during the positive deflection of the wave (the part of the wave above the zero line), so x-rays are only produced by the anode at that time. In order to improve image quality and increase x-ray production, most machines are able to multiply the electricity from the wall so there are three overlapping waveforms happening at the same time. This provides constant electron and x-ray production and can decrease the exposure time needed for imaging.

Film and Screens

X-ray film has emulsion on both sides, unlike standard photographic film that has the emulsion only on one side of the film. The emulsion is a thin coating of gelatin-containing silver halide particles that is bonded to a plastic sheet. Silver halide produces black-and-white images using the same technology as that used in black-and-white photography. The silver halide reacts to light to form an invisible latent image which must be processed with chemicals to give a lasting visible image.

Because silver halide reacts better to visual light than x-rays, special amplifying screens may be used. Screens are sheets of plastic or cardboard covered with an emulsion of phosphor crystals. These crystals are similar to the crystals found in glow-in-the-dark items and phosphorescent bacteria. They glow when they are bombarded by x-rays and the light produced is then transmitted to the film. This decreases the number of x-rays needed, which in turn decreases the radiation exposure (mAs) required. Because the particles are very small and the amount of light produced is also small, differential light and dark patterns will form depending on how many x-rays are absorbed or reflected by overlying tissues. Bone, for instance, reflects most of the x-rays, so those phosphor crystals underneath the bone will not react. This makes a white image on the film because the silver halide crystals haven't reacted to the light produced by the phosphor and are washed away during the developing process. Air density does not reflect any x-rays, so air-filled structures are seen as black on the film because all of the silver halide crystals have reacted and stick to the plastic base of the film during developing.

Screens come in varying speeds, which means that the number and size of the crystals varies. High-speed screens will provide very fast images, but the quality of the image may be low because the crystal size is larger. Low-speed screens require slightly longer exposure times, but the image quality is improved. It is important to use the correct film for the correct screen, because the wavelength of the light produced by the screen and the exposure time needed by the film is different depending on the speed and type of phosphor.

The film and screens are encased in a light-tight frame called a *cassette*. The cassette has a back lined with lead or other heavy metal and a bakelite or fiberglass front. The front of the cassette allows x-rays to penetrate to the screens and film. The lead absorbs x-rays, so the x-rays do not backscatter and decrease image quality. This will be covered in more detail in the section on Troubleshooting when Using Digital Radiography.

Nonscreen film (film that is used for direct reaction to x-rays) gives much higher detail, but requires longer exposure times. This is used for techniques such as dentistry, research applications, and some orthopedic imaging that requires extremely fine detail. The cassette for nonscreen film is an opaque plastic envelope. The film is sandwiched between layers of black paper. A thin sheet of lead is between the film and the back of the envelope. This lead sheet should be disposed of according to EPA requirements and should not be thrown in the trash. The lead may be reused to make more cassettes.

There are two types of light-sensitive films available: blue-light sensitive and green-light sensitive. The type of film should be decided based on the type of screen used. Green-light sensitive film should be used with rare earth screens. Blue-light sensitive film should be used with calcium tungstate screens.

Film Chemistry

The two chemicals used to process the film and form a permanent image are called the *chemistry*. Developer is used in the first step in film processing. The developer is an alkaline (basic) chemical solution that causes the silver halide crystals that have reacted to the light to form metallic silver, precipitate out of solution in the gelatin, and stick to the plastic base of the film.

The second step is rinsing the film with water (or an acetic acid and water mixture). This removes the excess developer. Adequate rinsing is important because it increases the life of the next chemical, the fixative. Together, the fixative and the developer are called the chemistry.

The fixative fixes the image to the plastic and prevents further reaction to the developing agent or light. The fixative is an acid that completely stops the chemical reaction from the developer and prevents any undeveloped silver halide from further reacting to light. It also removes all unreacted silver halide from the image and hardens the coating on the film to increase its longevity. In general, the fixative should be in contact with the film for twice as long as the developer time.

The unreacted silver comes off with the gelatin and goes into solution in the fixative. Used fixative should be disposed of according to EPA requirements and should not be flushed down the sink. Silver traps may be provided by x-ray machine inspection companies. The silver may be reused after it is recovered from the chemicals. In most states, silver recovery is required by law. Old radiographs should also be sent for silver recovery.

A final rinsing step with running water removes the fixative and prevents damage to the underlying plastic base of the image by the acid. The image should then be dried completely prior to viewing.

It is important *never* to allow fixative to go into the developer. Even a few drops of fixative will poison the developer and make it completely useless. Fixative is acidic and developer is alkaline, so, when the two are mixed, they will have an exothermic (heat producing) reaction.

Several factors are important to x-ray film developing: light, static electricity, temperature, and chemistry. Full-spectrum visible light will affect film at all stages from being removed from the package to entrance into the fixative. All film manipulation should be in the dark to prevent exposure to visible light. Exposure to light results in an artifact called

film fog. This term refers to dark areas on the developed film that may obscure the image. Luckily, x-ray film does not react to some light wavelengths. Dark red bulbs will not affect either the blue-light or the green-light sensitive types of film.

Static electricity can occur in very dry or cold weather. Static causes artifacts resembling black lightning bolts or trees on developed radiographs. Removal of film too quickly from the box, or failure to ground oneself prior to removing a film from the package, will cause these artifacts. Care should be taken to minimize static when environmental conditions are favorable for it to form.

Temperature has a huge effect on developing times. The chemical reaction of the developer is temperature dependent. Most developers work at 68°F for 5 minutes. Developing time should be increased or decreased by 30 seconds for every 2 degrees variation from 68°F. For instance, if the temperature of the developer solution is 76°F, the developing time should be 3 minutes:

$$\frac{76-68}{2\times30} = 4 \times 30 = 120 \text{ seconds} = 2 \text{ minutes}$$
5 minutes − 2 minutes = 3 minutes
developing time

With automatic processors, the developer is maintained at a constant temperature of 95°F. Special developer and fixative are manufactured specifically for these temperatures. Automatic processors also keep their chemicals in constant motion, reducing the possibility of biological overgrowth (algae and bacteria) that will decrease chemical longevity. Most also have the ability to replenish the chemistries by suction into the machine as needed. This makes upkeep much easier. It is very important not to try to process radiographs before the machine has reached the appropriate temperature because doing so will decrease film quality.

Technique and Quality Control

The technique for taking the image and the methods of quality control are very important both for improving image quality and for reducing exposure of the animal and the technician to radiation. Knowledge of the reasons for proper positioning, appropriate use of personal protective equipment (PPE), radiographic technique, and evaluation are all important in producing a diagnostic radiograph.

Heel Effect

The **heel effect** is the increased clarity and darkness of the side of the film closest to the cathode. This occurs because the number of x-rays will be larger closer to the place they are produced and diminished the farther they are away from the source. Always try to place the thickest part of the area of interest closest to the cathode end of the x-ray tube, so that the image clarity will be improved.

mAs versus kVp

mAs is the amount of electricity put through the cathode to cause the electrons to be released from the atoms. This produces an electron cloud along with a lot of heat. In order to prevent overheating the tube, the mAs should be kept as low as possible. Since the mAs determines the number of electrons available to strike the anode target, it determines the number of x-rays produced. This is seen as increased density on the film (the darkness of the overall film).

It is important to remember that the mA is the amount of electricity and the s is the time that the electricity is applied. In general, the mA should be high but the s should be as low as possible. This decreases the amount of heat generated by the cathode but increases the number of electrons produced. Many machines only allow the adjustment of mAs as a whole and do the adjustments internally.

The starting mAs to be used depends on the type of screen used and whether or not a grid is used. Grids will be discussed a little later on. The faster the screen, the lower the mAs required to produce the image.

SCREEN TYPE	mAs
Fast (high-speed screen)	2.5–10
Medium (par-speed screen)	5–12.5
Slow (high-detail screen)	30–40

If a grid is used, the exposure time(s) should be doubled, which also doubles the mAs. In other words, if the original mAs is 2.5 ($\frac{1}{120}$ second at 300 mA), the new mAs with a grid will be 5 ($\frac{1}{60}$ second at 300 mA).

The kVp is the intensity of the charge difference between the cathode and the anode. This determines the speed of the electron cloud as it crosses the gap and the energy of the x-rays produced. Higher energy x-rays have more penetrating power than lower energy x-rays. By increasing the kVp, the contrast (difference between levels of grey on the film) will be increased. Higher kVp can also increase density to a certain extent, so high kVp, low mAs techniques will produce less heat, have shorter exposure times, and give better contrasted images. Higher contrast usually implies higher quality.

The starting kVp can be estimated using Santes' rule, which states:

$$(2 \times \text{thickness of body part in centimeters}) + SID = kVp$$

Once the starting kVp and mAs are calculated, a technique chart can be made. A radiograph of the area is taken and the image is evaluated for quality, contrast, and density. If the density (darkness) is too much, the mAs should be decreased by 30 to 50%. If the film is too light, the mAs should be increased by 30 to 50%. The kVp may also be used to adjust the density. Decreasing the kVp by 10 to 15% will decrease density. Increasing the kVp by 10 to 15% will increase the density. The radiographs should also be assessed for contrast. If, for instance, the overall darkness (density) is too intense, but the grey scale is perfect, adjust the mAs only. If there is not enough contrast, the kVp should be adjusted.

Once the perfect film is obtained, a chart is generated by increasing or decreasing the kVp by 2 for each 1 cm measurement. Individual charts should be made for each body part because of the differences in density. The abdomen, for instance, is very dense and needs much higher mAs than the thorax which is not dense at all (contains air).

The *SID* (source image distance) is the distance between the film and the x-ray tube. Some x-ray machines are precalibrated with 2 SID measurement calibrations on the arm of the machine: one for tabletop views and the other for Bucky views. Generally, the desired SID will be 40 cm. The Bucky is a tray below the table that usually has a grid and is used for larger animals in order to improve film quality (see later in this chapter). The kVp calculated by Santes' rule is the one needed for tabletop views and must be adjusted (increased) if a grid or Bucky tray is used.

Personal Protective Equipment

Somatic damage is the damage to the body caused by radiation that manifests during the animal's or the person's lifetime. Most radiation damage can be repaired by the body, but large doses or repeated small doses of radiation can cause damage to DNA or RNA that may be beyond the body's capacity to heal. This may be genetic damage to the reproductive organs that may be passed to the offspring or it may be somatic damage to other organs that can result in cancer, bone marrow damage, or cataracts.

Direct radiation is the absorption of x-rays directly from the primary beam. These are the highest energy and penetration and highest speed x-rays. They can cause the most damage to DNA and RNA if they are stopped by the cell. They can be avoided by keeping body parts out of the lighted area and minimizing the animal's exposure by **collimating** the beam, or decreasing the size to the minimum acceptable for the image needed. The **primary beam** is contained within the lighted area when the beam is collimated.

Scatter radiation refers to the x-rays that have hit a surface (either the animal, the cassette, or the table) and been reflected. They may go in any direction from the surface. These x-rays are slower and will not penetrate as deeply into the body, but this does not make them less dangerous. Scatter that penetrates the skin is more likely to stick to cellular DNA and RNA instead of passing right through the cell, resulting in damage. Most veterinary technicians are aware of the damage that direct radiation can do to the body, but few consider scatter radiation to be a problem. Minimizing exposure to scatter radiation is best performed by the use of chemical restraint of the animal and remote positioning.

Lead is the best protection from radiation. Because of the density and atomic weight of lead, x-rays cannot penetrate a lead barrier easily. Most states require lead gowns and gloves be provided for the technician, but thyroid collars and lead-impregnated glasses should also be provided. A lead barrier wall is also useful.

Because most of the damage done to cells by x-rays involves rapidly dividing cells, pregnant women and children under the age of 18 should not be exposed to radiation in the performance of their duties (even with a lead barrier). Lead coverings will protect abdominal organs including ovaries and testicles in other employees.

The hands are the body part closest to the patient during manual restraint and positioning. Lead gloves will help decrease exposure to both primary and scatter radiation, but should not be relied on totally. Lead mitts that only cover the tops of the hands and allow the fingers to be free for better restraint and positioning will not protect against scatter radiation and should not be used.

Thyroid collars are important because one of the highest incidences of thyroid adenocarcinoma occurs among veterinary technicians (even radiology technicians do not have as high an incidence). The reason for this is the amount of scatter radiation exposure that vet techs can incur from manual restraint of patients for x-rays. Because the thyroid gland is rapidly dividing and superficially located in a potentially unprotected area (the throat), exposure to scatter radiation is likely.

Lead-impregnated glasses are important because there is a high incidence of cataract formation from x-rays. Cataracts are water bubbles in the lens of the eye. They can occur from scatter radiation because the lens epithelium is a rapidly dividing area that is superficial. Corneal squamous cell carcinoma and other ophthalmic cancers can also occur.

All radiation PPE should be checked occasionally to make sure the barrier is intact. Folding gloves or gowns, animal bites through lead gloves, and normal wear and tear can all make lead barriers ineffective over time. Gowns and gloves should be radiographed every 6 to 12 months to ensure effective coverage.

Dosimetry badges are not truly personal protective equipment. They do not protect against radiation, but they do monitor the radiation assumed to be absorbed by the body. The **maximum permissible dose** (MPD) is the maximum dose of radiation that an individual can receive over a given period. This is monitored by law. The best method of preventing overdose of radiation is to use the *as low as reasonably achievable* (**ALARA**) model. In some states, it is illegal to restrain animals manually for radiography. To assure that the MPD and ALARA are being met, dosimetry badges are issued to every employee involved in radiation techniques in the practice.

Dosimetry badges should be worn on the outside of the lead apron at the collar in an area not covered by the thyroid shield. If they are within the lead apron, a falsely low reading will occur. A dosimetry badge should be provided for (and worn by) each employee allowed in the x-ray imaging room. Badges should be monitored a minimum of once a year by a reputable company. The maximum permissible dose is 0.05 Sv per year (the equivalent of 5 rems per year).

Dosimetry rings may also be provided in some practices, especially practices performing nuclear scintigraphy or CT scans.

Grids

Scatter radiation not only causes somatic damage, it causes decreased image quality because bouncing radiation also activates the phosphors in the screens. To reduce the blurring effect of scatter radiation, grids are used. **Grids** are very thin strips of lead separated by sheets of paper or cardboard. The paper allows the x-ray photons to pass through unobstructed, but the lead sheets absorb the photons that are coming in at the wrong angle (scatter radiation). This will also improve contrast (along with the kVp). It is important to note that grids must be used for any technique where the area of interest is greater than 10 cm in thickness.

Grids may be focused or unfocused. *Unfocused grids* have the strips parallel to each other perpendicular to the base. *Focused grids* have strips that are placed at a slightly increasing angle as they go farther from the center to accommodate the fact that the light beams are coming in at an angle from the source the farther they get from the center of the beam. Unfocused grids can be placed over the cassette without regard to side. Focused grids must be placed with the appropriate side toward the beam or else a phenomenon called grid cutoff will occur. With grid cutoff, the center of the image will be present, but the image will be undeveloped at the edges. (See Figure 10.4.)

Grids also vary in their grid ratio and lines per centimeter. The **grid ratio** is determined by the height of the lead strip in relation to its width. An 8:1 grid ratio will not absorb as much scatter as a 16:1 grid ratio. Lines per centimeter is the distance between lead strips on the grid. Thinner strips mean that more lines per centimeter are present. This makes for a better image quality because thicker strips will show up on the film with a stationary grid (rather than a Bucky tray) as striations in the image. Both lines per centimeter and grid ratios are used to calculate the grid efficiency.

The *Bucky tray* (also called a **Potter-Bucky tray**) is usually placed beneath the table and is used for under-the-table techniques on larger patients. This tray contains a grid that will move back and forth rapidly. The advantage of a Bucky technique over a stationary grid is that there are no grid lines present on the finished film.

Using a grid (whether it is a Bucky or stationary) requires modification of Santes' rule:

$$(2 \times \text{thickness in cm}) + 40 + \text{grid ratio adjustment} = \text{kVp}$$

GRID RATIO	GRID RATIO ADJUSTMENT
5:1	6–8
8:1	8–10
12:1	10–15
16:1	15–20

Collimation

The collimator restricts the size of the x-ray beam leaving the tube. It is a set of 4 lead sheets that are adjustable via knobs on the tube housing. One set of 2 sheets controls the width of the beam, the other the length. Collimation of the beam reduces the radiation exposure of the patient and the technician. A light is

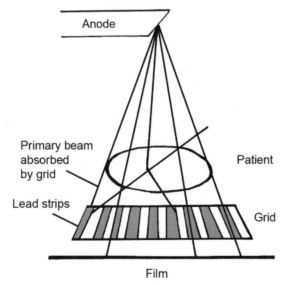

Figure 10.4 *Focused Grid*

usually present behind the collimator, enabling the technician to visualize the expected route of the primary beam. Collimation not only decreases exposure to the primary beam but reduces scatter radiation as well.

Film Labeling

Labeling of the film must be within the emulsion in order to be accepted as a legal image in a court of law. This may be done by writing directly on the undeveloped image with a pencil or exposing a lead marker on the cassette during the exposure. The minimum label for a radiograph should include the hospital's name and address, the first and last name of the patient, and the date. Many markers will also include the animal's age, sex, and breed. Additional markers should be in-

cluded if necessary (L and R, time markers, and so on). The **Orthopedic Foundation of America** (OFA) also requires that the breed identification number or microchip number be included on their films.

Artifact

Most artifacts are actually caused by human error while taking the radiograph or during the developing process. For these reasons, untrained personnel should not take radiographs. Human error may increase the number of radiographs needed and the radiation exposure of both patient and coworkers. The ALARA rule should be followed at all times.

Every film should be evaluated and trends noted so that troubleshooting of technique and maintenance of equipment can be performed early.

TROUBLESHOOTING ARTIFACTS			
ARTIFACT	**MACHINE CAUSES**	**HUMAN ERROR CAUSES**	**DEVELOPING CAUSES**
film too dark	machine timer out of calibration	kVp set too high mAs set too high SID too low	too much time in developer high developer temperature
Film too light	tube failure timer not calibrated drop in voltage from the wall	kVp set too low mAs set too low incorrect film with screen (blue-sensitive film with rare-earth screen, for example)	too little time in developer developer temperature too low developer exhausted developer poisoned with fixative developer diluted with water
Lack of contrast (uniform grey)		kVp set too high radiation fog increased temperature and humidity during film storage out-of-date film not using a grid with a high kVp double exposure safelight failure or light leakage in the darkroom	chemical fog (old chemicals, storage in high temperatures) increased developer time

(continued)

TROUBLESHOOTING ARTIFACTS (continued)

ARTIFACT	MACHINE CAUSES	HUMAN ERROR CAUSES	DEVELOPING CAUSES
Lack of detail	x-ray beam not directed at the film properly (may be machine problem or human error)	increased object–film distance patient motion double exposure	
Heavy lines on radiograph		grid out of proper focal distance grid out of alignment with beam grid upside down damaged grid	roller marks from jammed film or dirty rollers in the automatic processor
Inconsistent film density	pitted or damaged anode (target) Bucky not centered under primary beam (may be machine problem or human error)	poor cassette maintenance (improper screen-to-film contact, light leakage) cassette not locked into Bucky correctly improper collimation	
Black marks on film		folded or crimped film, fingernail marks static electricity developer on film prior to processing incorrect technique when loading cassette	films stuck together during processing (not waiting long enough between feeding films into processor or allowing film to touch each other in hand tank)
White marks on film		improper cassette maintenance (hair in cassette, scratched screen, contrast medium on cassette)	air bubble on film during processing film touching side of hand tank during processing fingerprints fixer splashing on film prior to developing
Yellow film			incorrect fixation (not fixed long enough, film sticking together during fixation, incomplete final wash)

Digital Radiography

Digital radiography is becoming increasingly common in veterinary medicine. Digital radiographs allow for increased storage space (film radiographs need to be kept for a minimum of several years after the date of imaging as a medical record, which varies by state), decreased plumbing problems, and decreased need for chemical and heavy metal disposal. Because images are adjustable on the computer, faulty technique can usually be compensated for and poor images salvaged without the need for further radiation exposure of the patient and the veterinary staff. Radiographic archives may be transmitted electronically to specialty practices for evaluation instead of copying or giving them to the client and hoping to have them returned to the medical record.

Two different types of digital radiography are available using different technologies: **computed radiography** (CR) and **direct digital radiography** (DDR). Many practices choose the CR because it can be used with only existing film radiographic equipment with only minor modifications.

Computed radiography requires an x-ray machine (with mAs and kVp adjustments, a timer, collimator, Bucky, and grid), an imaging plate, a plate reader, and a computer. CR does not require cassettes, film, or developing equipment. The imaging plate (IP) is used instead of the film to generate an image. The plate reader processes the latent image and turns the data into a digital signal. Software for the computer allows the image to be manipulated and enables data storage, retrieval, and transfer. The software packages are called PACS (picture archiving and communication systems) and differ among manufacturers.

The imaging plate has a layer of phosphor crystals that can store x-ray energy. It is equivalent to 200-speed film (medium speed). The x-rays cause the electrons in the crystals to move to a higher energy state. This change in configuration can then be read by the reader using a red laser light. When the light hits the crystals, the crystals with the high-energy electrons drop back to the normal state and phosphoresce (similar to intensifying screens in regular film imaging). The reader then gathers the light energy and converts it to a digital image which is then sent to a computer for further evaluation and analysis.

Direct digital radiography is similar to CR except that the image is acquired directly to the computer rather than via an image plate and reader. Currently, these machines are more expensive than the CR models and are not seen as frequently in veterinary medicine. They contain the x-ray machine, the digital image receptor, an image processing unit, and a computer with an image management system. The digital image receptor is the same as the imaging plate in the CR system. Instead of being read in a reader, however, the laser beam hits the image receptor directly and the information is received by the image processing unit. The advantages to this technique are that there is no movement of the plate, so the likelihood of phosphor damage is decreased.

Troubleshooting for Digital Radiography

Computed radiography and direct digital radiography can adjust for errors of exposure up to 20% by image manipulation on the computer. Image processing using the PACS system should only be performed by the veterinarian. Raw images should be stored on the computer to prevent artifacts from image processing that may occur due to overmanipulation of the images. The raw image is the original histogram, or greyscale graph, of the image. This is truly what is manipulated during image analysis and processing, not the image itself. Most machines have preset histograms for various techniques (abdomen vs. thorax, for example), so, with proper technique, the histogram should not need to be adjusted a great deal.

RADIOGRAPHIC TROUBLESHOOTING		
ARTIFACT	CAUSE IN CR	CAUSE IN DDR
Thin, white, jagged lines on perimeter of image	cracked imaging plate	
Fogging of image	backscatter (apply lead foil to the back of the plate) imaging plate not erased prior to exposure	receptor not erased prior to exposure
Multiple images	More than one imaging plate loaded into the cassette	
White line perpendicular to printed image sheet	laser printer problem	laser printer problem
White line across image	plate reader debris	reader debris
Curvy white lines	hair in image plate	
Moiré interference pattern on image (ripples or waves that appear to be optical illusions)	problem with the Bucky use of a grid with the same frequency of lines as the reader's scan lines incorrectly loaded image plate	problem with the Bucky use of a grid with the same frequency of lines as the reader's scan lines

Positioning

Positioning the animal for radiography is an art form. Proper positioning is critical to the veterinarian's ability to interpret a radiograph and diagnose pathology. Incorrect positioning is the most common cause of x-ray retakes in practice.

Proper positioning includes establishing the correct field of view, placing the animal and its limbs in the correct orientation, placing the cassette, film, or digital plate in the correct position, and proper collimation and placement of the beam.

Small Animals

Ideally, small animals such as dogs and cats should be anesthetized or heavily sedated for basic radiographs in order to minimize radiation exposure. In cases where this is not possible (many gastrointestinal studies must be performed on awake animals, for instance), care must be taken to ensure that the operator's body is out of the primary beam and heavily protected against scatter radiation.

Skull radiographs should always be performed on anesthetized or sedated animals for proper positioning. Perfect symmetry is important and minor changes can completely invalidate the film. Most skull series require a minimum of 3 views and may require up to 6 views. The 5 most common views are shown in the table. Right and left sides should be identified with a marker.

SKULL RADIOGRAPHS

VIEW	FIELD OF VIEW (AREA INCLUDED IN PRIMARY BEAM)	POSITION	BEAM CENTERING	OBJECT OF STUDY
Lateral skull	tip of nose, occiput, atlas, dorsal part of skull, ramus of the mandible	right lateral recumbency with legs pulled caudally; both sides of mandible superimposed; sponge placed under muzzle to allow midline of skull to be parallel with tabletop	medial canthus of the eye	nasal cavity, frontal sinuses, osseous bulla
Ventrodorsal (VD) skull	tip of nose, occiput, atlas, zeugmatic arches	dorsal recumbency (on its back) with head and neck extended and legs pulled caudally; hard palate and cervical spine parallel to the table (tape the maxilla to the table—tape should go through the mouth); sponge under the neck to extend the neck	on the midline between the medial acanthi of the eyes **note:** the endotracheal tube should be removed for this view	nasal cavity and nasal septum
Open-mouth VD skull	same as above	same as above except the mandible, endotracheal tube, and tongue are pulled back with a tape loop	angled 20 degrees from vertical so it is aimed into the mouth toward the base of the ears	frontal sinuses, caudal portion of the pharynx
Frontal or skyline view	bridge of the nose, zygomatic arches, base of skull	dorsal recumbency with forelimbs pulled caudally; nose is at a 90-degree angle to the table	centered over the frontal sinuses **note:** measure from the medial canthus of the eye to the tabletop	frontal sinuses
Open mouth tympanic bulla view	similar to the frontal view	dorsal recumbency with forelimbs pulled caudally; tape loops are placed around both the maxilla and the mandible and both should be at a 45-degree angle to vertical	the beam should be centered between the two angles (mandible and maxilla) and centered over the bullae **note:** measure at the commissure of the lips	osseous bullae (ear pathology)

Spinal radiographs should also be performed on anesthetized or heavily sedated patients because they allow proper positioning of the patient and decreased motion artifact. Spinal radiographs may be either plain films or with contrast (myelography). Myelography is performed in cases of suspected spinal cord or disc disease. It involves the injection of a water-soluble organic iodide into the epidural space. This allows the radiopaque material to migrate along the spine within the cerebrospinal fluid. Abnormalities in the ability of the material to migrate (masses, disc protrusion, and so on) will show as thin or absent areas of the contrast column. If a cerebrospinal fluid analysis is needed, it should always be performed prior to the myelography to prevent contamination of the sample.

The spine may be separated into segments for ease of discussion: cervical, thoracic, thoracolumbar, lumbar, and sacrococcygeal. Most spinal views will be performed in extension (with the spine straight). (Exceptions are noted in the table.) Collimation is necessary. Remember, the tighter the collimation, the less scatter and the clearer the image obtained. Pads, troughs, and tape are needed for proper positioning and should be readily available.

SPINAL RADIOGRAPHS

VIEW	FIELD OF VIEW	POSITION	BEAM CENTER	OBJECT OF STUDY
Lateral cervical	occiput to the spine of the scapula; view should include all the structures of the neck	Lateral recumbency with forelimbs pulled caudally; neck should be straight; pads under jaw and cervical spine will keep structures parallel to the tabletop	over the spine midway between atlas and spine of the scapula	cervical spine
VD cervical spine	same landmarks as above	dorsal recumbency with forelimbs pulled caudally; no padding is needed for this view, but it is important to keep the landmarks parallel to each other and perpendicular to the beam	same as above **note:** take measurement at the manubrium (most cranial portion of the sternum)	same as above
Flexed lateral cervical spine	same landmarks as above	right lateral recumbency with limbs in a natural position, head should be flexed (pulled toward the chest) ventrally	same as above	same as above; this may be dangerous in animals with abnormalities of the cervial spine
Lateral thoracic spine	spine of the scapula to the last rib; collimate beam to the dorsal portion of the back to midway through the ribcage ventrally	right lateral recumbency with limbs extended cranially; pad should be placed under the sternum to maintain the spine parallel to the tabletop	midthoracic region **note:** measure at the highest point of the ribcage	thoracic disc spaces

(continued)

SPINAL RADIOGRAPHS (continued)

VIEW	FIELD OF VIEW	POSITION	BEAM CENTER	OBJECT OF STUDY
VD thoracic spine	spine of the scapula/ thoracic inlet to the last rib; collimate to include the middle third of the thorax	dorsal recumbency with limbs extended cranially; it is very important to have the spine and the sternum superimposed on the radiograph	sternum note: measure at the highest point of the sternum	thoracic disc spaces
Lateral thoracolumbar spine	midthorax to midlumbar region	lateral recumbency with padding under the sternum; it is very important that the spine be parallel to the tabletop	beam should be centered over the anticlinal vertebrae (the dip in the spine on palpation) note: measure at the highest point of the ribcage	thoracolumbar junction is the most common area of injury in the canine
Ventrodorsal thoracolumbar spine	same as above	dorsal recumbency with legs extended cranially, spine and sternum superimposed	same as above	thoracolumbar junction
Lateral lumbar spine	last ribs to wings of the ilium; collimate to include midway down the abdomen	lateral recumbency with forelegs in a natural position; pads should be under sternum and between rear legs to maintain ilium and spine parallel to the tabletop	center over the middle of the lumbar region note: measure over the area of the anticlinal vertebra	lumbar spine
VD lumbar spine	last ribs to wings of the ilium	dorsal recumbency with wings of ilium parallel to each other and spine straight	center over the midlumbar region note: measure over the area of the anticlinal vertebrae	lumbar spine
Lateral lumbosacral	last three lumbar vertebrae to first few coccygeal vertebrae	lateral recumbency with forelegs in a natural position; pads should be under sternum and between rear legs to maintain ilium and spine parallel to the tabletop	center over the wings of the ilium note: measure at the highest point of the hip region	lumbosacral spine and sacrum

VIEW	FIELD OF VIEW	POSITION	BEAM CENTER	OBJECT OF STUDY
SPINAL RADIOGRAPHS *(continued)*				
VD lumbosacral	same as above	dorsal recumbency with rear legs extended caudally; obturator foramen should be equal in size on resulting radiograph	see above	see above

Thoracic radiographs will not require as high a setting on mAs because of the amount of air present. In other words, there is less soft tissue for the beam to penetrate, so fewer electrons will be needed. In general, a grid will not be required for a thoracic radiograph on an animal that is less than 15 cm thickness (for other areas, use a grid if the animal is greater than 10 cm). This is because the amount of soft tissue in the thorax is minimal, so there is less material to cause scatter.

The type of thoracic studies done will depend on the condition of the animal. An animal in respiratory distress should never be placed in dorsal recumbency. Dorsal recumbency will cause interference with activity of the diaphragm because of the weight of the liver and other viscera. Animals coming in for cancer surveys should have a minimum of 2 lateral views (right and left) and a ventrodorsal (VD) or a dorsoventral (DV) view. This allows the veterinarian to see potentially hidden metastases.

VIEW	FIELD OF VIEW	POSITION	BEAM CENTER	OBJECT OF STUDY
THORACIC RADIOGRAPHS				
Lateral thorax (usually right lateral, may also use left lateral for metastasis checks)	manubrium, last rib including the dorsal and ventral surfaces of the animal	right (or left) lateral recumbency with legs extended cranially, sternum should be parallel to the tabletop	heart base	lungs, heart, trachea, esophagus, metastasis check
VD thorax	manubrium, last rib, lateral chest walls should be included in the view; ideally, a portion of the cervical trachea should be included	dorsal recumbency, front legs extended cranially, rear legs in natural position, sternum and spine should be superimposed	heart base	same as above
Dorsoventral (DV) thorax	same as above	sternal recumbency, front legs slightly extended and elbows rotated medially, rear legs in natural position, spine and sternum superimposed	heart base	same as above

note: this view will show the thoracic blood vessels very well; also good for pneumothorax |

Because the abdomen has so many different densities, it is best to use a high kVp, low mAs technique for abdominal radiographs. This will give the maximum amount of contrast and minimize radiation. In deep-chested dogs such as greyhounds, using 2 different plates (one the cranial abdomen and one the caudal abdomen) will be helpful. If two different plates are not used, the cranial portion of the abdomen will be underexposed and the caudal portion overexposed. In these cases, measure over the 13th rib for the cranial portion of the abdomen and over the femoral head for the caudal portion. For all other animals, measurement of the abdomen over the 13th rib should provide adequate density of the image.

ABDOMINAL RADIOGRAPHS				
VIEW	FIELD OF VIEW	POSITION	BEAM CENTER	OBJECT OF STUDY
Lateral abdomen	13th rib cranially, femoral heads caudally, dorsal surface and ventral surface of the animal	right lateral recumbency (this puts the fundus of the stomach toward the beam); use pad under sternum to keep spine parallel to tabletop	caudal to last rib	liver, spleen, gastrointestinal organs, reproductive organs, kidneys, bladder
VD abdomen	same as above	dorsal recumbency with forelegs and hindlegs extended and stifles internally rotated so that the patellas are centered in the trochlea	same as above	same as above

If the study is of a joint, the bone above and below the joint of interest should be included in radiographs of the appendages. If the study is of a bone, the joints above and below the bone of interest should be included in the field of view. All radiographs of limbs should be labeled as to side (R or L).

Note: The Orthopedic Foundation of America (OFA) is a certifying organization that was formed to try to reduce the incidence of hereditary abnormalities in purebred dogs (especially hip dysplasia). The organization includes radiologists, statisticians, and geneticists and currently certifies animals for a large number of genetic diseases including cardiomyopathy, deafness, closed angle glaucoma, elbow dysplasia, patellar luxation, and thyroid. The OFA's requirements can be accessed at www.offa.org/hdappbw.pdf. Dogs to be assessed for hip dysplasia must be ≥2 years of age. All required information including the animal's AKC registration name, number, and breed must be included within the emulsion of the film. The view for OFA hip certification is the VD pelvis with legs extended and must include the entire pelvis and the stifles. Obturator foramina must be equal in size on the radiograph and the patellas must be in the middle of the trochlear ridge or evaluation is impossible. OFA readings are purely subjective (a board of board-certified veterinary radiologists evaluates every film and gives it a score of excellent to poor and a grade of 1 to 4 depending on the severity of dysplasia). Another measure of hip dysplasia is the PennHIP evaluation.

HINDLIMB VIEWS				
VIEW	FIELD OF VIEW	POSITION	BEAM CENTER	OBJECT OF STUDY
Lateral pelvis	cranial portion of the wings of the ilium to the caudal border of the ischium	right lateral recumbency with the down leg pulled cranially and the up leg pulled caudally slightly; a pad should be placed under the up leg to ensure that the spine remains parallel to the tabletop; the acetabula should be superimposed on the image	hip joint measure at the thickest portion of the area	pelvis, acetabula
Flexed VD pelvis	wings of the ilium to caudal border of ischium	dorsal recumbency with legs in a frog-legged position (stifles should be cranial to the hip joint)	center of the pelvis measure at the thickest portion of the area (over the acetabula)	pelvis, hip joints
Extended VD pelvis	wings of the ilium to proximal tibia (should include patellas)	dorsal recumbency with rear legs extended (hold at the tarsus) and stifles rotated inward so that the patella lies in the middle of the trochlear groove; femurs should be parallel to each other on the image	caudal pelvis (ischium) note: measure at the stifle with legs in full extension	hip joints, pelvis, femur note: this is the view used for OFA hip studies (see text following)
Lateral femur	the ventral part of the pelvis including the acetabulum proximally to the proximal tibia distally	lateral recumbency (depending on side of interest) with up leg abducted; leg of interest should be on the plate in a natural position	centered over midfemur note: measure over thickest portion of the thigh; L/R markers should be used	femur (diaphysis)
Craniocaudal femur	hip joint to stifle	dorsal recumbency with leg extended and as close to parallel to the plate as possible; patella should be centered in trochlear groove on image	midfemur note: measure over thickest portion of the thigh; L/R markers should be used	femur (diaphysis)
Lateral stifle	distal femur to proximal tibia	lateral recumbency with leg of interest in natural position and up leg pulled out of the way	stifle joint (medial side) measure over thickest point of area of interest	stifle joint

(continued)

VIEW	FIELD OF VIEW	POSITION	BEAM CENTER	OBJECT OF STUDY
HINDLIMB VIEWS *(continued)*				
Caudocranial stifle	Distal femur to proximal tibia	ventral recumbency with leg of interest in extension caudally; patella should be on the plate	stifle joint note: measure over the distal femur	stifle joint
Lateral tibia/fibula	stifle joint proximally to tarsus distally	lateral recumbency similar to lateral stifle; plate should be placed more distally	tibia/fibula (medial side) note: measure over thickest region of gastrocnemius	tibia/fibula diaphyses
Caudocranial tibia/fibula	stifle joint proximally to tarsus distally	ventral recumbency similar to caudocranial stifle	tibia/fibula note: measure over stifle joint	tibia/fibula diaphyses
Lateral tarsus	distal tibia to proximal metatarsals	lateral recumbency (see stifle and lateral tibia); plate should be under the area of interest	tarsus (medial side) note: measure at the tarsus	tarsus
Plantarodorsal tarsus	distal tibia to proximal metatarsals	ventral recumbency (see caudocranial stifle and tibia); dorsal surface of foot in contact with plate	tarsus note: measure at the tarsus	tarsus
Dorsoplantar tarsus	distal tibia to proximal metatarsals	ventral recumbency, but foot pulled cranially and rear of tarsus (calcaneus) is in contact with the plate	tarsus note: measure at tarsus	tarsus
Lateral metatarso-phalangeal	distal tibia to last phalanx of longest digit	lateral recumbency	metatarsal bones (medial side)	metatarsal bones
Oblique metatarso-phalangeal	same as above	lateral recumbency, foot may either be spread with a paddle or held at a 45-degree angle to the plate	metatarsal bones note: measure at the thickest portion	metatarsal and phalangeal bones
Dorsoplantar metatarso-phalangeal	same as above	see dorsoplantar tarsus	metatarsal bones note: measure at the thickest portion	same as above

	FORELIMB VIEWS			
VIEW	**FIELD OF VIEW**	**POSITION**	**BEAM CENTER**	**OBJECT OF STUDY**
Lateral scapula	dorsal border of the scapula to the shoulder joint	lateral recumbency with down leg extended cranially and up leg extended caudally; head should be extended dorsally note: measure over thickest portion	scapula	down scapula
Caudocranial scapula (PA)	sternum to the lateral portion of the spine of the scapula; shoulder joint and caudal border of the scapula should be included	dorsal recumbency with legs extended cranially; head should be rolled away from the side of interest	scapula note: measure to the sternum	spine of scapula and medial border of scapula
Lateral shoulder	distal portion of scapula, proximal portion of humerus	lateral recumbency with shoulder of interest on the table pulled cranially; other leg is pulled caudally; head and neck are extended dorsally	shoulder joint (medial side) note: measure to sternum	shoulder joint
Caudocranial shoulder (PA)	sternum to proximal humerus	dorsal recumbency (see caudocranial scapula)	shoulder joint note: this view is rarely used	shoulder joint
Lateral humerus	distal scapula to proximal radius/ulna	lateral recumbency	humerus (medial side)	humerus (diaphysis)
Caudocranial humerus (PA)	same as above	dorsal recumbency with both forelimbs extended cranially	humerus (caudal side) note: this view will cause elongation of the image because of the increased distance (OFD) between the humerus and the film	humerus (diaphysis)
Lateral elbow	distal humerus, proximal radius, and ulna	lateral recumbency with foreleg in natural position	elbow note: measure over the epicondyles of the humerus	elbow
90-degree flexion elbow	same as above	same as above except the elbow should be flexed to 90 degrees	same as above	elbow; excellent for visualization of the anconeus

(continued)

FORELIMB VIEWS *(continued)*				
VIEW	**FIELD OF VIEW**	**POSITION**	**BEAM CENTER**	**OBJECT OF STUDY**
Craniocaudal elbow (AP)	same as above	sternal recumbency with forelimbs extended cranially	elbow note: measure over mid bicipital region	elbow (condyles of the humerus)
Lateral radius/ulna	elbow to carpus	lateral recumbency with foreleg in natural position	radius, ulna note: be sure to include entire olecranon	radius and ulna
Craniocaudal radius/ulna (AP)	same as above	sternal recumbency with forelimbs extended cranially	same as above	radius and ulna
Lateral carpus	distal radius and ulna to proximal metacarpals	lateral recumbency with carpus in extended position	carpus	carpus
Flexed lateral carpus	same as above	lateral recumbency with carpus in flexed lateral position	carpus	carpus (may be better for visualization of slab fractures)
Dorsopalmar carpus (AP)	same as above	sternal recumbency with carpus extended	carpus	carpus
Medial and lateral oblique carpus	same as above	same as above although foot is either supinated or pronated 45 degrees for view	carpus	carpus

*Metacarpal and phalangeal views are generally the same for both fore- and hindlimbs. In the forelimbs, the palmarodorsal view is rarely used. Refer to metatarsal and phalangeal views described earlier.

PennHIP is a determination of the distraction index of the hip joint. The distraction index is the ability of the femoral head to be subluxated (completely or partially dislocated) out of the acetabulum. Whereas any veterinary hospital is capable of taking an adequate OFA film, only veterinarians certified in the techniques are able to do PennHIP studies. The advantage of PennHIP over OFA is that earlier diagnosis of the potential for hip dysplasia is possible (animals may be tested at 6 months of age). Animals must be anesthetized for this procedure.

Large Animals

Large-animal radiography generally involves only the extremities and the skull unless taken with the sophisticated equipment available at a university teaching hospital. Because of the large size of the animal, the generation of adequately penetrating x-rays is almost impossible. If enough radiation were produced, the risk of radiation damage to the personnel would be large. Forelimb views may be taken as far proximal as the elbow joint. Hindlimb views may be taken as far proximal as the stifle joint.

Most radiology units used for large animals are portable with fixed anodes. This is important because overheating of the machinery can occur. Safety of personnel is very important. Hands should not be used to hold cassettes in place. Cassette holders with long poles are used for placement. Positioning for large animals can be facilitated with wooden blocks.

Horses' legs are shaped like cylinders. This allows various views to be taken in order to get a 360-degree evaluation of the joint. This is very important for prepurchase exams of valuable horses. Missing a small bone chip can result in huge loss of income for clients and the possibility of litigation for the veterinarian. The remaining views from the metacarpus distal to the hoof are the same as for the foreleg.

LARGE ANIMAL FORELIMBS				
VIEW	FIELD OF VIEW	POSITION	BEAM CENTER	OBJECT OF STUDY
Craniocaudal (AP) elbow	distal humerus, proximal radius	plate should be placed caudal to the elbow, animal should be weight-bearing but slightly abducted	elbow joint perpendicular to plate from the cranial side	elbow
Mediolateral elbow	same as above	the limb of interest should be extended cranially, the plate should be placed on the lateral side of the joint	on the elbow, source should be from medial side	elbow
Dorsopalmar (AP) carpus	distal radius to proximal metacarpals	the horse should be weight-bearing on both legs (square); the plate should be caudal/palmar to the carpus	carpus; the source should be cranial to the carpus at a 90-degree angle to the plate	carpus
Lateromedial carpus	same as above	the plate should be on the medial side of the carpus	carpus; the source should be lateral to the carpus at a 90-degree angle to the plate	carpus
Dorsolateral-palmeromedial oblique carpus	same as above	the plate should be on the palmeromedial surface of the carpus	carpus; the source should be on the craniolateral side of the carpus	carpus
Dorsomedial-palmerolateral oblique carpus	same as above	the plate should be on the palmerolateral surface of the carpus	the source should be on the craniomedial side of the carpus	carpus

(continued)

LARGE ANIMAL FORELIMBS (continued)

VIEW	FIELD OF VIEW	POSITION	BEAM CENTER	OBJECT OF STUDY
Flexed lateromedial carpus	same as above	position is with the leg flexed at the carpus (knee); the plate is placed medial to the carpus	the source is lateral to the carpus	carpus
Dorsoproximal 60-degree dorsodistal oblique (skyline) carpus	the cranial surface of the carpus	the leg should be flexed at the knee with the cannon bone (metacarpus) parallel to the ground; the plate should be placed directly against the dorsal surface of the cannon bone	the beam should be angled at a 60- to 65-degree angle to the plate through the carpus	looks at the first line of carpal bones
Dorsoproximal 20-degree dorsodistal oblique (skyline) carpus	the cranial surface of the carpus	same position as above	the beam should be angled at a 20- to 25-degree angle to the plate through the carpus	looks at the second/distal row of carpal bones
Dorsopalmar metacarpus (AP)	carpus proximally, fetlock distally	plate should be caudal/palmar to the metacarpus	source should be from cranial/dorsal surface perpendicular to the plate	metacarpal bones (MC 2–4)
Lateromedial metacarpus	same as above	plate should be placed medial to the metacarpus	source should be lateral to the metacarpus perpendicular to the plate	metacarpal bones (MC 2–4)
Dorsolateral-palmaromedial oblique metacarpus	same as above	plate should be placed on palmaromedial surface (caudomedial)	source should be dorsolateral to the metacarpus perpendicular to the plate	metacarpal bones (MC 2–4)
Dorsomedial-palmarolateral oblique metacarpus	same as above	plate should be placed on the palmarolateral surface (caudolateral)	source should be dorsomedial to the metacarpus, perpendicular to the plate	metacarpal bones (MC 2–4)
Dorsopalmar fetlock (AP)	distal metacarpus to proximal long pastern (P1)	plate should be placed on the palmar (caudal) surface of the fetlock (metacarpophalangeal joint)	source should be dorsal to the fetlock perpendicular to the plate	metacarpophalangeal joint (fetlock)
Lateromedial fetlock	same as above	plate should be placed medial to the fetlock	source should be lateral to the fetlock perpendicular to the plate	metacarpophalangeal joint (fetlock)
Dorsolateral-palmaromedial oblique fetlock	same as above	plate should be placed on the caudomedial (palmaromedial) surface of the fetlock	source should be dorsolateral (craniolateral) to the fetlock perpendicular to the plate	metacarpophalangeal joint (fetlock)

	LARGE ANIMAL FORELIMBS *(continued)*			
VIEW	**FIELD OF VIEW**	**POSITION**	**BEAM CENTER**	**OBJECT OF STUDY**
Dorsomedial-palmarolateral oblique fetlock	same as above	plate should be placed on the caudolateral (palmarolateral) surface of the fetlock	source should be dorsomedial (craniolateral) to the fetlock, perpendicular to the plate	metacarpophalangeal joint (fetlock)
Dorsopalmar pastern (AP)	distal P1 to proximal P2 (short pastern)	plate should be on the caudal/palmar surface of the lower leg, parallel to the axis of the lower leg; place the plate against the fetlock and heels of the hoof	source should be dorsal to the lower leg; beam should be angled so that it is perpendicular to the axis of the pasterns	long pastern (P1) and interphalangeal joint (pastern joint)
Lateromedial pastern	same as above	plate should be on the medial surface of the lower leg	source should be lateral to the lower leg	same as above
Lateromedial hoof	P2 and hoof	plate should be directly medial to the lower leg	source should be directly lateral to the lower leg	coffin bone (P3)
Dorsopalmar hoof	same as above	hoof should sit on the plate (volar surface should contact plate surface)	beam should be angled 45-degrees from vertical	coffin bone (P3)
Dorsolateral-palmaromedial oblique hoof	same as above	same as above	beam should come from the lateral side at 45 degrees from vertical	coffin bone (P3)
Dorsomedial-palmarolateral oblique hoof	same as above	same as above	beam should come from the medial side at 45 degrees from vertical	coffin bone (P3)
Dorsoproximal-palmarodistal oblique navicular	same as above	requires a navicular block positioner; the hoof is placed at a 45-degree angle from vertical to the plate	the beam comes in perpendicular to the plate	navicular bone
Palmaroproximal-dorsodistal oblique navicular	same as above	hoof surface contacts the plate	the beam comes from the caudal/palmar surface at a 45-degree angle from horizontal	navicular bone

LARGE ANIMAL HINDLIMBS				
VIEW	FIELD OF VIEW	POSITION	BEAM CENTER	OBJECT OF STUDY
Caudocranial stifle (PA)	distal femur to proximal tibia	plate placed cranial to joint	source caudal to joint perpendicular to plate	stifle
Lateromedial stifle	same as above	plate placed medial to stifle	source lateral to stifle, perpendicular to plate	stifle
Dorsoplantar tarsus (AP)	distal tibia to proximal metacarpus	plate should be plantar/caudal to the hock	source should be cranial to the hock at a perpendicular angle to the plate	tarsus/hock
Lateromedial tarsus	same as above	plate should be medial to the hock	source should be lateral to the hock at a perpendicular angle to the plate	tarsus/hock
Dorsolateral-plantaromedial oblique tarsus	same as above	plate should be plantaromedial to the hock	source should be cranial and lateral to the hock	tarsus/hock
Doromedial-plantarolateral oblique tarsus	same as above	plate should be plantarolateral to the hock	source should be cranial and medial to the hock	tarsus/hock
Flexed dorsoplantar tarsus	same as above	hock should be in flexed position and the plate should be on the plantar surface	source should be caudal and dorsal to the hock and the beam should be directed at a 60-degree angle to perpendicular through the joint	calcaneus

Exotics and Pocket Pets

Pocket pets, reptiles, and birds are generally imaged as *crittergraphs*: whole-body images of the animal in DV/VD or right lateral recumbency. For birds, restraint boards are available that make positioning easier. Many snakes, rodents, and rabbits can be positioned with a restraint tube. All other small exotic species can be restrained with a combination of sedation/anesthesia and masking tape. Other types of tape will remove plumage, scales, and fur and may make temperature control difficult in already compromised patients. Use of a dental radiography machine can increase the clarity of images in very small patients.

Turtles and tortoises should have a skyline radiograph performed to assess the lung fields as well as a DV and lateral. Tortoises can be placed on a coffee can or box that brings the animal off the surface of the table. This will allow the tortoise to move its legs without being able to move away. The radiograph is then taken against a wall with the x-ray tube in the horizontal position. The beam should go from the head of the tortoise through the tail in a cranial to caudal direction. Many exotic animal practices have wall-mounted Buckys especially for taking horizontal views.

Contrast Studies

Contrast studies may be used to improve images from various areas that might not be easily seen on plain films. The same techniques are used for plain films and contrast studies except for the use of contrast media. Contrast studies can help show variations in the walls of tubular organs such as the gastrointestinal system and the urinary tract, help show obstructions or masses, and help to determine the extent of fistulas (draining tracts). Contrast is also used in myelography to assess the spinal cord. Two general types of contrast media are used: positive and negative contrast. Positive contrast media shows up as **radiodense** (white) on the x-ray. Examples of positive contrast media are barium sulfate and organic iodides. Negative contrast media show up as **radiolucent** (black) on the image. Gases such as room air, oxygen, and carbon dioxide are usually used. Double contrast studies can also be used. This usually involves the use of an organic iodide and a gas.

Barium is generally used for gastrointestinal (GI) studies (barium swallow for upper-GI and barium enema for lower-GI studies) because it is not affected by digestive enzymes or acids. Studies can take up to 3 hours to clear through the GI tract, so multiple views over a long time period must be taken. In general, GI studies are performed on awake or mildly sedated animals because anesthesia affects gastrointestinal motility. This causes increased exposure of veterinary staff to x-rays. If perforation of the gastrointestinal tract is suspected or vomiting is a problem, barium should not be used because it causes peritoneal inflammation and severe aspiration pneumonia, which can be fatal. Barium should never be used for bladder studies. Barium is generally dosed at 3 to 5 ml/lb for upper-GI studies and 5 to 7 ml/lb for lower-GI studies.

Varying forms of organic iodides may be used for different types of contrast studies. Ionic solutions of organic iodides are used for GI studies with suspected GI perforation. They do not show up on radiographs as well as barium and should only be used if perforation is suspected. Ionic solutions may also be used for IV injection (cardiovascular studies, kidney studies, and so on) or injection into the bladder for positive contrast. Ionic solutions should never be used for myelographic studies because they cause meningeal inflammation. Organic iodides are generally dosed at 1 ml/lb for upper-GI studies, 3 to 5 ml/lb for cystography (bladder evaluation), and 1 ml/lb for IV injection.

Nonionic iodides should be used for myelography. They may also be used for IV studies, as with ionic solutions, but they are very expensive. Nonionic iodides should be dosed at 1 ml/lb for myelography.

Organic iodides can cause acute anaphylaxis and renal failure in susceptible humans, but are generally well tolerated in animals. People with shellfish allergies should be careful when handling organic iodides.

When negative contrast media such as carbon dioxide, oxygen, and air are used, care must be taken not to overinflate the bladder or the rectum because the gases may be absorbed across the mucosa or even rupture the organ and cause embolisms (gas in the arteries of the brain or the heart). Gas should be injected until the organ has some resistance to palpation.

Double contrast studies are a combination of gas and iodine. Usually gas is added first followed by a small amount of organic iodine (if gas is added second, bubbles may form that can confuse the image). A total of 1 to 3 cc of iodine (3–5 ml/lb) should be added to the gas-inflated bladder.

Generally, contrast studies of any type should be performed on fasted animals. Enemas may be needed to clear the lower gastrointestinal system.

Ultrasound

Ultrasound is the production and reception of high-frequency, short wavelength sound waves. Audible sound is in the 20 KHz range (20,000 cycles/second). Ultrasound is generated at 2 to 10 million Hz (2 to 10 MHz). The computer in an ultrasound machine makes two calculations. The first is the distance traveled by the sound to the source and back to the **transducer** head. This gives a measure of the depth of the structure in the animal. The next is the impedance. The impedance is the ability of the object to stop and reflect the sound wave. The percentage of sound waves that are reflected back to the ultrasound head from the various tissues is received by the head (transducer) and interpreted by the computer as varying shades of white, grey, and black. It may even be used to determine the motion of an object (such as a needle being inserted into a body cavity or a visceral organ). Ultrasound has become increasingly important in veterinary medicine as both a diagnostic tool and an aid to laboratory testing.

Air and bone have the highest impedance (reflect more sound) and are seen as white or **hyperechoic**. Pure liquid has the lowest impedance to sound and is seen as black or **hypoechoic**. Fat is usually **isoechoic** (has the same reflection as surrounding tissues) unless it is diseased (saponified or calcified fat will show up as hyperechoic). When there is a difference between the impedance of two types of tissues, this shows as a change in density on the image and allows the veterinarian to differentiate tissues and organs. The spleen, for instance, is usually hyperechoic because of the amount of dense connective tissue. The bladder is hypoechoic because it contains urine, but it is surrounded by a relatively hyperechoic bladder wall.

History

Diagnostic ultrasound has been used in medicine since the 1950s. It is viewed as a safe diagnostic test because it does not cause disruption of the DNA or radiation poisoning. However, it can cause cell damage and increased cellular heat if used incorrectly. Cell damage occurs via a process called cavitation. Cavitation occurs when heat is produced within cells, causing intracellular gas pockets to form and explode the cells. This is very rare with modern diagnostic ultrasound, but is common with therapeutic ultrasound units used in physical therapy. It is also the mechanism that causes plaque destruction with dental ultrasound units.

A few studies documenting the prenatal effects of diagnostic ultrasound on brain development in animals show that there are changes in neural development in animals that receive 30 minutes of ultrasound. This may indicate that excessive use of prenatal ultrasonography might contribute to mental retardation and autism. Most practitioners, however, feel that the benefits outweigh the risks.

A more sophisticated type of ultrasound, Doppler sonography, is increasingly used to diagnose heart disease and blood vessel abnormalities such as aneurysms. Doppler analyzes the speed and pattern of blood flow and looks for turbulence (interruption of flow). This is especially useful in veterinary medicine when diagnosing cardiac valve abnormalities.

Ultrasound machines are regulated by the USDA and the FDA. Regulation is based on the mechanical index (a measure of cavitation) and the thermal index (a measure of tissue heating produced by the machine). Machines must be calibrated to conform to the appropriate standard and should be serviced by reputable companies.

Technique and Quality Control

Patient preparation for ultrasound is relatively simple. For abdominal ultrasound techniques, the animal should be fasted to minimize ingesta (substances inegested) and gas in the gut, which might interfere with imaging. In animals, the area should be shaved to enable better contact of the transducer to the skin (remember, air will reflect sound waves). This area is called the acoustic window. Ultrasound acoustic coupling gel is then used to create a fluid interface between the transducer and the patient. The acoustic window should be wiped with alcohol as a degreaser prior to this step. The transducer is then moved over the area of interest and images are assessed.

Various adjustments can be made to assess different items. Controls found on the ultrasound machine include brightness, contrast, depth, gain, output, and time gain compensation. If any of these controls are not properly set, the image quality and diagnostic usefulness will be decreased.

Brightness adjusts the histogram (adjusts the amplitude or height of the histogram) to increase or decrease the total brightness of the image. None of the other controls can compensate for incorrect brightness settings. Contrast adjusts the greyscale of the image, which is the differentiation between various levels of grey. These two controls should be adjusted so that all levels of grey including white and black may be seen.

Depth is an indication of the amount of tissue that is displayed on the monitor in centimeters (cm). Ideally, this should be adjusted so that the area or organ of interest occupies two thirds of the image. The image is seen as a wedge with 9 sectors. The 3 sectors closest to the transducer are called the near zones. The next 3 sectors are the mid zones and the farthest sectors are called the far zones. The 3 sectors in each zone are called right, center, and left. This allows the ultrasonographer to identify the areas analyzed and photographed for future analysis if the veterinarian is not present at the time of the study.

Gain increases the sensitivity of the transducer to the reflected sound waves, which causes the image to become brighter. The output or power increases the intensity of sound produced by the transducer. Because the sound waves are higher in intensity, the reflections will be more intense and cause a brighter image as well. These two controls cannot compensate for brightness and contrast mistakes, however.

The time gain compensation compensates for the loss of energy of the sound waves reflected from areas very deep to the transducer head. This means that the lobes of the liver on the dorsal side of the animal (far sector) will have the same echogenicity as the lobes on the ventral side (near sector). This is an advantage when assessing relative echogenicity of tissues. If this control is incorrectly set, nonexistent pathologies may be diagnosed.

Artifacts with Ultrasonography

Some ultrasound artifacts are actually useful, but most are not. Useful artifacts include acoustic shadowing and distant enhancement. Other artifacts that can confuse the image and diagnosis are slice thickness artifact, reverberation, mirror image, and refraction.

Acoustic shadowing occurs when all the sound is reflected at an interface between two different densities. This happens with bone, urinary calculi (stones), mineralization, and saponified fat (pancreatitis).

Distant enhancement occurs when the sound waves go through a fluid-filled cyst or an organ. The image will show a hyperechoic area far to the fluid-filled object. This confirms that the organ or cyst contains fluid.

Slice thickness artifact will show a thickened area if it cannot interpret the echoes correctly. This is common if the gain is set too high.

Reverberation artifact happens when there is a very reflective interface (air to tissue or fluid to bone). The sound waves bounce back and forth between the surfaces and produce horizontal lines on the image near the area of reflection.

Mirror image artifact happens when there is a highly reflective surface present. The transducer receives the reflection from the tissue plus the reflection from the other surface. This can be compensated for by decreasing the depth setting.

Refraction artifact will create shadows on the image. It is the result of sound waves that do not reflect straight back at the transducer but rather come in at an oblique angle.

Other Imaging Techniques

Many other imaging techniques are becoming more commonly used in veterinary medicine within the last 10 years. With the increase in the importance of the human-animal bond and the perception by most Americans that the family pet is a member of the family, clients are more willing to do advanced diagnostic procedures and surgical interventions than in the past. These techniques have enabled diagnosis of previously mysterious diseases and improved patient care and prognosis.

Magnetic Resonance Imaging
Magnetic resonance imaging (MRI) uses nonionizing radio frequencies to acquire images. It works best for

soft-tissue analysis. The machine generates multiple 2-dimensional cross sections, or slices, of tissues in any plane. Many different tissue properties may be assessed by altering scanning parameters or using heavy metal dye contrast media.

The T2 weighted scan shows fat, water, and fluid bright and bone dark. The FLAIR scan shows edematous tissues bright, but free water dark, and can be weighted for assessing cerebral blood flow or neural activity.

Safety is a major concern with MRI as is the expense of the studies. The procedure may require long time periods (hours) to perform a complete study with the animal completely immobile (anesthesia is required). This exposes employees to anesthetic gases and can pose anesthetic risks to the patient.

Other safety concerns involve the high-powered magnet used in the MRI. All personnel in the room should remove any metal from their person prior to operating the machine. People and animals with pacemakers or stainless steel sutures or hemoclips should not be in the room while the magnet is in use. The magnet is very powerful and could displace any magnetic metal foreign object in the room.

The last safety concern is the liquid nitrogen that is used to cool the machine. In rare cases, overheating of the machine or a nitrogen leak can cause complete replacement of all the oxygen in the room, causing the death of everyone in it.

MRI has not been shown to damage developing fetuses, so pregnancy is not a contraindication.

Computerized Axial Tomography

Computerized axial tomography (CAT or CT) is used primarily for central nervous system (brain, spinal column) and nasal cavity diagnostics. The CT is basically a very high-powered x-ray machine that takes images from multiple angles and organizes them into 2-dimensional slices (similar to MRI images). The advantages of CT over plain radiographs are that there is no superimposition of densities and there is high contrast resolution. Minor density dif-

ferences are much easier to distinguish on a CT than on a plain radiograph.

The x-ray source and target of a CT are located on a ring around a moving gantry (table). The ring rotates around the patient. Sensors are located on the opposite side of the ring and the image is collected for analysis by a computer to form a tomographic reconstruction. This forms a virtual slice of the image. The gantry is advanced and the process is repeated until the desired area has been fully imaged. These slices may be stacked into a 3-dimensional reconstruction. The display has the same density gradient as a radiograph. Bone appears white, gas black, tissue grey.

As with MRI, anesthesia is required for a CT study, so anesthetic risks must be evaluated prior to proceeding with the study.

Other risks include the massive doses of x-rays that may be needed during a study. Pregnant women should never be in the room during CT scans. One x-ray image requires 0.02 scan dose while the average head CT requires 1.5 scan doses and a cardiac CT requires 13 scan doses of radiation.

Many CT scans require contrast agents that can cause complications in some patients. Radioiodine can cause anaphylaxis or renal failure and gas studies can cause air embolisms just as in film radiography.

Nuclear Scintigraphy

Nuclear scintigraphy is used primarily for function studies of organs. Scintigraphy uses a small amount of a radioactive isotope tracer called technetium 99m (^{99m}Tc), which emits gamma rays that can be read by a gamma scintillation camera. The technetium is compounded to a substance required by the target organ (iodine in hyperthyroid cats) and is injected into the animal. The gamma scintillation camera then scans the animal for several minutes, and areas of increased uptake can be seen on the image. Technetium will also have increased uptake in any area with increased blood flow. Animals are usually sedated for the procedure, but usually do not require general anesthesia.

The images obtained from nuclear scintigraphy differ from other modes of imaging in that surrounding tissue detail is weak or completely absent. Only the areas of uptake will be visible as a series or cloud of small dots.

Safety issues relate to the radioisotope and gamma ray emissions. Technetium has a half life of 6 hours, so animals can generally be released to their owners within 1 to 3 days. Technician safety includes minimizing exposure to animals during and after testing, wearing appropriate PPE to prevent contamination, and proper disposal of urine and feces after treatment.

Practice Questions

1. What are the subatomic particles involved in the generation of x-rays?
   a. gamma rays
   b. electrons
   c. protons
   d. neutrons

2. What does ALARA stand for?
   a. as little as reasonably accessible
   b. as low as reasonably achievable
   c. as little as Roentgen allows
   d. as low as reasonably allowable

3. Which of the following is NOT important in radiology?
   a. piezoelectric effect
   b. magnetic field production
   c. heat production
   d. scatter radiation

4. Which of the following is *false* about personal protective equipment for radiology?
   a. it should be used by everyone in the x-ray room
   b. it should contain lead
   c. it is fully protective against radiation from the primary beam
   d. it protects against somatic damage and genetic damage

5. Which of the following is NOT a radiographic artifact?
   a. static electricity
   b. film fog
   c. impedance
   d. fingerprints

6. Which of the following is a possible hazard with MRI?
   a. pacemaker electrode relocation
   b. somatic damage
   c. cavitation
   d. radiation burns

7. Which of the following is true of CT scans?
   a. They can be performed on pregnant animals without risk to the fetus.
   b. They are 3-dimensional radiographs.
   c. They allow visualization of metabolic activity.
   d. They use sound waves for imaging.

8. The kVp
   a. affects the number of electrons produced by the cathode.
   b. affects the speed of the x-rays produced by the anode.
   c. should be set as low as possible to prevent overheating the tube.
   d. should be increased or decreased at the same rate as the mAs.

9. Scatter radiation is
   a. the radiation that is produced by the edge of the target.
   b. the radiation that is produced within the primary beam.
   c. the radiation that is produced when the beam hits a target and is reflected.
   d. responsible for the image produced on the film.

10. Mirror image artifact is common in
    a. radiography.
    b. ultrasound.
    c. MRI.
    d. CT scan.

11. Which of the following is Santes' rule?
    a. (temperature in Fahrenheit – 68) ÷ 2 × 30
    b. (2 × thickness of body part in cm) + SID = kVp
    c. A grid must be used for any body part greater than 15 cm in thickness.
    d. All radiographs must be labeled within the emulsion in order to be considered a legal record.

12. Which of the following is *false* about OFA films for hip dysplasia evaluation?
    a. The AKC registration number must be included in the label.
    b. Films may be evaluated as early as 6 months of age.
    c. OFA film evaluation is a subjective assessment by a panel of experts.
    d. Perfect positioning is required for evaluation.

13. Which of the following is *false* about equine radiology?
    a. A minimum of 4 films is required for the proper evaluation of a joint.
    b. Films taken in the field usually use a stationary anode.
    c. It is acceptable for the technician or assistant to hold the plate or the cassette in position.
    d. Blocks may be used to aid in proper positioning.

14. The formation of water bubbles within cells that explode and destroy the cell is called
    a. cavitation.
    b. quenching.
    c. impedance.
    d. somatic damage.

15. mA affects
    a. the speed of the electrons.
    b. the amount of gamma radiation.
    c. the number of electrons.
    d. the contrast of the finished film.

16. A dog with pneumonia and a broken right (R) femur presents at your clinic. Which of the following films would NOT be appropriate?
    a. right lateral femur
    b. right lateral thorax
    c. VD thorax
    d. right lateral pelvis

17. A dog presents with a melanoma on his right front first digit. Which of the following would be appropriate?
    a. VD thorax
    b. right dorsopalmar phalanx
    c. both of the above
    d. neither of the above

18. Which of the following would require the highest kVp?
   a. lateral thorax
   b. lateral abdomen
   c. skull
   d. distal extremity

19. Which of the following is true regarding an anterior posterior view of the stifle?
   a. You will get better detail on the radiograph than with the PA view.
   b. The image of the joint will appear larger on the AP film than on the PA view.
   c. There will be increased scatter radiation with this view.
   d. This is a better view for assessing the patella.

20. Which of the following is the best view for assessing the anconeal process?
   a. lateral elbow
   b. 90-degree flexion elbow
   c. craniocaudal elbow
   d. none of the above

21. Which of the following is the best view for assessing the lateral femoral condyle?
   a. lateral stifle
   b. lateral elbow
   c. craniocaudal stifle
   d. caudocranial stifle

22. Which of the following is the best view for assessing the distal row of the carpus for a slab fracture?
   a. lateromedial carpus
   b. oblique carpus (either dorsomedial or dorsolateral view)
   c. dorsoproximal 20-degree dorsodistal oblique
   d. dorsoproximal 60-degree dorsodistal oblique

23. Which of the following is the best view for assessing a tortoise for pneumonia of the left lung?
   a. dorsoventral
   b. lateral
   c. ventrodorsal
   d. skyline

24. A dog comes in for severe ear infection on the right side. Which of the following is the most important view?
   a. right lateral
   b. entrodorsal
   c. frontal
   d. open-mouth view

25. A dog comes in with a facial fracture of the zygomatic arch. Which of the following is the view that will show the fracture best?
   a. right lateral
   b. ventrodorsal
   c. frontal
   d. open-mouth view

26. You are performing a flexed cervical radiograph. Which of the following is *false*?
   a. The median plane of the head and neck should be parallel to the tabletop.
   b. The forelimbs should be pulled caudally.
   c. The measurement should be taken at the widest part of the skull.
   d. The beam should be centered on the cervical spine between the back of the skull and the spine of the scapula.

27. Which of the following is *false* concerning radiographs of the abdomen?
   a. One large plate is adequate when taking VD radiographs of deep-chested dogs.
   b. Measurements should be over the thickest region (usually the last few ribs).
   c. A grid should be used for all animals over 10 cm in thickness.
   d. DV radiographs put all the abdominal viscera in the anatomic orientation.

28. Which of the following types of contrast media should be used to visualize a radiolucent bladder stone?
   a. barium sulfate
   b. air
   c. ionic organic iodides
   d. nonionic organic iodides

29. Which of the following is a possible complication for barium sulfate as a contrast medium?
   a. air embolism
   b. anaphylaxis
   c. aspiration pneumonia
   d. cavitation

30. How long does it take for contrast to traverse the upper GI tract?
   a. 15 minutes
   b. 30 minutes
   c. 1 hour
   d. 3 hours

31. What is the dosage for barium for a lower-GI series?
   a. 1 to 2 ml/lb
   b. 3 to 5 ml/lb
   c. 1 to 2 ml/kg
   d. 3 to 5 ml/kg

32. Which of the following is true for an upper abdominal series?
   a. The machine should be set for high kVp, low mAs.
   b. The animal should be fasted for 3 hours prior to the procedure.
   c. The animal should be sedated or anesthetized.
   d. Radiographs should be taken prior to the contrast, then every hour until the contrast passes in the stool.

33. Which of the following is true of a VD pelvis?
   a. The stifles should be in a natural position.
   b. The ilium should be parallel to the tabletop.
   c. The patellas should be centered in the trochlear grooves on the radiograph.
   d. The field view should be collimated to include the ilium, ischium, and proximal femur.

34. Which of the following is *false* about PennHIP?
   a. Only practitioners certified in the technique are allowed to perform this procedure.
   b. Animals can be assessed for hip dysplasia as young as 6 months of age.
   c. This procedure can be performed on awake animals.
   d. PennHIP evaluation tests the laxity of the hip joint.

35. Which of the following is true of thoracic radiographs?
   a. There is more scatter radiation generated from thoracic films than from skull films.
   b. A grid is required for any thorax greater than 15 cm in thickness.
   c. High mAs is usually needed.
   d. VD films will allow visualization of the heart base and blood vessels.

36. An animal is brought in with suspected pneumothorax. Which of the following will show this the best?
a. right lateral
b. DV
c. VD
d. left lateral

37. A film comes through the automatic processor. Half the film is black, the rest is readable. Which of the following is a likely cause?
a. film fog
b. two films in the same cassette
c. poorly aimed beam
d. improper collimation

38. A film comes through the automatic processor. There are several black crescents on the film. Which of the following is a likely cause?
a. film fog
b. bent film
c. static
d. contrast material on the dog's coat

39. A film comes through the automatic processor and there are lightning-shaped black areas all over the film. Which of the following is a likely cause?
a. film fog
b. bent film
c. static
d. contrast material on the dog's coat

40. A film comes through the automatic processor. There are blobs of white areas all over the film. Which of the following is a likely cause?
a. film fog
b. bent film
c. static
d. contrast material on the dog's coat

41. You have just purchased a new cassette with rare-earth screens. Which of the following is true?
a. You should use blue-light sensitive film.
b. You should use green-light sensitive film.
c. You should have a purple light in the developing room.
d. You should have a yellow light in the developing room.

42. Double contrast imaging is usually performed on which organ?
a. stomach
b. kidneys
c. colon
d. bladder

43. A film is processed and reveals a central circular area that is well developed surrounded by a white area. Which of the following artifacts is possible?
a. upside-down focused grid
b. collimation too narrow
c. grid line artifact
d. dirty screens

44. Which of the following can cause a film to be too dark?
a. a temperature of 75° in the developing bath
b. mAs set too low
c. old fixative chemical
d. inadequate final rinse

45. Which of the following can cause decreased longevity of film?
a. a temperature of 75° in the developing bath
b. mAs set too high
c. inadequate first rinse
d. old fixative chemical

46. What is the chemical compound that allows film to respond to light?
    a. calcium tungstate
    b. silver halide
    c. phosphor crystals
    d. elemental silver

47. Most states have a requirement to trap elemental silver from which chemicals after processing?
    a. developer
    b. fixative
    c. rinse
    d. surfactant

48. How long must x-ray films be maintained?
    a. 1 year
    b. 2 years
    c. 5 years
    d. varies by state

49. Which of the following is NOT necessary for film labeling?
    a. patient name
    b. client name
    c. hospital name
    d. date of birth

50. Which of the following methods is best for diagnosing an aneurysm in the abdomen?
    a. radiographs
    b. MRI
    c. Doppler ultrasound
    d. CT

Answers and Explanations

1. b. Electrons are produced by the cathode and strike the tungsten anode to produce x-rays and heat. Gamma rays are pure energy, protons are positively charged particles, and neutrons are neutrally charged. The electromagnetic field does not have the correct polarity to attract the protons, and neutrons would not move in either direction because they have no charge.

2. b. ALARA means as low as reasonably achievable. The goal of radiography is to reduce x-ray exposure to as low as reasonably achievable levels in order to reduce somatic damage.

3. a. The piezoelectric effect is important to ultrasound. It refers to the ability of the crystals in the transducer to give off ultrasonic frequencies. Magnetic field production is important to the generation of the electron stream and the production of x-rays. Heat is also produced by this process. Scatter radiation is produced when x-rays strike and reflect from a target.

4. c. Personal protective equipment should never be relied upon to protect the operator from the primary beam. It protects better against scatter radiation. All PPE for radiography should contain lead and be used by everyone in the x-ray room. The purpose of PPE is to reduce the possibility of somatic and genetic damage.

5. c. Impedance is an ultrasonographic artifact. Static electricity, film fog, and fingerprints are all radiographic artifacts.

6. a. Pacemaker electrodes may be magnetic and be moved by the powerful electromagnetic field produced by the MRI. Somatic damage and radiation burns may occur secondary to CT scans, radiography, and scintigraphy. Cavitation is a possibility with ultrasonography.

7. b. CT scans are 2 to 3 dimensional radiographs. The beam irradiates a circle around the patient (also called a slice) giving a 2-dimensional image. Several 2-dimensional slices may be stacked together and analyzed using image analysis. CT should be avoided with pregnant animals because the amount of x-rays produced is much higher than with traditional radiography. Metabolic activity can be assessed using scintigraphy. Ultrasonography uses sound waves for imaging.

8. b. The kVp affects the speed of the electrons and the speed of the x-rays, while the mAs affects the number of electrons. The kVp should be set high and the mAs should be set low in order to reduce heat production in the tube. KVp is inversely proportional to mAs.

9. c. Scatter radiation is produced when the primary beam hits the patient, the table, or another object and is reflected in a different direction. Scatter will decrease film quality.

10. b. Mirror image artifact occurs in ultrasound when the wave bounces off a reflective surface (such as the diaphragm). The only other way that mirror imaging can occur is if the film is folded within the cassette in radiography, but this is rare.

11. b. Santes' rule is (2 × thickness of body part) + SID = kVp. This is the rule that is used to calculate a starting kVp for making a radiographic technique chart. Answer choice **a** is the formula for calculating developing time depending on temperature variation. Choices **c** and **d** are procedural rules for radiology that do not have names.

12. b. OFA films will not be accepted for final evaluation until the animal is more than 2 years of age. OFA requires that the AKC registration number be included in the film label and perfect positioning with the femurs parallel and obturator foramens equal in size be maintained. The OFA is a subjective analysis of hip films by a panel of board-certified veterinary radiologists.

13. c. It is never acceptable for a technician, staff, or owner to place any part of their body within the primary beam. The other statements are true: 4 films is the minimum required for proper joint evaluation in the horse, the usual x-ray machine in the field is a stationary anode, and blocks are often used to aid in the positioning of horses.

14. a. Cavitation is the formation of water bubbles that causes cellular disruption to occur. Quenching and impedance are other terms used in ultrasonography and somatic damage is a possibility in radiography.

15. c. mA is the amount of energy put through the cathode. This increases the number of electrons produced. mA affects the overall lightness and darkness of the film (density); kVp affects the speed of the electrons and the contrast of the film.

16. c. VD thorax would cause respiratory distress to an animal with pneumonia. A better option would be a DV thorax, which would not compromise the action of the diaphragm. All the other listed views would be appropriate for the case.

17. c. Both of the above are appropriate. VD thorax (as well as a right and left lateral thorax) should be performed to check for metastasis since melanomas are likely to metastasize. The dorsopalmar phalanx as well as a spread lateral foot should be performed to assess the digits.

18. b. Lateral abdomen. KVp is responsible for contrast and there are a lot of soft tissue structures that must be differentiated in the abdomen. The thorax would require the least because of the amount of air density. The skull and distal extremity would not need as much contrast definition as the abdomen.

19. b. The image of the joint will appear larger on the AP film than on the PA film because of the increased object film distance. This may cause a loss of detail. Since the patella is farther away from the film, it will be less clear on an AP film.

20. b. 90-degree flexion elbow opens up the joint and allows a better view of the anconeal process than with the lateral view alone. Craniocaudal elbow will not give much detail. The flexed elbow is the view of choice for UAP (ununited anconeal process).

21. d. The caudocranial stifle will have the least amount of magnification and the best detail of the condyle. The lateral view should have the condyles overlapping and will not give an adequate picture. Both views should be taken, however, to assess the joint completely.

22. c. Dorsoproximal 20-degree dorsodistal oblique will give the best view of the fronts of the distal row of the carpal bones. A lateromedial carpus may also show a slab fracture, although identifying which of the bones are involved may be difficult. The 60-degree dorsodistal oblique will give a better assessment of the first row of carpal bones.

23. d. A skyline (craniocaudal) view of a tortoise will enable the best visualization of pneumonia. The lungs lie dorsally under the carapace and a VD or DV view will be complicated by the presence of viscera. A lateral view may be helpful, although figuring out which lung is involved will be difficult.

24. d. Open-mouth rostrocaudal view is the best for visualization of the osseus bullae. The frontal view is best for the frontal sinuses, the lateral will show the bullae, but they will be superimposed. The VD view will be complicated by overlying structures.

25. b. Visualization of the zygomatic arch is best performed on a VD view. This will give an unobstructed view of the arches.

26. c. The measurement should be taken over the manubrium. The other answers are true (median plane of the head and neck should be parallel to the tabletop, the forelimbs should be pulled slightly caudally, the beam should be centered on the midcervical region).

27. a. In large, deep-chested dogs, the difference between measurement at the xiphoid and the pelvis is very large, so two plates are needed for adequate visualization of the viscera. Measurements should be taken over the thickest region, with a grid if the animal is greater than 10 cm thickness. DV radiographs put the organs in anatomic orientation, but many veterinarians still prefer to read VD films.

28. c. Ionic iodides are the best for this case. Radiolucent stones require positive contrast media. Nonionic iodides are generally used for myelography and are expensive. Barium should never be used in the bladder and air is a negative contrast medium.

29. c. Aspiration pneumonia is a possible complication if used in a vomiting animal. Air embolism can occur if air, oxygen, or carbon dioxide is used as a negative contrast medium; anaphylaxis can occur with organic iodides.

30. d. Barium can take up to 3 hours to traverse the upper GI tract.

31. b. The dosage for barium for a lower GI series is 3 to 5 ml/lb by enema.

32. a. The machine should be set for high kVp, low mAs. The animal should be fasted for 12 hours prior to the procedure and an enema given to empty the tract completely. The animal should not be sedated or anesthetized because that will interfere with gastrointestinal motility. Radiographs should be taken prior to contrast, at 15 and 30 minutes, then every 30 minutes until the contrast has left the small bowel.

33. c. The patellas should be centered in the trochlear grooves. This means that the femurs should be parallel to each other and extended (slightly internally rotated). The field of view should generally include the entire femur.

34. c. PennHIP must be performed on anesthetized or heavily sedated animals in order for proper positioning and assessment of laxity to be achieved. Animals as young as 6 months of age may be assessed. Assessment is by certified practitioners only.

35. b. Grids are used for animals greater than 15 cm thickness (greater than 10 cm for any other portion of the body). Lower mAs is needed for thoracic films and less scatter is produced because of the small amount of soft tissue present. DV films are used for the best visualization of the heart base and blood vessels.

36. b. Pneumothorax will usually show up best on DV films because gas rises. It may be difficult to visualize on the other types of thoracic radiographs if it is mild.

37. a. Film fog is the most likely cause. This happens because of exposure of the film to light, which could have occurred either because the light box was opened or the cassette was not closed correctly. Two films in the same cassette should have shown either a doubled image, films stuck together in the processor, and so on. A poorly aimed beam would have shown part of the film to be unexposed and improper collimation would have shown the image to be missized.

38. b. Black crescents on the film would normally indicate bent film. Static would be shaped like lightning bolts, film fog would look like a black bar across the film, contrast material would look like white spots on the film.

39. c. Static appears as black lightning- or tree-shaped marks on the film. See answer 38 for descriptions of other common artifacts.

40. d. Contrast material on the animal's coat. See answer 38 for descriptions of other common artifacts.

41. b. Green-light sensitive film should go with rare-earth screens. Blue-light sensitive films should go with calcium tungstate screens. Red lights are always preferred in the darkroom.

42. d. Double contrast imaging is most commonly performed on the bladder. Positive contrast is generally used for imaging the stomach, kidneys, and colon.

43. a. An upside-down focused grid will produce that artifact. Narrow collimation would be rectangular in shape. Grid line artifact is seen with stationary grids (not Bucky grids) and appear as a series of thin lines across the entire film. Dirty screens will generally show up as different areas of decreased contrast.

44. a. A temperature of 75° in the developing bath is 10° higher than the optimum for developer. This means that the developing time should have been decreased (see answer 11). Low mAs would have given a film that was not dark enough; old fixative and inadequate final rinse would not have affected the darkness.

45. d. Old fixative would not have been as effective in hardening the image and fixing it to the film base. The first 3 answers would have affected the darkness of the image, not the longevity.

46. b. The light-responsive chemical in x-ray film is silver halide. Calcium tungstate and phosphor crystals are in the screens and elemental silver is what is produced after the developing process.

47. b. Fixative is the chemical that should be trapped for retrieval of elemental silver. The developer converts silver halide to elemental silver, the rinse just rinses the chemicals off the film, and the surfactant stabilizes the film (if used).

48. d. The amount of time that films must be kept on record varies by state, but is usually several years.

49. d. Date of birth is not necessary for proper film labeling. Patient name, client last name, the name of the hospital, and the date of the radiograph are all required information.

50. c. Doppler ultrasound is the best method for diagnosing an aneurysm in the abdomen because it evaluates turbulent blood flow. Radiographs would only see a very large aneurysm, abdominal CT is expensive and has increased radiation risk, and MRI is also expensive.

11 ▶ ANESTHESIA AND ANALGESIA

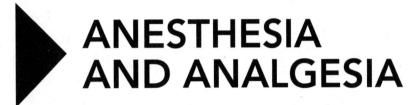

CHAPTER OVERVIEW

This chapter aims to prepare veterinary technician students for the VTNE by organizing the topic of anesthesia into manageable pieces. Anesthetizing a patient is a serious matter. With all there is to know about anesthesia, veterinary technicians can find their job quite daunting. Successful patient anesthesia is a skill that is developed with time and practice. Veterinary technicians must be experts at inducing, maintaining, and recovering anesthetized patients. A good veterinary technician, or veterinarian for that matter, should never be complacent with an anesthetized patient. A technician should be alert and recognize changes in a patient's anesthetic depth as well as spotting patient or equipment abnormalities that must be quickly resolved.

A technician's knowledge should include correct anesthetic equipment use, selection, and maintenance. To do all of this a technician needs to know common categories of preanesthetic drugs, anesthetics, analgesics, emergency drugs, monitoring equipment, anesthesia systems, and patient monitoring techniques. These will be reviewed in this chapter and will provide the basic knowledge needed to be successful on the VTNE and in practice.

Key Terms

agonist

alveoli

analgesia

antagonist

antitussive

apnea

arrhythmia

aspiration

atelectasis

auscultation

bradycardia

canthus

depolarization

diastole

edema

embolus

emesis

endogenous

eupnea

hemostasis

hypercapnia or hypercarbia

hypoxemia or hypoxia

intubation

miosis

murmur

mydriasis

myelinated nerve

nephrotoxic

nystagmus

parenteral

paresis

positive-pressure ventilation

precipitate

repolarization

respiratory minute volume

systole

thromboembolism

thrombus

vagal tone

ventricular premature contractions (VPC)

Concepts and Skills

Anesthesia can be broken down into five main topics:

- **Anesthetic Agents.** These are drugs that are used for preanesthetics, induction, or maintenance during anesthesia. These drugs come in two forms: injectable and inhalant gas.
- **Anesthetic Machines.** Gas anesthesia is delivered to the patient by means of anesthetic machines. Two types of breathing systems are connected to anesthetic machines for use with veterinary patients: rebreathing and nonrebreathing systems.
- **Anesthetic Monitoring.** The depth of anesthesia can be determined by closely monitoring a patient's physical parameters, using specialized monitoring equipment.
- **Analgesia.** Pain is an undesirable and often detrimental side effect of surgery, which is why anesthesia is generally used. Providing pain relief perioperatively (before, during, and after procedures) is not only humane, but it can also help a patient's healing and recovery.
- **Emergency and Critical Care Drugs.** In a life-threatening situation a veterinary technician's knowledge of and quick access to these drugs may mean the difference between life and death.

Anesthetic Agents

General anesthesia is a state of reversible unconsciousness, analgesia, amnesia, and decreased or absent reflexes. The most common reason to place a patient under general anesthesia is for surgery to be performed. Putting a patient under general anesthesia is called induction and can be done by using many drugs and/or gases. Combining multiple drugs and gases is called balanced anesthesia, and is often preferred over the use of a single drug or gas. The premise for using balanced anesthesia is that the combination of two or more drugs (known as a *drug cocktail*) maximizes the advantages, but not the disadvantages, of the individual components.

Most veterinary practices will not use all of the anesthetic agents available, but instead become proficient with a handful of them. A veterinary technician should still be familiar and stay current with other anesthetic agents. It will help to be familiar with the different anesthetic drug categories and their typical advantages and disadvantages, and to know the names of some common examples in each category.

Anesthetic agents come in two forms: injectables and inhalants. The former are usually given intravenously, intramuscularly, or subcutaneously, and the latter are gases that are inhaled.

Injectables

Injectables are drugs that are usually given by intravenous, intramuscular, or subcutaneous injection. The injectable agents used in anesthesia can be grouped as preanesthetics, induction, and maintenance drugs.

Preanesthetic Drugs

Preanesthetic drugs are given prior to anesthesia induction. The same drug can be designated as a preanesthetic if given prior to anesthesia or called an anesthetic if given to induce anesthesia. Labeling a drug as a preanesthetic is only related to the |point at which it is given. In general, drugs are used as preanesthetics for one or more of the following reasons.

To Tranquilize or Sedate an Animal

Drugs such as diazepam (Valium) not only tranquilize but also have an antianxiety affect. Providing antianxiety has additional benefits for patients that are in an unknown situation and are nervous, anxious, and afraid. It takes more anesthetic drug to bring a patient from an excited state to a sleeping state than it would to bring a patient from a tranquil state to a sleeping state. In other words, a smaller amount of drug is needed to get the same effect. Also, a tranquil patient is easier to restrain for an IV catheter placement. Excessive catecholamines (epinephrine) are produced when an animal is excited and fearful. These endogenous catecholamines can induce heart arrhythmias in combination with certain anesthetic agents like halothane and pentothal.

To Decrease the Dose of Maintenance Anesthetic Drugs

Agents that are used to keep a patient under general anesthesia are called maintenance anesthetic drugs. Minimizing the amount of any one drug given limits its adverse affects while maintaining its beneficial effects. A preanesthetic that tranquilizes, sedates, and/or provides analgesia also allows less maintenance anesthetic drug to be given and thus decreases the adverse affects of the latter.

To Provide Smoother Induction and Recovery

As a patient becomes anesthetized, it goes through progressively deeper stages of unconsciousness and anesthesia. This is reversed as the patient starts to wake up from anesthesia. The earlier stages, particularly stage II, of anesthesia can be difficult for the patient and for the people working with the patient. As they progress through stage II, animals can become very agitated and excited, even more so than before induction. Many animals in this semiconscious stage will vocalize (howl or whine), paddle their legs, struggle, and have increased heart and respiratory rates. Due to their loss of neurologic inhibition, animals in this excitement stage may be stronger and are harder to restrain than before the anesthetics were given. Stage II excitement is similar to the sudden involuntary movement or tremor that can happen to a person on the verge of falling asleep. The awake patient's natural inhibitory actions are being suppressed during anesthesia induction. These abrupt physical outbursts subside as the patient enters deeper stages of unconsciousness and anesthesia. The stage II excitement will also occur as part of the patient's recovery from anesthesia. Preanesthetics that help inhibit the physical excitement will help prevent the violent movements and vocalization associated with stage II excitement upon induction and recovery.

To Provide Analgesia

The term **analgesia** comes from the Greek meaning *without pain*. Certain preanesthetics will provide pain relief, or analgesia. If a general anesthetic does not also provide analgesia, it only prevents the perception of pain, not the physiological changes caused by pain, which has many deleterious effects on patients. There are several ways to relieve and prevent pain. It is good practice to limit pain by using several of these methods at the same time. This is called multimodal pain relief. Once an animal recovers from general anesthesia, its brain perceives the pain. Having another analgesic currently in the body that prevents or limits pain in a different way than general anesthesia will be beneficial. Pain can be prevented or limited by using local anesthetics (numbing agents), nonsteroidal anti-inflammatory drugs (NSAIDs), corticosteroids, narcotics, and other methods such as massage or acupuncture. Preanesthetic drugs that have analgesic affects have the benefits of minimizing windup or hyperesthesia, and can also allow for less general anesthetic to be given and still provide pain control.

To Prevent Problems

Several other problems associated with general anesthesia can be prevented or limited by using preanesthetics. For example, **emesis** (vomiting) can be either induced or prevented by the use of preanesthetics. If a patient is not fasted prior to anesthesia, **aspiration** (inhaling foreign substances) of stomach contents may occur. The chances of aspiration can be decreased by the use of a preanesthetic either to cause vomiting prior to induction or to decrease the likelihood of vomiting while under anesthesia. Preanesthetics can also limit **bradycardia** (abnormally slow heart beat) in situations that cause vagal stimulation such as intubation, handling of viscera, or eye surgery. Another situation requiring preanesthetics is decreasing salivation to prevent airway obstruction or for easier intubation. GI tract motility can be decreased to prevent vomiting and diarrhea. Using the right preanesthetic drugs will prevent seizures before, during, and after a surgery.

Drugs Commonly Used as Preanesthetics

The autonomic nervous system is the sympathetic or adrenergic system that regulates the fight-or-flight response. It is the body's involuntary response to fear. What does your body turn on and off for fight or flight? The sympathetic nervous system turns on more blood flow to muscles, lungs, and heart; airways dilate; pupils dilate (mydriasis); heart and respiratory rates increase; but it turns off the GI tract, salivation, and tearing. Drugs that mimic this are called sympathomimetics (sympathetic-mimickers). The parasympathetic or cholinergic system has the opposite effect. That system regulates rest and rejuvenation. Drugs in this category are called parasympathomimetics, and they increase tear flow, salivation, gastric juices, and digestion and decrease pupil size (**miosis**).

The following are common examples of preanesthetic drugs that are used in veterinary medicine.

Atropine and **glycopyrrolate** are drugs that are classified as anticholinergic or antiparasympathetic. They prevent rest and rejuvenation. They also prevent vagal affects: administration causes decreased GI tract function, salivation, and tearing; it prevents bradycardia (slow heart beat) and causes mydriasis (pupil dilation). Glycopyrrolate will last longer than atropine and does not cross the blood–brain or placental barriers. It can be mixed in the same syringe with acepromazine, and it can be used as an antidote for organophosphate toxicity. It should not be used in patients with tachycardia, constipation, GI tract obstruction, or glaucoma.

Acepromazine is classified as a phenothiazine derivative; it has sedative effects and prevents nausea (known as antiemetic effect). It can be mixed with atropine in the same syringe. It causes vasodilation, which can lead to hypotension (low blood pressure). This drug also lowers the brain's seizure threshold, which can allow a seizure-prone patient to start seizing. It should not be used in patients concurrently using organophosphates, or with a known history of seizures, head trauma, hypothermia, or hypotension. Boxers and sight hounds are very sensitive to acepromazine. Acepromazine should be avoided in patients with vWD (von Willebrand's disease).

Diazepam (Valium) is a widely known drug classified as a benzodiazepine. It is used for its sedation effects, and as an alternative to acepromazine in high-risk patients. It has anticonvulsant, antianxiety, and appetite-stimulating effects. It can be mixed with ketamine in the same syringe, but should not be mixed with other drugs or they will precipitate out of solution. It should not be stored in plastic syringes because the plastic will bind it, and it is light sensitive. Diazepam is a controlled substance.

Xylazine (Rompun®) is classified as an alpha-2 agonist. It has sedative and anesthetic effects depending on the amount given (dose dependant); it also has analgesic effects. It has emetic effects when given intravenously, especially in cats, and it normally causes horses to sweat and have muscle twitches. It should be used only in healthy animals, due to its cardiovascular depression effects, such as hypotension, bradycardia, and pale mucous membrane color. It causes diuresis, so bladders will fill up quickly, and it decreases gastrointestinal motility in ruminants, which can lead to bloating, salivation, and regurgitation. The reversal agent is yohimbine (an **antagonist** to the agonist effects of xylazine).

Medetomidine (Domitor®, Dexdomitor®) is classified as an alpha-2 agonist and has similar effects to xylazine. Its sedative and anesthetic effects depend on the amount given (it is dose dependent). It also has analgesic effects. It should be used only in healthy animals, due to its cardiovascular depression effects, such as hypotension, bradycardia, and pale mucous membrane color. It causes diuresis, so bladders will fill up quickly. The reversal agent is Atipamezole (Antisedan®). The pharmaceutical company has made it easy to calculate the amount of atipamezole needed for reversal. The amount equals the amount of medetomidine already given.

Detomidine (Dormosedan®) is classified as an alpha-2 agonist, and has similar effects to xylazine. It is used primarily in horses and has sedative and anesthetic effects depending on the amount given (it is dose dependent). Like medetomidine, it also has analgesic effects, and should be used only in healthy animals, due to its cardiovascular depression effects, such as hypotension, bradycardia, and pale mucous membrane color. It also causes diuresis, so bladders will fill up quickly. The reversal agent for this drug is also yohimbine.

Alpha-2 agonists, which include the three drugs just described (xylazine, medetomidine, and detomidine) should only be used for patients with normal cardiovascular systems and normal liver function and who are between the ages of 4 months and 6 years. An anticholinergic should *not* be given after the drug has taken effect. Normal patient monitoring parameters are different when these drugs are used. Heart rates of 40 to 60 beats per minute (bpm), peripheral pulses that are hard to feel, or mucous membranes that are pale or bluish are all considered normal for patients using an alpha-2 agonist.

Narcotics (opioids) are a class of drugs that in general have the following characteristics. They are controlled substances. They are dose dependent. They have analgesic effects. They can cause extreme excitement, or *morphine mania*, rather than sedation in some cats and horses. They have emetic effects; for example, morphine is often given as a preanesthetic to cause vomiting in order to empty the stomach of any food that could be aspirated while the animal is anesthetized. They can cause constipation, which results from bowel peristalsis becoming segmented.

The digesta in the bowel are churned in the same location without progressive movement through the intestines.

Narcotics are respiratory depressants, so veterinary technicians must be prepared to assist ventilation with techniques such as bagging the patient or **positive-pressure ventilation**. Naloxone can be used as a reversal agent for many narcotics. Narcotics produce their effect by stimulating one or more of 4 different receptors: mu, kappa, sigma, and delta. Receptors are locations on cells or neurons that specifically link to these chemicals. Two common narcotics used in veterinary medicine are morphine and oxymorphine. Morphine is the oldest, and least potent of the class, but it is the drug to which all others in the class are compared. Oxymorphone is a more potent morphine, so less volume is needed to get the same effect.

Butorphanol (Torbugesic®, Torbutrol®) has **antitussive** (anticough) effects. Codeine is another narcotic with antitussive effects. However, codeine has only one-tenth the potency of morphine, so it is seldom used as a preanesthetic. Butorphanol has both agonist and antagonist effects, giving this drug a ceiling effect, which means that the effects are limited and will top out; adding more drug will not cause an increased effect.

Induction or Maintenance Injectable Agents

Certain drugs are commonly used in veterinary medicine to take an animal from an awake state to general anesthesia. Many of them can be given during general anesthesia to keep a patient anesthetized longer or deeper (*topped off*). These drugs include ketamine, tiletamine and zolazepam, propofol, and thiopental (pentothal). A combination of drugs can be used to produce a state called neuroleptanalgesia in a patient.

Ketamine (Vetaset®, Ketaset®)

Ketamine is classified as a dissociative anesthetic and is a controlled substance. It can produce anesthesia and provides somatic analgesia (pain relief to the body's outer shell and extremities), but not visceral

analgesia (pain relief to the body organs). Surgeries, such as spays, should include additional analgesia to prevent visceral pain.

Ketamine has some stimulating effects to increase muscle tone, salivation, and cardiac output. The patient's swallow reflex is retained longer than with other induction agents. This can make intubation a challenge, but it also decreases the chance of aspiration. The drug can cause muscle rigidity (catalepsy), which is why sedative and muscle-relaxing drugs such as diazepam or acepromazine are combined as a cocktail with ketamine. Ketamine can induce apnea as well as seizures.

Tiletamine and Zolazepam (Telazol®)

Tiletamine and zolazepam are controlled substances. Tiletamine is a dissociative drug and zolazepam is a benzodiazepine. This mixture is similar to the combination of ketamine (a dissociative drug) with diazepam (a benzodiazepine) with similar effects as those individual drugs. The tiletamine-zolazepam cocktail will have a smoother recovery in cats than in dogs. In cats, the tiletamine (dissociative anesthetic) wears off first, while in dogs it is the zolazepam (sedative) that wears off first. On recovery, dissociative anesthetics can cause hallucinations, delirium, excitement, disorientation, and confusion when no other drug is on board to provide sedation.

Propofol

Propofol is a milky liquid that is an exception to the rule that only clear liquids should be given by an intravenous route. Propofol has an egg base and contains no preservative. This is a good medium for microbial growth once the seal is broken. This limits its shelf life to several hours after it has been opened. It should be administered by IV slowly over 60 to 90 seconds. It causes apnea when given too quickly, and prevents a surgical plane of anesthesia if give too slowly. A unique benefit is that recovery is not prolonged by topping off, in part because it is rapidly metabolized by muscle.

Thiopental (Pentothal)

Classified as a barbiturate and considered ultra short-acting, this drug is a chemical with a sulfur side chain that allows it to be metabolized more quickly. Most other drugs in the barbiturate class have an oxygen side chain, causing them to stay in the tissues longer. This drug usually comes in a powder form (usually 5 grams) which needs to be reconstituted to either 2.5% or 5% strength by adding 200 cc or 100 cc of sterile water respectively.

Like all barbiturates (and many other drugs as well), pentothal is a hepatic enzyme inducer, which means that it can induce intolerance or resistance to a drug by increasing the speed of its metabolism by the liver. For example, if a dog is on phenobarbital to prevent seizures and induction is done using pentothal, the patient would need more pentothal than usual to become anesthetized. That is because the patient has developed a tolerance to all drugs that are metabolized by the hepatic enzyme system.

This drug depresses respiratory and cardiovascular systems. It is highly protein bound, and a low total protein would essentially increase the free circulating levels of barbiturates. It is very lipid soluble, in fact, ultra short-acting barbiturates are the most lipid soluble. The drug is fast acting, because it crosses the blood–brain barrier quicker than barbiturates in the long- and short-acting groups.

The drug quickly redistributes to fat from the circulation. However, subsequent injections can saturate the fat, which leads to more drug being left in the circulation. As a result, the patient will have a prolonged recovery because circulating barbiturates take a relatively long time to be metabolized by the liver. Patients with very little fat may easily be overdosed because there is little fat reservoir for the circulating pentothal to go to. That is why animals such as sighthounds, which are very lean, should not by anesthesized with barbiturates. Methohexital (a barbiturate used in human medicine) has been used as a safer substitute for pentothal in sighthounds.

Pentothal is given IV by injecting one-third to one-half the calculated dose in a bolus, after which the patient is observed to see what stage of anesthesia is induced. The drug must be given time to equilibrate with fat before more is administered to the desired effect. This is called *titrating* the dose.

Neuroleptanalgesia

Neuroleptanalgesia is not a drug. It is a term used to describe a patient with profound sedation and analgesia. The patient is not under general anesthesia, but rather under neuroleptanalgesia. The disadvantages of general anesthesia are lessened, yet minor surgical procedures can still be done. Neuroleptanalgesia is achieved by combining a sedative and a narcotic. One example is Droperidol plus Fentanyl (Innovar-Vet®), but other combinations of sedatives and narcotics can be used as well to produce profound sedation and analgesia effects.

Inhalants

Inhalants are gaseous agents that are absorbed into the body through the lungs. Historically, there have been a number of anesthetic inhalants, such as ether, most of which are no longer used. Gases that are used in veterinary medicine include halogenated hydrocarbons and nitrous oxide.

Inhalant anesthetics come in different potencies, measured by their minimum alveolar concentration (MAC). This is a number given to all inhalant gases that indicates its potency. MAC is defined as the lowest concentration of gas anesthetic within the alveoli that prevents movement in 50% of the patients when pain is induced. (Of course, movement does not necessarily mean awareness of pain.) The lower the MAC number, the higher the potency of the gas (less has to be given to get the same effect) and the higher the solubility in water (in this case the bloodstream). Most anesthetized patients are maintained at a gas percentage that is 1.5 to 2 times the MAC number.

Halogenated Hydrocarbons

Halogenated hydrocarbons are the most common group of inhalant gas anesthetics. They are liquid at room temperature, but they evaporate very quickly.

They require the use of a vaporizer to regulate the speed at which they evaporate. These inhalant gases include a bromine or fluorine molecule (these are halogens). Halogenated gases are less flammable than nonhalogenated gases. Common veterinary inhalant gases include halothane (Fluothane®), isoflurane (AErrane®), and sevoflurane (SevoFlo®). These are listed from the lowest MAC to the highest MAC. These gases have progressively less induction time, recovery time, and metabolism as the MAC gets larger.

Halothane (Fluothane®)

Halothane has been associated with hepatotoxicity with prolonged exposure, and it can induce arrhythmias such as ventricular premature contractions (VPCs) when combined with epinephrine (adrenaline) or barbiturates. It can cause malignant hyperthermia in pigs, people, and dogs (particularly doberman pinschers). Malignant hyperthermia is a rapidly elevated, life-threatening temperature increase that is due to a reaction to the gas. This gas has also been implicated in increased abortion rates in humans working in surgery and anesthesia.

Isoflurane (Aerrane®)

Isoflurane is the leading anesthetic inhalant gas used in veterinary medicine. It has a strong odor that irritates many patients, causing them to struggle when only using a mask or induction tank and no preanesthetic drugs. The good news is that it has low, if any, toxicities.

Sevoflurane (SevoFlo®)

Of the gases discussed, sevoflurane is the least metabolized and has the fastest induction and recovery. This is due to its high MAC, low potency, and low water solubility. It is easily blown off (exhaled) and does not stay in the blood to be metabolized by the body. This means that the anesthetic machine dial needs to be set to a higher gas percentage than the other listed gases in order to maintain anesthesia.

Nitrous Oxide (N₂O)

Commonly known as laughing gas for its euphoric effects on humans, nitrous oxide is still used in human dentistry. However, it does not have general anesthetic effects in animals, because the MAC is much too high and it is not very water soluble. Unlike halogenated hydrocarbons, N_2O needs no vaporizer, as it evaporates slowly enough on its own; it is supplied in a pressurized gas tank. In the N_2O tank, which is blue, it is in both a liquid and a gas state. This results in a constant pressure, which can be determined by the pressure dial on the tank, and will not decrease until the tank is nearly empty. As a result, the pressure dial cannot be used to determine the amount of N_2O that is left in the tank as can be done with other tanks of gas such as oxygen. Like oxygen, N_2O needs a flow meter. Flow meters are gas specific, and as such are only made to be used with one particular gas.

The only reason N_2O is used in veterinary medicine is to take advantage of the second-gas effect. The second-gas effect lowers the total amount of anesthetic gas needed to achieve general anesthesia. This was more important when inhalant gases were more potent and fat soluble, and induction and recovery times were much longer. When older halogenated hydrocarbons, such as halothane and an even older gas called methoxyflurane (metofane), were the standard gas anesthetic used, N_2O could be given at the same time to decrease the amount of halogenated hydrocarbons given to the patient. Essentially, the second-gas effect allowed a patient to receive less anesthetic gas to get the same effect. Newer halogenated hydrocarbons have been developed that have less induction and recovery times, and there is little benefit to using N_2O with them.

Diffusion hypoxia is a concern when a patient is recovering from N_2O. N_2O has such a high MAC value that it will diffuse out of the blood into the lungs very quickly and displace the oxygen. This is life threatening. To help prevent diffusion hypoxia, the recovering patient should be given 100% O_2 for at least 10 minutes, with the oxygen flow rate set to at least twice that of the N_2O flow rate.

Anesthetic Machines

Anesthetic machines are used in one of two ways: either total or partial rebreathing or nonrebreathing. Although anesthetic machines come in a mind-boggling number of varieties, they are all essentially the same. They all have the same parts, but the shapes and arrangements of the parts varies. Anesthetic machines are used to deliver inhalant gases and oxygen to a patient. The key to understanding any anesthetic machine is to follow the path of an oxygen molecule from the source all the way to the patient.

Common Parts
The following parts are found on all complete anesthetic machines: the oxygen source, a gas tank pressure gauge, a pressure regulator valve, an oxygen flow meter, an oxygen flush valve, and a vaporizer. The machine will connect to the patient as well as to a scavenging system. Each part is reviewed in more detail in the sections that follow.

Oxygen Source
Before a surgery is started, the total oxygen supply should be sufficient for the surgery, including a backup source. In the United States, oxygen comes in green tanks. Oxygen tanks, like other tanks of different gases (such as CO_2, N_2O, and helium), are color coded and have a pin system that prevents a tank of the wrong gas from connecting to the anesthetic machine. This safety feature combines three pins that stick out from the tank's nozzle in such a way that they form a different-shaped triangle for each type of gas. This makes it impossible to connect the wrong gas to the machine by accident. A tank's neck or nozzle is connected to the machine at its yoke. If a central oxygen tank (large, centralized tank providing oxygen to an entire facility) is being used, there is no tank in the yoke of the anesthetic machine.

Oxygen tanks hold compressed gas. Their sizes are designated by a letter. Two common tank sizes in veterinary medicine are E and H. An E tank holds approximately 660 liters while an H tank holds approximately 7,000 liters, and each starts out at a pressure of approximately 2,100 psi (pounds per square inch). The tremendous pressure in these tanks makes them dangerous if they are punctured or fall over and break open. Pressurized gas tanks should be securely connected to a wall.

Unlike N_2O, the pressure in an oxygen tank decreases proportionately to the amount of gas that is being removed from the tank. Estimating the remaining amount of oxygen left in a tank can be done by determining the psi inside the tank. If the pressure gauge shows a psi of 2,100 when an E tank is full with 700 liters of oxygen, then a tank that has half the pressure is half full, or 1,050 psi = 350 liters. For an E tank, multiply the psi by 0.333 to estimate the number of liters left in the tank. For an H tank, multiply the psi by 3.333 to estimate the number of liters left in the tank. For example, 1,050 psi × 0.333 = 349.65 liters of O_2 left in an E tank. If oxygen is used at a flow rate of 1L/min, this tank would last about 349.65 minutes or about 5.83 hours (or 5 hours and 50 minutes).

Gas Tank Pressure Gauge
The gas tank pressure gauge is a dial connected to the top of a tank of gas. It measures the psi in the tank.

Pressure Regulator Valve
The pressure regulator valve is located between the pressure gauge and the outlet of the oxygen tank. It makes sure that the oxygen pressure does not exceed 50 psi as it leaves the tank and enters the anesthetic machine. This regulates the pressure exiting the tank so that the anesthetic machine and tubing do not rupture. This automatic safety feature is built into all

oxygen tank connections. Some connections have two pressure dials: one that measures the pressure in the tank itself and one that measures the pressure leaving the tank (which should never be greater than 50 psi).

Oxygen Flow Meter

Oxygen flow is measured in liters per minute (LPM). An oxygen flow meter is used to set the amount of oxygen that is delivered to the patient. Gas flow meters are made to work with only one type of gas (gas specific). A common source of leaks in an anesthetic machine can be traced to a cracked flow meter's glass tube or to damage to a gasket from overtightening the knob. For measuring the flow rate, a bobbin or ball is used as a float in the glass tube. When reading the oxygen level using a bobbin, read it at the top edge. When reading the oxygen level using a ball, read it at the ball's diameter, the widest part of the ball.

Oxygen Flush Valve

Activating the oxygen flush valve allows pure oxygen to be delivered to the patient, bypassing the anesthetic vaporizer as well as the oxygen flow meter. The advantage of this is that an animal that needs pure oxygen and not anesthetic gas can have it delivered by using the oxygen flush valve. However, there are disadvantages to using it as well. The pure oxygen from the oxygen flush valve comes out much faster than it does through the flow meter. There is a real risk of overfilling the animal's airways with too much pressure. The lungs can be damaged very easily with pressures greater than 20 cm H_2O (see Manometer). The oxygen flush valve should always be used with the pop-off valve open (see Positive Pressure Relief Valve). The oxygen flush valve must be used briefly in short quick bursts to avoid increasing the airway pressure too much. Patients can be disconnected from the anesthetic machine during the use of the oxygen flush valve to avoid lung damage from excessive pressure.

Besides excessive pressure, another disadvantage of using the oxygen flush valve is the dilution of anesthetic gas every time it is used. Too often it happens that the reservoir bag is empty and the oxygen flush valve is used to fill it. The result is an animal that becomes less anesthetized and starts to wake up due to the diluted anesthetic gas. To compensate, the anesthetic gas gets turned up. The patient then gets too deep. Anesthetized patients should be handled according to their individual needs, but during most anesthesia the amount of anesthetic gas required for maintenance does not change much. The oxygen flush valve should be used when pure oxygen is needed, but that should not be necessary during most surgeries. Double checking the oxygen flow rate and making sure that it is set high enough will usually prevent overuse of the oxygen flush valve.

Vaporizer

The vaporizer is usually the most expensive part of an anesthetic machine. It is a canister that holds the volatile liquid inhalant anesthetic and regulates its evaporation rate. Factors affecting the evaporation rate of any liquid (including anesthetic gases) include temperature, humidity, and air flow. In a nonprecision vaporizer (VIC, or vaporizer in the circle), these factors *will* affect the liquid. In a precision vaporizer (VOC, or vaporizer out of the circle), on the other hand, these factors *will not* affect the liquid.

Nonprecision Vaporizer

The nonprecision vaporizer is located in the circle (VIC). The amount of the anesthetic gas delivered is set by turning a dial. This dial does not have units but rather is marked with numbers from 0 to 10. Ten is the setting that is all the way open and 5 would mean it is halfway open. A nonprecision vaporizer is affected by temperature, oxygen flow rate, and humidity. Therefore, the amount of vaporization that occurs when the dial is at 5 on one day will be different from the amount of vaporization that occurs on another day, when temperature, oxygen flow rate, and humidity are different. The amount will even change as the oxygen flow is adjusted during anesthesia. Nonprecision vaporizers are usually used with low-volatile anesthetic liquids, such as methoxyflurane (metaphane). Non-precision vaporizers with methoxyflurane (metaphane) are an older technology that is rarely used in current veterinary medicine.

Precision Vaporizer

The precision vaporizer is located out of the circle (VOC). The amount of the anesthetic gas delivered is set by turning a dial to a percent (%). The percentage of anesthetic gas is mixed with oxygen coming t hrough the flow meter. A precision vaporizer delivers the precise percentage of anesthetic gas from its outlet port regardless of the temperature, oxygen flow rate, and humidity. Precision vaporizers are gas specific and can accurately deliver only the anesthetic gas they are made to vaporize. Familiarization with each vaporizer in a clinic is important and will include knowing how to adjust the dial to the desired percentage of gas, where to fill it, and how to drain it. It is important not to overfill or tip vaporizers because the liquid anesthetic might enter parts of the vaporizer that should not get wet. It takes some time to dry, and until it does the vaporizer will not function accurately. It is also recommended that vaporizers be turned off when they are being filled. Do not fill a vaporizer while a patient is connected. Prior to every surgery the amount of liquid anesthetic in the vaporizer should be checked and filled as needed. This should be routinely done along with checking the machine for leaks and making sure the oxygen tanks are adequately full and turned on. Gases exit the vaporizor at the common gas outlet. The common gases are oxygen and the anesthetic gas. The common gas outlet will be connected to one of two breathing systems: a rebreathing system or a nonrebreathing system.

Breathing Systems

Breathing systems are connected between the common gas outlet of precision vaporizers and the patient. The parts of a breathing system depend on whether the patient is rebreathing its own unused exhaled air or not. Breathing systems may be either rebreathing or nonrebreathing systems.

Rebreathing System

The rebreathing system is also called a circle system. In this type of system, the fresh gases coming from the common gas outlet enter the circle at the place where exhaled gases from the patient are circulating. There is no actual visible circle, but the parts of the circle are all connected together so that gases flow in one direction over and over again. There are some advantages to having fresh gases and exhaled gases mixing together. Exhaled gases will warm and moisten the fresh gases. The gases that an animal exhales will include unused oxygen and anesthetic gas. These gases get recirculated and rebreathed so the amount of the fresh gases supplied can be turned down. In this way a rebreathing system conserves oxygen and anesthetic gases. However, there are also some disadvantages to having fresh gases and exhaled gases mixing together. Adding more gases to the exhaled gases increases the pressure in the breathing tubes, thus adding resistance to breathing. Also, the exhaled carbon dioxide (CO_2) can build up. Elevated CO_2 in the blood is called **hypercapnia** or **hypercarbia**. An additional disadvantage is that it will take longer to change the patient's depth of anesthesia after the anesthetic gas percentage is changed. Since there is a lot of dead space (the room or space in the tubes that contributes to stagnant gases), the newly changed gases need to combine with the older gases in the circle. It will take time for this mixture to approach the percentage of anesthesia set on the dial of the vaporizer. Veterinary technicians will need to plan ahead and determine in advance when to increase or decrease the percentage of anesthetic gas needed because the patient will not respond right away.

The following parts are included in the circle of a rebreathing system: manometer, breathing tubes, reservoir bags, pop-off valve, and CO_2 absorber. Even the patient can be considered part of the circle. These parts, as well as the operation of a rebreathing system as an open, semiopen, or closed circuit, are reviewed in more detail in the sections that follow.

Manometer

The manometer measures the pressure within the breathing circle (also called a *breathing circuit*). Since the animal's lungs are part of the breathing circuit, the manometer also measures pressure in the lungs. Manometers use one of two different units of measure. The most common unit is cmH_2O (centimeters of water). This really measures how much pressure it takes to move water one centimeter. The second, and less common, unit is mmHg (millimeters of mercury). During anesthesia and routine patient breathing the manometer should not exceed pressures of 4 cmH_2O (~2–3mmHg). Higher pressures than this can prevent an anesthetized patient from breathing. When manually ventilating (often called bagging), keep the pressures at or below 20 cmH_2O (~14 mmHg). Higher pressures can damage the **alveoli** (air sacs in the lungs).

Breathing Tubes

The breathing tubes connect the patient's endotracheal tube or face mask to the machine. Two common breathing tubes are the Y tube and the universal F tube. The Y tube is shaped like the letter Y. The universal F tube has a tube within a tube. The inspired air is in the inner tube and is surrounded by a tube that contains exhaled air. This can help warm the inspired air. The technician must connect the universal F tube correctly to the proper inhalation and exhalation ports.

One-Way Inhalation and Exhalation Valves

These only allow gases to travel in one direction through the circle. These valves are incorporated into the inhalation and exhalation ports, which are the openings where the breathing tubes are connected. Veterinary technicians must be able to determine which port has the inhalation valve and which port has the exhalation valve.

Reservoir Bag

The reservoir bag (or Rebreathing Bag) is used for reserve breathing capacity (such as when a patient needs to take a deep breath), and for positive pressure ventilation (or *bagging*). Watching the reservoir bag can also help monitor a patient's respiratory rate as well as the quality of respirations. In general, 6 times the tidal volume (10 ml/kg) is the minimum size bag to use. Tidal volume is defined as the volume of air exchange during normal breathing (**eupnea**). Always use the next size up if the animal is between bag sizes. A significantly larger bag will not inflate as much (making it hard to see the respirations) and there is increased dead space (making it take longer to change the percentage of anesthesia), but there is less chance of increased breathing pressure and there will be plenty of reserve air for a patient to take a deep breath. When giving a breath to (bagging) the patient, the pop-off valve (positive pressure relief valve) must be completely closed. Doing this during anesthesia every 5 to 20 minutes will prevent **atelectasis** (collapsing of the alveoli) and flush the stagnating CO_2 from the alveoli, airways, and breathing tubes. Flushing will help prevent hypercapnia, hypoxia, and respiratory acidosis. The reservoir bag is also used in critical situations when the animal stops breathing (**apnea**) to provide artificial respiration.

Pop-Off Valve

The pop-off valve (or Positive Pressure Relief Valve) can be thought of as a hole that vents gases and pressure from the circle. This hole should be connected to some kind of scavenging system so that the waste gases are not exhausted into the room. The only time the pop-off valve should be closed is when the patient is being bagged. On occasion, a veterinarian may use *low-flo* or a closed system and partially or completely close the pop-off valve during surgery. In these cases, it is critical continuously to monitor the bag size and manometer pressure, and adjust the oxygen flow rate. However, more routinely and for safety, the pop-off valve should remain all the way or partially open, except when giving a patient a breath.

Carbon Dioxide Absorbent

Gases in the circle that do not exit through the pop-off valve will need to go through a container of CO_2 absorbent. CO_2 absorbents include soda lime and barium hydroxide lime. A chemical reaction takes place when CO_2 percolates through and comes in contact with granules of the CO_2 absorbent. The CO_2 molecules are converted into heat and water. The canister may become warm, and water is captured in a trap at the bottom of the canister. It is important to understand that soda lime and barium hydroxide lime are used up (exhausted) whether the anesthetic machine is in use or not. The CO_2 absorbent granules will be used up and not able to absorb CO_2 when they change color, become hard, and when they reach a specified age.

Changing color is pH dependent. Purple is a typical color change indicating exhausted absorbent, but there are other colors depending on the variety of the absorbent used. Since the color change fades with time, the absence of a color change is not a reliable way to tell whether the granules are exhausted or not. If one-third to one-half of the CO_2 absorbent in the canister turns color during a surgery, it should all be replaced before the next surgery.

Fresh granules are easily pulverized between your fingers. Old and exhausted granules, even those without a color change, are much harder. Over time, CO_2 in the air will exhaust the absorbent ability of the granules, regardless of anesthetic use. Set a regular time interval for discarding the CO_2 canister. Every 1 to 4 weeks is a typical range. Use the hardness test to determine the correct interval for every different CO_2 canister and machine.

Open, Semiopen, and Closed Anesthetic Circuits

Rebreathing systems can be operated in one of three ways: as a closed, a semiclosed, or an open circuit (or circle).

In a closed circuit, the oxygen supply equals the patient's metabolic consumption of oxygen, which is approximately 4 to 8 ml/kg/min. Essentially, there is a low level of oxygen flow so that there is no extra or wasted unused gas. The advantages of a closed circuit are that it is economical: it retains more heat and humidity, and causes the least amount of environmental pollution. The term *closed circuit* does not come from the fact that the pop-off valve is closed but because theoretically the gases in and out are equal, so there is no need for extra gas from the outside and no influence on the outside by waste gas. It is difficult to provide anesthesia using a closed circuit. The patient's gas requirements will change throughout surgery and changing the oxygen flow to match the animal's precise needs is very difficult.

In a semiclosed circuit, the oxygen delivered exceeds the patient's oxygen consumption and excess gases are continually eliminated through the pop-off valve. Depending on how much the patient's oxygen requirements are exceeded, a semiclosed circuit can be deemed as a low-flow, a medium-flow, or a high-flow semiclosed circuit. The advantages of using a semiclosed circuit with medium and high flows are that it is safer for the animal because it does not run low on oxygen, and there is a more rapid change in anesthetic concentration than with low flows (or even closed circuits). However, with the excess oxygen flow there is more potential for increased pressure, more waste and pollution, and it is less economical.

An open circuit provides gas anesthesia to the patient via a mask or an induction chamber. It is considered open because there is no tight seal. There are several disadvantages to using an open circuit:

- It takes longer to induce a patient due to the increased dead space within a mask or an induction chamber.
- Stage II excitement phase is more apt to happen, and lasts longer than if an injectable anesthetic is used first. The vocalization and struggling that occurs with Stage II excitement can be troubling.
- Monitoring the patient is more difficult. CRTs and gum color cannot be checked when a mask is on. When an animal is in an induction chamber, monitoring other vital signs is difficult.

- There is an increase in waste gases, and the wasted gas cannot be efficiently scavenged. This exposes the humans present to the waste gas anesthetic.

Regardless, an open circuit is often used in small or fractious patients.

Nonrebreathing Systems

The nonrebreathing system does not have a circle and the patient breathes only fresh gases. When operated correctly, this system does not have the disadvantages of a rebreathing system: CO_2 or pressure buildup in the breathing tubes or a delayed patient response to changes in the delivered anesthetic gas. However, fresh oxygen can be cold and dry, even to the point of causing dehydration and hypothermia in small patients. There are no exhaled gases in this system to warm or humidify the incoming fresh gas. Due to the built-in loss of exhaled gases, the oxygen and anesthetic gas need to be delivered at increased rates when compared to a rebreathing system. Thus, more gas is wasted with this system. A nonrebreathing system will benefit smaller animals the most, typically those at or under 15 pounds. If it is used on larger patients the high flow rates of gas would cause a lot of wasted gas. With large animals, the flow rate required may exceed the anesthetic machine's capabilities.

Basically a nonrebreathing system consists of a set of tubing, a pop-off or exit port or vent, and a reservoir bag. Because there is no rebreathing (or recirculation) of gases there is no need for CO_2 absorbents or one-way exhalation and inhalation ports or valves. Because the pop-off is always open (unless the patient is being bagged) there is no backup of pressure and no need for a manometer. Nonrebreathing tubes connect directly to the endotracheal tube so there is no need for other breathing tubes. However, there is still a need to retain a reservoir bag and a pop-off-like vent (which is not really a valve and not actually a pop-off valve).

All rebreathing apparatuses have three openings to connect. One attaches to the fresh gases at the common gas outlet, one attaches to the scavenging system, and one attaches to the patient's endotracheal tube. There is very little dead space between the attached endotracheal tube and the nonrebreathing apparatus. This is beneficial for small patients with small tidal volumes. It could take a significant number of breaths for a ferret to receive fresh gases if it were attached to a 2-foot long Y breathing tube.

Scavenging System

Once gases have exited the pop-off valve or the exit port (on a nonrebreathing system) they are considered waste gases that should be removed, or scavenged, so that the people and the animal in the room will not be exposed to them. As mentioned before, hepatic problems and abortions have been associated with people who are chronically exposed to certain anesthetic gases. An older inhalant gas called methoxyflurane (metaphane) is nephrotoxic. Waste gases can also cause dizziness, nausea, and headaches in people. The scavenged gases are not returned to the circle, but instead are directed either out of the room or through a filter. The scavenged gas and the scavenging system that is used to remove the waste gases are not included as part of the circle.

Scavenging systems vary. They can be a tube that connects the pop-off valve (or exit port) to a vent leading outside (a passive scavenging system), they can be suctioned away (an active scavenging system), or even filtered. A filter, like an F/air canister, uses activated charcoal to filter out halogenated hydrocarbons. These filters do not filter out CO_2 or N_2O, only halogenated hydrocarbons. Filters have a time limit for use, and they gain weight as the inhaled gas collects in the filter. When there is a certain weight gained, or the time of use has lapsed, the filter is full. For an F/air canister the limits are 12 hours of use or 50 grams of weight gained, whichever comes first. When a scavenging system cannot be used, human exposure to anesthetic gas cannot be avoided, such as during patient recovery, when emptying or filling the vaporizer, when there is a leak in the system, and when using an open rebreathing system. In these cases it is wise to be in a well-ventilated room.

Anesthetic Monitoring

The best monitor is a well-trained and alert veterinary technician. Veterinary technicians should know their monitoring equipment's limitations and be able to judge for themselves the patient's status, regardless of what a monitor is showing. A veterinary technician should be familiar with what is normal and be able to judge what is normal for this patient, in this particular situation, and at this moment. What is normal for an animal at rest is not the same as what is normal for this same animal during an exam or on a surgery table. A veterinary technician should continually observe an anesthetized patient, keeping his or her hands on the patient rather than monitoring from afar. Connecting with the patient should become second nature so that minor changes in muscle tone, respiratory quality, reflexes, and other factors will be noticed.

Despite each patient's relative normal values, a veterinary technician should know some general normal and abnormal values in order to gauge the different depths of general anesthesia. A patient slides in and out of different levels of anesthesia (called *stages* and *planes*) at varying speeds. The drugs used as preanesthetics, analgesics, and anesthetics can alter the parameters used to determine a patient's stage and plane. Monitoring a patient can be approached in two ways: hands-on monitoring and monitoring with equipment.

Hands-On Monitoring

Anesthesia monitoring requires a veterinary technician to get their hands on the patient. No patient can be accurately assessed by just looking at a monitor or by checking any one parameter. What follows are several hands-on monitoring parameters that every technician should observe during anesthesia.

Heart Rate

The veterinary technician should determine the patient's heart rate (HR), measured in terms of beats per minute (bpm). An anesthetized patient would normally have a lower HR, as would a sleeping patient. However, the HR may be elevated more than expected or even more than normal. Sometimes the drugs administered can elevate the HR above what would be expected. For example, when atropine is used lower HRs are prevented, so a higher than expected HR may be seen. Or, when ketamine is used, since it does not depress cardiac output like many other anesthetics do, a higher than expected HR may be seen. Sometimes drugs are not the reason for a higher than expected HR. When a patient loses blood pressure (BP) the HR elevates to compensate. Lower than expected HRs may also be considered normal. The HR is expected to be lower in patients given an alpha-2 agonist. A patient with medetomidine on board and an HR of 60 would be considered normal, yet if this patient had been given propofol this would be considered bradycardic. Also, expect lower HRs when surgery stimulates vagal tone. This is a stimulation of the parasympathetic system (rest and relaxation) and results in a slower HR. Procedures that stimulate vagal tone include ocular surgeries and GI tract surgeries. Even placing an endotracheal tube can stimulate vagal tone and result in a lower than expected HR. Plan ahead for these procedures and administer, or be ready to administer, an anticholinergic drug to prevent too much parasympathetic stimulation.

The veterinary technician should also take into account the species and size of the patient when assessing HR. In general, the smaller the patient, the higher its HR, and conversely the larger the patient, the lower its HR. An anesthetized miniature pinscher may have an HR of 120 and a St. Bernard (given the same anesthetic and at the same stage and plane of anesthesia) may have an HR of 70, and both could be considered normal. The reverse would not typically be true. Keep these variations in mind while learning normal values and when studying the chart on stages and planes.

An HR is not necessarily the same as the pulse rate. The heart rate is determined at the heart by **auscultation**, by precordial palpation, and by visualization (although this is uncommon). Pulse rates are found by palpating an animal's peripheral arteries, which is why they are called peripheral pulses. A technician should use the appropriate terms. Monitors attached to an appendage provide a pulse rate. Auscultation of the heart with a stethoscope provides an HR. The HR should be the same as the pulse rate, but that is not always the case. If the HR and the pulse rate are not equal when taken simultaneously, this is called a pulse deficit.

Besides determining the HR or pulse rate, a veterinary technician should also judge the quality of the HR or pulse rate. A pulse rate of 100 may fall within normal for the situation, but if it is weak or thready the quality is not good. Describing the pulse quality can also include terms like *bounding* or *snappy*, which describe an abnormally strong pulse quality. An HR may be 100, but if there are arrhythmias, where beats are skipped, delayed, or premature, then the quality is not good. The other monitoring parameters listed in the following sections also need the same consideration regarding the variation of what are considered normal levels as well as judging their quality.

Respiratory Rate

The veterinary technician also determines the respiratory rate (RR). An anesthetized patient would normally have a lower RR. However, drugs that are administered can decrease the RR even more than would be expected for an anesthetized patient. Narcotics in general are respiratory depressants. Several other drugs can be expected to cause apnea when initially given intravenously, such as ketamine, thiopental, and propofol (some are dose related and/or rate related). The quality of respirations is as important as the RR. If a patient has 16 bpm but has long pauses followed by quick and/or shallow breaths, then this is poorer quality respiration than that of a patient with 8 bpm whose breaths are deep and consistently spaced. Abdominal breaths and agonal breaths are not considered good quality breaths. Abdominal breaths look like a hiccup with a sudden jerky abdominal contraction in order to expand the diaphragm to breathe. Abdominal breaths occur during very deep anesthesia when the diaphragm and thoracic muscles are not coordinating the breaths. An agonal breath is a sudden inspiration that looks similar to a gasp, yet there is no expiration. This can be considered the body's last gasp in a reflex attempt to get a last breath. Patients showing abdominal breathing or an agonal breath are in serious trouble or even terminal.

Perfusion

Perfusion is the oxygenated blood flow to tissues. When perfusion is bad, the tissues do not receive the amount of blood flow or the amount of oxygen required to sustain them. This results in tissue death, whether of a few cells or of an entire organ. We may assume that the perfusion we are able to check is similar to that of the perfusion in tissues that we cannot check. For example, if perfusion to the patient's gums is judged to be good then the perfusion is assumed to be good to other tissues such as the brain or kidneys. Perfusion is judged by looking at several parameters at the same time.

Peripheral Pulse

The peripheral pulse was covered in more detail under the heading Heart Rate. If the quality or rate of the pulse is poor, then oxygenated blood flow to the tissues is most likely poor as well. Peripheral locations that can be used to determine pulse quality and rate include the femoral artery, the lingual artery, and the pedal arteries. A peripheral pulse should be obtained in conjunction with an HR to detect the presence of pulse deficits.

Capillary Refill Time

Capillary refill time (CRT) is determined by blanching out the mucous membrane color on the buccal surface of the gums. This is done using momentary finger or thumb pressure on the gum. The typical location is over the maxillary canine root, although this can be done elsewhere if the gum color is black and obscures the normal pink color. The time it takes for the blanched gum to return to its initial color is estimated. The normal range of time for this to occur is 1 to 2 seconds. If CRT is less than 1 second, the refill is fast and may indicate hypertension (high blood pressure) or compensatory shock. If CRT is longer than 2 seconds, it is prolonged and perfusion may be poor, which may indicate hypotension (low blood pressure), hypovolemia (low blood volume), or cardiac output problems.

Blood Pressure

Blood pressure (BP) can be estimated by feeling peripheral pulses. The pressure that is felt is the difference between the systolic and the diastolic pressure. Palpable peripheral pulses are lost below an MAP of 70 mmHg. To accurately determine a patient's BP, a monitor will have to be used.

Mucous Membrane Color

Normal mucous membranes (mm) are moist and pink tissues found in the mouth, eyelids, prepuce, penis, and vulva. During anesthesia some of these locations may not be accessible to check due to the sterile field. A veterinary technician should be accomplished at determining the mm color at any location. Mucous membrane color can be used to assess the patient's perfusion, but it can sometimes be deceptive and not accurately indicate the patient's true perfusion status. For example, pale mm may indicate shock or hemorrhage (and thus poor perfusion), but pale mm can also occur as a result of edema, or gums that are flooded with water during a dental procedure. Blue mm color can indicate hypoxia, but when it appears there may have been a lack of oxygen for too long already. Bright red, brick red, or cherry red gums may give a false sense of good perfusion because these colors can be caused by carbon monoxide, septic shock, or endotoxic shock.

Body Temperature

To monitor body temperature effectively, the changes in body temperature should be tracked. Changes in an anesthetized patient's temperature are to be expected. Usually, any one temperature or any one external site where the temperature is taken cannot be the sole determiner of the patient's temperature status. As expected with any sleeping animal, the temperature of an anesthetized animal will decrease from the preanesthetic temperature. The degree to which it changes is what is of concern.

An animal's temperature is most commonly taken rectally. Rectal temperatures may not accurately reflection the core body temperature in an anesthetized animal. Anal tone decreases as a patient gets deeper under anesthesia. This allows room air to enter the colon, decreasing the temperature. In addition, as the colon relaxes, fecal material moves down to the rectum. A rectal temperature can be inaccurate if the thermometer is placed in the middle of fecal material or if there is room air in the rectum. Rather than relying only on a rectal temperature, also feel the extremities. The paws and ears can help assess the temperature. Avoid feeling areas that may be in the spotlights or in contact with a heat source. Feeling the paws and ears can also help indirectly to determine the patient's perfusion.

Good perfusion is required to keep extremities warm. Body temperature will decrease under anesthesia, and a source of external heat is required. A decrease in a patient's temperature of more than

2 degrees, or a temperature below 99°F, should prompt the use of additional sources of heat. Heat sources can include warm circulating water blankets, warm air pillows, warmed IV fluids, warm rice socks, and warm towels. Electric heating pads made for human use are not a good heat source as they can result in thermal burns. Use microwaves to heat items with caution. Microwaves can unevenly heat items, resulting in hot spots that are too hot for a patient. When fluids are microwaved, mix them first before using. Malignant hyperthermia is a special condition to be aware of. Anesthetized patients can have a reaction to some anesthetics, especially halothane. Halothane can cause a sharp spike in temperature. If an anesthetized patient's temperature rises more than 2 degrees due to an anesthetic reaction, then the halothane should be discontinued.

Reflexes

As a patient goes deeper and deeper under general anesthesia, its normal reflexes diminish or disappear in a predictable order. Knowing which reflexes are still present can help determine a patient's stage and plane of anesthesia. A patient loses the following 4 reflexes in the order listed, and they return in the reverse order as the patient awakens.

Swallow

The swallow reflex is also called the cough or gag reflex. This is the first reflex to be lost and the last one to return during general anesthesia. In order for an endotracheal tube to be placed, this reflex must be significantly diminished or gone. When an animal swallows, material goes down the esophagus, which is not the correct place for an endotracheal tube. Without a swallow reflex, material like saliva, water, food, or digesta can go down the trachea. This is called aspiration. Aspiration into the lungs, or aspiration pneumonia, is a life-threatening condition. It is always a good idea to seal the trachea by placing an endotracheal tube whenever the swallow reflex is lost.

Pedal

Pronounced *peedle*, the pedal reflex is a withdrawal of a leg or other movement as a reaction to a significant toe pinch. It is an indicator of deep pain. The toe pinch is done by digging a thumbnail into the dorsal surface of a phalangeal bone (top of the toe), not from the pad side of the toe nor in the webbing between the toes. The nail needs to dig in hard enough to at least blanch your thumbnail in an attempt to elicit a pain response from an anesthetized patient. If not properly done, the patient may be judged to be absent of deep pain, and the error not discovered until the surgeon uses the scalpel blade.

Palpebral

The palpebral reflex is a blink response to protect the eye. Using a finger to lightly touch the eyelashes and medial and lateral **canthus** will cause a blinking response in an animal that has maintained its palpebral reflex. Even a slight twitch or movement of the eyelids, brow, or cheek means this reflex is present.

Corneal

The corneal reflex is also a blink response to protect the eye. There should be a reflexive blink when something touches the cornea. To test this reflex, a finger is used to touch the cornea lightly. Lack of a blink or twitch means that the corneal reflex is lost. The corneal reflex should not be checked routinely on an animal because it can cause corneal injury. The corneal reflex should only be checked when the palpebral reflex is gone and there are other indications that the patient is too deep. The loss of the corneal reflex is not desired and, as can be seen on the chart of anesthetic stages and planes, it indicates the patient is in a critical situation.

Eye Monitoring

Monitoring the rotation of the eye in the orbit (globe position) and the pupils' response to light can help determine a patient's depth of anesthesia.

Globe Position

The eye, or globe, is considered central when the full pupil is visible. The eye is considered ventromedial when the pupil has moved so that it is in the medial canthus of the orbit (or cross-eyed). The eye does not go from perfectly central to ventromedial in one fast motion. There is a continuum of movement. with the central eye being analogous to the noon sun and the ventromedial eye being like the setting sun. The stages and planes chart uses +/− to indicate that the eye is in transition, with the words central or ventral used to indicate which way it is headed. A patient with a completely central globe is not in a surgical plane of anesthesia. The animal may be either too light or too deep, and neither is a good surgical plane of anesthesia.

Pupillary Light Reflex

Pupillary light reflex (PLR) is determined by shining a light into the pupils and noting whether the pupils constrict (miosis). This is not routinely done during anesthesia, but it can be done to help judge whether a patient is entering a critical stage and plane.

Muscle Tone

In general, muscle tone will become progressively more relaxed the deeper a patient gets. A veterinary technician should compare the patient's muscle tone to assess change indicating lesser or greater anesthetic depth. Muscle tone should be judged by comparing later tone to earlier tone in the same patient. Do not compare muscle tone between patients. Jaw tone and anal tone are used to judge a patient's muscle tone.

Jaw Tone

Spreading the mandible and the maxilla with just a finger and thumb is a very sensitive way to tell whether the muscle tone has changed.

Anal Tone

Ana tone is a visual assessment of the anus. Compare the anal opening size as the patient becomes anesthetized or wakes up. The anus will be closed at relatively light anesthetic depths and more open at deeper anesthetic depths.

STAGES AND PLANES OF ANESTHESIA

STAGES AND PLANES OF ANESTHESIA	BEHAVIOR OR STATUS OF PATIENT	RESPIRATION	CARDIOVASCULAR	REFLEXES				RESPONSE TO SURGERY	EYEBALL POSITION
				CORNEAL REFLEX	PALPEBRAL	PEDAL	GAG AND SWALLOW		
I. Voluntary excitement	drowsy, disoriented, struggles	normal to panting	HR unchanged	+	+	+	+	struggles	central
II. Involuntary excitement, or excitement stage	appears excited, limbs padding, vocalization, yawning	irregular, from hyperventilation to apnea	HR may increase	+	+	+	+	struggles	± nystagmus
III. Anesthetic Planes Plane 1	light anesthesia	slow and regular ≈ 12–20 BPM	HR > 90 BPM, pulse strong, CRT ≤ 2 sec	+	+	+	–	movement	± ventral
Plane 2	medium anesthesia, or surgical anesthesia	slow and regular, possibly shallow ≈ 12–16 BPM	HR > 90 BPM, pulse strong, CRT ≤ 2 sec	+	+	–	–	HR and RR may increase	ventral
Plane 3	deep anesthesia, or surgical anesthesia for only the most severe surgery	shallow < 12 BPM, some abdominal breathing	HR 60–90 BPM, CRT increased, weakened pulse	+	–	–	–	none	± central
Plane 4	too deep, anesthetic emergency, overdose	shallow and all abdominal breathing jerky	HR < 60 BPM, CRT prolonged, weak pulse, pale mm	–	–	–	–	none PLR absent	central
IV. Danger	moribund (dying)	respiratory failure	cardiovascular collapse, shock, cardiac arrest	–	–	–	–	none	central

Anesthetic Monitoring Equipment

Monitoring equipment is often used to supplement a veterinary technician's abilities to assess an anesthetized patient physically. The following are common types of equipment currently used in veterinary medicine. Many of these monitors can be either standalone or combined into one unit.

Audio Patient Monitor

The audio patient monitor (APM) is essentially a speaker that amplifies heart and lung sounds. The APM is connected to the patient through an esophageal stethoscope. The sounds heard are the same that can be heard when ausculting the chest using a stethoscope.

Esophageal Stethoscope

An esophageal stethoscope is a hollow tube that is placed into the esophagus with its distal end over the base of the heart. Different sizes are available for the variety of patient sizes seen in veterinary medicine. An esophageal stethoscope can also be attached to an ordinary stethoscope so that you can monitor the patient without having to place the large diaphragm or bell on the thoracic wall, which could prevent contamination of the sterile field during a surgery.

Electrocardiogram

An electrocardiogram (ECG) provides an image of the heart's electrical activity. Using lead II is best for determining heart rate and rhythm. Use the ECG's display or paper printout to count the number of complexes per minute to determine the heart rate. Noticing patterns or the lack of them, plus changes in the waves or complexes, can indicate arrhythmias. A normal ECG will have waves that are above or below the baseline. There are normally 5 waves, each of which is identified by letters starting with *P* and ending with *T*. The P wave indicates atrial depolarization, which results in atrial chamber contraction, atrioventricular (AV) valves opening, the first heart sound (S1), and the ventricles filling with blood. Cardiologists would examine each of the next 3 waves (Q, R, and S) individually. However, a veterinary technician should look at them together and call them by one name, the QRS complex. The QRS complex indicates ventricular depolarization, which results in ventricle chamber contraction (**systole**), semilunar valves opening, the second heart sound (S2), blood being pushed through the pulmonary and aortic arteries, and the filling of the atrial chambers. The T wave is an indication of ventricular repolarization, which can be thought of as ventricular diastole. The atria also repolarize, but this happens during the QRS complex. Due to the sheer mass of the ventricles compared to the atrium's, the electrical waves of the ventricle depolarization overshadow the waves of the atrial repolarization. When an anesthetized patient is being monitored, a missing or abnormally shaped wave can indicate that part of the heart is having electrical problems. If it is the P wave, consider the atrium as having a problem. If it is the QRS complex, consider the ventricle as having a problem.

Blood Pressure Monitors

Blood pressure (BP) is given in two numbers (and a third can be extrapolated from these two numbers). Systolic BP is the higher of the two numbers and occurs when the ventricles are contracting. The diastolic BP is the lower of the two numbers and occurs when the ventricles are filling. The atria do the opposite of what the ventricles are doing. A mean arterial pressure (MAP) of 60 mmHg is considered the minimum to perfuse the major organs, and in an anesthetized patient a MAP of 70 to 90 mmHg is desirable. BP does not necessarily mean that blood is flowing well to the tissues, so it is only one of the types of data used to determine perfusion. For example, when the BP is elevated due to vasoconstriction the actual amount of blood flow to peripheral tissues is decreased. In an anesthetized patient, monitor the BP changes over time rather than relying on a single reading to indicate the patient's status. BP is monitored using either direct or indirect methods.

Direct Blood Pressure

This method of obtaining BP is invasive and requires a catheter to be placed. In veterinary medicine, direct BP is done less frequently than indirect BP. There is a risk of hematoma and infection, but the readings are continuous and the most accurate. Two ways of obtaining a direct BP are by using arterial or central venous pressures.

In the arterial method, the peripheral arteries are used to place a catheter. The femoral or dorsal pedal arteries are commonly used. A catheter is placed in the artery and is directly connected to a BP dial.

The central venous pressure provides a pressure (in units of cmH_2O) of the blood returning to the heart. An accurate pressure can be done by placing a catheter in the vena cava with its tip close to the right atrium. The pressure is measured by a tube of water and the meniscus will rise and fall with each breath. In dogs and cats, less than 8 cmH_2O, measured on exhalation, is considered normal.

Indirect Blood Pressure

The indirect method of obtaining a blood pressure (BP) is not invasive and uses a sensor or probe plus a cuff placed on the surface of a limb or on the tail. In order to compare a patient's BP over time it is important that the same site be used and in the same position. BP variances will occur when using different sites, different positions, and even with different operators. Doing the procedure the same way every time is important for consistent readings. Two ways of obtaining an indirect BP are by using Doppler or oscillometric methods.

The Doppler method is a manual method that uses an ultrasound probe, which converts the pulse waves into an audible sound. The probe must be positioned over an artery with blood flow. The sound can be described as a swish or a whoosh. The probe, coated with ultrasound gel, can be placed over an artery on a distal limb or ventral tail and carefully held, or taped in place. Too much pressure will alter the blood flow and the BP readings. The correct size cuff is chosen by its width. The width should be about 40% of the site's circumference, or the BP readings will be altered. The cuff is placed proximal to the probe and inflated until there is no more audible whoosh sound. The cuff's pressure is released slowly until the whooshing sound is heard. The pressure dial, which is attached to the cuff, is read at the point the whoosh returns. This is the systolic BP. The pressure dial should be held and read at the level of the patient's heart. The BP reading may be falsely low if the pressure dial is held higher than the level of the patient's heart, as much as 1 mmHg for every inch change. The opposite is true if the pressure dial is held below the level of the patient's heart. Take several readings and average them. In addition, a cat's Doppler BP readings are about 14 mmHg less than they actually are when compared with direct BP methods. Take all of these factors into account when determining the systolic BP with a Doppler.

The oscillometer method uses a digital readout for the BP, and can be generated automatically. A cuff that can sense the pulsating (oscillating) blood flow and limb size is used on a limb or the tail. It is important to familiarize yourself with each machine's cuffs; lengthwise measurements are marked on them for correct matching with the patient's size. The systolic, diastolic, and MAP pressures are automatically displayed. Like the Doppler, the systolic pressure is underestimated. An oscillometer's MAP is the most accurate reading of all the types of BP methods.

Pulse Oximetry

A pulse oximeter (pulse ox) measures the patient's saturation percent of hemoglobin with oxygen (the percentage of hemoglobin bound with oxygen). Keep in mind that this is not a blood gas measurement, which measures partial pressure of oxygen (PaO_2) in units of mmHg. Pulse oximeter oxygen saturation (SpO_2) is given in percentages. No measurement of SpO_2 will be greater than 100%. An SpO_2 below 90% indicates hypoxia. In a normal awake or anesthetized patient the SpO_2 would be greater than 95%. A pulse ox probe (or clip) is placed across a thin area of tissue such as the ear, tongue, webbing between the toes, a pinch of the skin, or the lip, and there are even rectal probes. A wavelength of light in the red spectrum is emitted from the probe and the amount not absorbed (reflected back) by the hemoglobin is measured. Attachment to darkly pigmented tissues should be avoided. Probe selection is also important for accurate readings. A clip should be used so that the two sides are parallel when tissue is between them. Thicker tissues require a wider clip. Pulse ox monitors will also display pulse rates, although they may indicate HR on the display screen.

Capnography

A capnograph measures the amount of carbon dioxide (CO_2) in the breathing tubes. Essentially this is the same amount in the lungs and in the blood. It is measured using units of mmHg. Normally during inspiration, CO_2 levels in the breathing tubes should be close to zero (unless CO_2 absorbent is exhausted or there is a relative increase in dead space). The patient exhales CO_2 and the levels will then increase. The CO_2 is best measured at the end of expiration when it would be at its highest level. This is called end tidal CO_2 ($ETCO_2$).

During anesthesia, $ETCO_2$ levels above 40 to 45 mmHg constitute hypercapnia, and levels below 25 to 35 mmHg constitute hypocapnia. A veterinary technician should manually ventilate (bag) the patient when hypercapnia occurs (assuming the CO_2 absorbent and breathing circuit size is correct). If a patient is hypocapnic, the most likely cause is that the patient has been hyperventilating. The increase in CO_2 is what causes the brain to signal respiration, not the lack of oxygen. A patient can have a normal oxygen level and a high or low CO_2 level. They are independent of each other.

Analgesia

Analgesia means without pain. Anesthesia alone is not pain control. Anesthesia is typically used so that a patient will not perceive pain during surgery while in an unconscious state. This does not mean that pain is not occurring. The nerve endings (called nociceptors) sense the pain, and the spinal cord is delivered these pain sensations and delivers them further to the brain. While under general anesthesia, the brain does not perceive the pain being sent its way, but the other tissues sense the pain and have physiologic changes.

Pain Physiology

Because pain can cause many deleterious effects and manifest in many different ways, it benefits the veterinary team to provide patients with analgesia. Analgesia can be achieved when pain is prevented, lessened, blocked, or not perceived along the nerve pathways. When analgesia is used in more than one of these ways it is called multimodal analgesia. Using analgesics (pain relievers) to prevent pain before it happens is called preemptive analgesia. There are at least two types of sensory pain neurons: a-delta fibers and c-fibers.

A-Delta Fibers

A-delta fibers are pain sensory neurons having the following characteristics: They transmit sharp pain sensations; they easily localize the source of pain; and they conduct signals relatively rapidly because they are large myelinated nerves.

C-Fibers

C-fibers are pain sensory neurons having the following characteristics: They transmit dull, aching, throbbing pain; it is difficult to localize the source of pain; and they are smaller, nonmyelinated nerves with slower conduction.

Visceral pain originates from the inner organs. C-fibers primarily transmit the pain that arises from the viscera. Usually organ pain is hard to localize and is typified by cramping, burning, and pressure. For example, a patient with kidney pain may appear to have back pain. Somatic pain originates from the body's outer shell, which includes the skin, muscles, bones, and joints. Somatic pain can usually be localized to the exact spot and is characterized by a sharp, stabbing sensation. An example of somatic pain would be an injection site. Both A-delta fibers and C-fibers can be found in the somatic tissue. Thus, pain that is dull, aching, and throbbing can be felt after the sharp stab of pain from an injection. These nerve fibers conduct the pain impulse to the dorsal root of the spinal cord.

The use of preemptive and multimodal analgesia can decrease phenomena such as hyperesthesia and wind-up. Pain at the periphery, especially if chronic, can lead to increased sensitivity to a stimulus such as touch, heat, and cold. This phenomenon is termed hyperesthesia. During surgery, when pain is not perceived, the pain impulses traveling to the spinal cord can lead to a build-up of chemical mediators that intensify the pain upon recovery. This phenomenon is termed wind-up. Analgesia produced at the level of the nociceptors can decrease hyperesthesia. Analgesia produced at the level of the spinal cord can decrease wind-up.

Alternatives to Pharmaceutical Analgesics

It is a good practice to provide analgesia multi-modally by incorporating methods other than drugs. Methods other than drugs can include environment manipulation, acupuncture, massage, manipulation, friendly human contact, and nursing care.

Environment Manipulation

Manipulation of the environment can include such things as providing familiar toys, providing a quiet environment away from loud animals, or decreasing fear and anxiety in order to decrease the perception of pain.

Acupuncture

In human medicine, the ancient art of Chinese medine has included such techniques as acupuncture. While the benefits can be debated, there is reasonable evidence to show that analgesia is a major benefit of acupuncture. Acupuncture is being incorporated into veterinary medicine as well. Many veterinarians and veterinary technicians have learned and used an acupressure point that is found on the rostral midline of the nose (the location of GV-26) of mammals. Insertion of a hypodermic needle at this point does not provide analgesia, but studies have shown that in dogs and cats it can stimulate respiration if the patient is not breathing. Training in acupuncture is available for veterinarians. Surprisingly, animal patients accept acupuncture very well. Anecdotally, animals have been known to fall asleep during acupuncture therapy, perhaps indicating that acupuncture is relaxing, and provides pain relief.

Warm/Cold Compresses

Cold compresses can reduce pain, bleeding, and inflammation immediately postoperatively. Warm compresses can also provide relief during the healing process.

Massage and Movement

Physical therapy for animal patients is becoming more available as veterinarians and veterinary technicians become certified in this specialty. Massage and movement can decrease edema, inflammation, and the associated pain by mobilizing lymphatics and blood supply. Select postoperative orthopedic patients can benefit from physical therapy, which increases range of motion and prevents muscle atrophy.

Friendly Human Contact

Positive contact with humans will help the healing process in companion animals. Have owners visit patients in the hospital. Make interactions with staff as positive as possible. Reinforce positive messages with talking and petting. From the animal's perspective, not everything associated with the veterinary treatment should be unpleasant or painful.

Nursing Care

Veterinary technicians have more contact with the patient than anyone else. As such, they have an extraordinary role in the recovery process. Schedule the least number of interruptions. Combine monitoring, medicines, temperatures, and moving the patient. Allow frequent walk times for elimination, fresh air, and exercise. Since the cage is the animal's home while hospitalized, avoid performing unpleasant procedures such as rectal temperatures and injections in the cage. The patient will be less stressed, tense, and uncomfortable while in the cage if it feels safe and pain free there.

Pharmaceutical Analgesia

There is also a pharmaceutical approach to analgesia. Remember that drugs that offer analgesia also have other affects; some of them undesirable or even harmful. This may partially explain why there are so many analgesics to choose from. The following categories and associated drugs are frequently used for analgesia.

Opioids

As stated earlier in this chapter, there are four types of opioid receptors: mu, kappa, delta, and sigma. The opioids have different degrees of receptor activity, and this may be the reason for choosing one over another. In general, however, all opioids typically produce some degree of analgesia, respiratory depression, sedation, euphoria, and addiction. The section on Preanesthetic Drugs earlier in this chapter offers more details about many of these drugs.

- **Morphine** is the standard to which all other narcotics are compared.
- **Oxymorphone** acts much like morphine, but it is several times more potent so a much smaller quantity is used to achieve the same effect.
- **Butorphanol** and **buprenorphine** both have agonist and antagonist affects (ceiling effect) so their analgesic effects will top out and any additional amount given will not provide any stronger analgesia.
- **Fentanyl** comes in a bottle to be injected into a patient, and is also available as a dermal patch.

The patch is placed on the skin where the fentanyl is then absorbed transdermally (across the skin).

- **Meperidine (Demerol)** is less potent than morphine and has a short duration of analgesia. Repeated doses can cause toxicity. Although this drug is commonly used in humans, this opioid is infrequently used in veterinary medicine.
- **Codeine** is less potent than morphine. Although this drug is commonly used as an analgesic in humans as well as in animals, this opioid is frequently used as an antitussive in veterinary medicine.

Nonsteroidal Anti-Inflammatory Drugs

Nonsteroidal anti-inflammatory drugs (NSAIDs) comprise the largest class of analgesics used. They are thought to block two (or more) enzymes called COX1 and COX2. The COX1 and COX2 enzymes convert arachidonic acid, one of the essential fatty acids, into prostaglandins. COX-1 is always present in the blood as a good enzyme protecting the kidneys, platelets, and the lining of the GI tract. When NSAIDs block COX1, the body's protective mechanism is blocked, which can result in gastrointestinal ulcers, bleeding, and renal failure. COX-2 is produced in the blood when there is tissue injury, resulting in inflammation and pain. When NSAIDs block COX2, inflammation and pain are blocked. NSAIDs that do not block COX1 should have fewer side effects related to GI tract upset, ulceration, bleeding, and renal failure. The ideal NSAID would block only the bad effects of pain and inflammation and not block the body's protective mechanisms. In other words, block COX2 but spare COX1. It is important to note that acetaminophen (Tylenol®) is not an NSAID and that it is particularly toxic to cats. The following NSAIDs are commonly used in veterinary medicine:

- **aspirin (acetylsalicylic acid)**
- **flunixin meglumine (Banamine®)**
- **phenylbutazone (Butazolidine®)**
- **ketoprofen (Ketofen®)**

- carprophen (Rimadyl®)
- etodolac (EtoGesic®)
- meloxicam (Metacam®)
- deracoxib (Deramaxx®)

Alpha-2 Agonists

The drugs classified as alpha-2 agonists have analgesic benefits in addition to their sedative and anesthetic effects. The section on Preanesthetic Drugs earlier in this chapter offers more details about these drugs.

- medetomidine (Domitor®, Dexdomitor®)
- detomidine (Dormosedan®)
- xylazine (Rompun®)

Adjunctive Analgesics

Adjunctive analgesics have analgesic effects, but they are rarely used as pain relievers in and of themselves:

- **Ketamine**—The Preanesthetic Drugs section earlier in this chapter offers more details about this drug.
- **Prednisolone or other corticosteroids**—Corticosteroids have anti-inflammatory effects, and pain is one of the cardinal signs of inflammation. Administering corticosteroids decreases the pain associated with inflammation. It is important to remember that NSAIDs should not be used routinely in conjunction with corticosteroids. Together corticosteroids and NSAIDs potentiate gastric mucosal damage, ulceration, and bleeding. Use cautiously postoperatively as they delay healing.

Local Analgesics

Local analgesics are also called local anesthetics or topical anesthetics. In general they work by preventing conduction of nerve impulses from the site of pain. Local analgesics dripped onto an incision site are called a splash block. When they are injected around nerves, they are referred to as local or regional nerve blocks. There are many types of nerve blocks done in veterinary medicine, including blocks for dentals (infraobital/mandibular), declaws, forelimbs (brachial plexus block), thoracotomys (intercostal nerve block), and epidurals. Many different agents are available; most of their names end in -*caine*.

- Lidocaine—Lidocaine is commercially available in combination with epinephrine. The vasoconstriction effects of epinephrine helps decrease bleeding and slows the lidocaine travel away from the local site. This provides hemostasis and results in longer local analgesia.
- Bupivacaine (Marcaine®)—Longer onset of action but much longer duration of action than lidocaine. Often used in combination.

Emergency and Critical Care Drugs

Anesthesia places veterinary patients in a state that approaches death. Being prepared for an emergency in case an animal *crashes*, or *codes*, is a necessity. Every veterinary technician should be familiar with commonly used emergency drugs, what they are used for, and where they are kept. It is wise to have all emergency drugs and supplies that a veterinarian wants readily available and portable. Crash carts or crash boxes can be moved or picked up at a moment's notice. Keep in mind that in an emergency you want to find things fast, so being organized is important. To keep a hospital's crash box uncluttered, consider what is really necessary to keep in it, and then have everything else close at hand. All crash boxes need a quick-reference chart for finding drug doses in a hurry.

Emergency Drugs

Emergency drugs should be administered so that they have the fastest effect. They should be given IV (intravenous), IC (intracardiac), or intratracheal. Intratracheal administration, which is through an endotracheal tube, is viable if an IV is not available and IC is not desired. The respiratory track's mucous membranes will absorb the drugs relatively quickly. Drugs administered intratracheally should be given at double their IV dose, and followed by manual ventilation. The ventilation can help distribute the drug more quickly.

Drugs to Include in a Crash Box

Emergency drugs to have on hand include epinephrine, atropine, lidocaine, corticosteroids, calcium gluconate, doxapram (Dopram®-V), and any reversal agents, such as flumazenil, naloxone, yohimbine, Antisedan®.

Epinephrine (Adrenaline)

Epinephrine, or adrenaline, is known as a sympathomimetic, adrenergic, or catecholamine. It is used to treat cardiopulmonary arrest and anaphylactic reactions or shock. It stimulates alpha and beta receptors. The beta responses are desired in an emergency. Beta-1 receptor stimulation increases heart rate and contractility. Increasing contractility of the cardiac muscle is known as having a positive inotropic effect. This jump-starts the heart for patients in cardiac arrest. Beta-2 receptor stimulation causes dilation of skeletal muscle vessels and bronchi. Dilating the bronchi is desired when treating airway constriction due to a reaction or asthma.

Alpha-1 receptor stimulation causes arteriole vasoconstriction. This helps to stop bleeding from peripheral sites. Alpha-2 receptor stimulation increases skeletal muscle contraction and strength. Epinephrine comes in either a 1:1,000 or a 1:10,000 dilution, so the emergency quick-reference chart must reflect the correct concentration that is being used. It can come with or without lidocaine mixed in. Do *not* use the epinephrine mixed with lidocaine in a crash box. See the section on Local Analgesics for the correct use of the lidocaine and epinephrine combination. Lidocaine and epinephrine should both be kept in the crash box, but they should be in separate bottles, not mixed together.

Atropine

Atropine is an anticholinergic drug that can be used to increase the HR. Atropine does not jump-start the heart the way epinephrine does; instead it prevents the HR from decreasing. It is used when bradycardia is a concern. It is also an antidote for organophosphate (an insecticide) toxicity.

Lidocaine

Lidocaine is given to treat ventricular premature contractions (VPCs). Heart arrhythmias are often due to an irritated, aggravated, hypoxic, or toxic cardiac muscle. If the cardiac muscle can be numbed to the irritation, then VPC arrhythmias can be stopped.

Corticosteroids

Some common examples of corticosteroids found in a crash box include dexamethasone sodium phosphate, dexamethasone solution (Azium®), and Solu-Delta-Cortef® (a form of prednisolone). Any one of these corticosteroids should be included in a crash box because they have anti-inflammatory effects, they can counteract shock, and they help relieve pain. As an added benefit, they give the patient a sense of euphoria, or well-being. Corticosteroids are used in emergencies such as cerebrovascular accidents (cva), spinal vascular accidents (sva), and intervertebral disc rupture. These are more commonly referred to as strokes and herniated discs. A **thromboembolism**, **thrombus**, or **embolus** (these terms are often used synonymously) is a clot or blockage in the blood vessels that causes the vascular accidents.

Calcium Gluconate

Calcium gluconate is a source of calcium for patients with hypocalcemia. It treats eclampsia, which is also known as hypocalcemia, postparturient paresis, milk fever, or postparturient tetani. Early signs of eclampsia in small animals are muscle rigidity and stiff gait. These can progress to seizures and death. The patient's history usually includes a recent parturition and lactation. Calcium is an electrolyte required for correct nerve impulses and muscle contractions, even cardiac muscle. Patients in cardiac arrest can be given calcium gluconate to help heart contractility. Calcium can be given IV and IC, but this must be done slowly since it can cause cardiac arrest. Auscultate the heart for any arrhythmias while giving it. Stop administration if arrhythmias occur. In large animals, such as cows and goats, milk fever signs are weakness, hypothermia, bloat, and constipation.

Doxapram

Doxapram (Dopram®-V) is a CNS stimulant of the brain stem, the primitive part of the brain that controls vital functions such as respiration. This drug stimulates respiration. It can be used to counter apnea during anesthesia. It can be given to newborns following C-section or dystocia to stimulate breathing. It can be administered transgingivally or IV. Transgingival administration is done by placing 1 to 5 drops of the drug under the tongue, where it is absorbed into the bloodstream. Due to its CNS stimulation, doxapram should not be given to seizure patients.

Reversal Agents

If anesthesia or sedation is performed using a reversible drug, include the reversal agent in the crash box. Narcotics such as morphine can have their effects reversed by using naloxone. Alpha-2 agonists such as xylazine and dexdomitor can have their effects reversed by yohimbine and Antisedan®, respectively. An anesthetized patient may need to be reversed immediately if it is too deep, or losing perfusion due to the effects of a reversible drug. Reversing the negative effects may be wanted in an emergency, but keep in mind that the positive effects, like pain relief, will also be reversed.

Drugs to Be Kept Close

The following drugs may not be best suited for a crash box, but they should be readily available in a critical situation:

- **Diazepam (Valium)** is given IV to stop seizures. Since this is a controlled substance, it should not be stored in a crash box. Generally speaking, controlled substances should be stored in a locked and secured cabinet. However, it is acceptable to keep diazepam out of a locked cabinet and readily at hand during normal operating hours at a veterinary practice.
- **Emetics** can be used in cases of toxin ingestion. Some toxins take effect very quickly (for example, ethylene glycol) and vomiting should be induced as soon as possible. Some commonly used emetics include syrup of ipecac, hydrogen peroxide, apomorphine, and xylazine (in cats). Never induce vomiting in a suspected ingestion of a caustic or corrosive agent (this includes most cleaners) because this can damage the esophagus. Never induce vomiting in an unconscious patient because of the risk of aspiration of the stomach contents into the lungs.
- **Activated charcoal** is given orally for adsorption (molecules adhere to it) of ingested toxins. It is available in a powder (to be mixed into a slurry), a premixed slurry, and tablets. Administration must be done after any emetics have lost their effect. The activated charcoal can adsorb to toxins that still remain in the GI tract after emesis.

Other crash box contents that may be included, space permitting, are an assortment of endotracheal tubes, an Ambu® bag, IV catheters, heparin flush, syringes, IV fluids, an infusion set, roll gauze, gauze sponges, tape, and other soft goods. Add only what will be necessary in an emergency situation, and keep the crash box orderly and stocked with currently dated drugs. Many crash boxes are used infrequently and the drugs are typically outdated before they are ever used. No anesthetic emergency is ever planned for, but a prepared veterinary technician can mean the difference between a patient's life and death.

Practice Questions

1. A 44-pound (20 kg) dog is being anesthetized using gas anesthesia. Which size reservoir bag would be the best choice?
   a. 1 L
   b. 2 L
   c. 3 L
   d. 4 L

2. Which of the following is NOT an advantage of using a rebreathing system over a nonrebreathing system for anesthesia?
   a. There is a lower chance of pressure build-up in the breathing tubes.
   b. It provides warmer gases to the patient.
   c. There is less wasted gas.
   d. It provides moister gases to the patient.

3. Which statement about an emetic is correct?
   a. It should be given after giving activated charcoal in order to remove a toxin from the stomach.
   b. It should be given to patient in a coma that occurred after ingestion of ethylene glycol.
   c. It can be useful in emptying the stomach of a recently ingested noncaustic substance.
   d. It is most effective if given preventatively prior to toxin ingestion.

4. An oxygen tank holds 700 L of oxygen. Using an oxygen flow rate of 10 ml/pound/minute and only dogs that weigh 25 pounds, how long will the oxygen last before the tank is completely empty?
   a. 700 hours
   b. 1,200 hours
   c. 1,800 hours
   d. 2,800 hours

5. Which of these is an alpha-2 agonist?
   a. ketamine
   b. morphine
   c. butorphanol
   d. medetomidine

6. When diazepam is mixed with any other drug besides ketamine, what happens?
   a. It becomes toxic.
   b. It precipitates.
   c. It loses effectiveness.
   d. It is considered illegal.

7. What does a pulse oximeter do?
   a. It measures the quantity of oxygen in the blood.
   b. It measures the percent of hemoglobin that is carrying oxygen.
   c. It determines the body's perfusion status.
   d. It provides the patient's heart rate.

8. Which of the following is not in the circle of a rebreathing anesthetic system?
   a. the patient
   b. the manometer
   c. the CO_2 absorbent canister
   d. the scavenging system

9. In cats recovering from anesthesia, when should the endotracheal tube be removed?
   a. when the palpebral reflex returns
   b. when the eye position becomes central
   c. when the swallow reflex returns
   d. when the anesthetic gas is turned off

10. Which of the following has a positive inotropic effect?
   a. dexamethasone
   b. xylazine
   c. epinephrine
   d. lidocaine

11. An indwelling catheter in a vessel being used to measure blood pressure would be
   a. indirect blood pressure monitoring.
   b. central venous pressure monitoring.
   c. venous pressure monitoring.
   d. measured in units of psi.

12. Atropine is kept in a crash cart to treat
   a. epileptic seizures.
   b. hyperkalemia.
   c. a vagal induced bradycardia.
   d. a rapid heartbeat.

13. All of the following are potential effects of using barbiturates *except*
   a. arrhythmias.
   b. analgesia.
   c. cardiac depression.
   d. drug tolerance.

14. Epinephrine increases heart rate and contractility by
   a. stimulating alpha-1 receptors.
   b. stimulating alpha-2 receptors.
   c. stimulating beta-1 receptors.
   d. stimulating beta-2 receptors.

15. Why is Solu-Delta-Cortef® kept in a crash box?
   a. for its anti-inflammatory effect
   b. for its pain relief
   c. to use as a diuretic
   d. for the sense of euphoria

16. Which of the following is true regarding calcium gluconate?
   a. It is used to treat hypercalcemia.
   b. It is used to correct hypoglycemia.
   c. It is used to treat hypokalemia.
   d. It is used to treat eclampsia.

17. An anesthetic gas with a high MAC value requires
   a. a higher flow of oxygen for maintenance level.
   b. a nonprecision vaporizer.
   c. a lower flow of oxygen for maintenance level.
   d. a higher percent gas for maintenance level.

18. Which anesthetic stage and plane best describe a patient that has a corneal reflex, no palpebral reflex, shallow respiration with some abdominal breathing, and an increased CRT?
   a. stage III plane 1
   b. stage III plane 2
   c. stage III plane 3
   d. stage III plane 4

19. Which of the following is an indicator of cardiovascular function in an anesthetized patient?
   a. a peripheral pulse
   b. the jaw tone
   c. respiratory rate and quality
   d. the pedal reflex

20. To maintain general anesthesia, the vaporizer setting should be
   a. kept constant to provide a smooth procedure with no patient movement.
   b. adjusted as needed throughout the procedure to provide the optimum level of anesthesia.
   c. periodically turned to zero to minimize accumulation of anesthetic in the patient's lungs.
   d. set at a level that is calculated based on the animal's weight.

21. Which of the following drugs does NOT typically cause apnea or respiratory depression?
a. propofol
b. ketamine
c. diazepam
d. morphine

22. Which of the following drugs is the most appropriate to administer to a greyhound with a history of seizures?
a. acepromazine
b. propofol
c. ketamine
d. thiopental

23. Induction
a. precedes intubation.
b. follows intubation.
c. requires an endotracheal tube be placed.
d. requires a gas anesthetic.

24. Which of the following preserves the swallow reflex the most when used for general anesthesia?
a. isoflurane
b. ketamine
c. xylazine
d. thiopental

25. A prolonged CRT is indicative of which of the following?
a. hypertension
b. liver problems
c. CNS problems
d. hypovolemia

26. The use of nitrous oxide in veterinary anesthesia
a. increases the amount of inhalant anesthetic agent required.
b. decreases the amount of inhalant anesthetic agent required.
c. can achieve a surgical plane of anesthesia as the sole agent.
d. effectively increases the MAC of the anesthetic agent.

27. Which of the following drugs has an antianxiety effect?
a. ketamine
b. carprofen
c. diazepam
d. telazol

28. If the rebreathing bag remains empty during anesthesia, which of the following would NOT be the cause?
a. The oxygen flow is too low.
b. The oxygen flow is too high.
c. The CO_2 absorbent canister may be leaking.
d. There is a leak in the circle.

29. Which of the following drugs would counteract the vagal effects of applying pressure to the globe of the eye?
a. epinephrine
b. zolazepam
c. glycopyrrolate
d. yohimbine

30. The approximate volume of oxygen in an E tank is
a. 70 L.
b. 660 L.
c. 7,000 L.
d. 2,100 L.

31. A sympathomimetic drug would NOT
  a. dilate bronchi.
  b. increase skeletal muscle contraction.
  c. increase salivation.
  d. increase cardiac muscle contractility.

32. Of the following gases, which one goes through the most metabolization in the body?
  a. nitrous oxide
  b. halothane
  c. sevoflurane
  d. isoflurane

33. Epinephrine with a 1:1,000 concentration contains how many milligrams in each milliliter?
  a. 1.0 mg
  b. 0.01 mg
  c. 0.1 mg
  d. 10 mg

34. Which of the following drugs is used to counteract apnea?
  a. naloxone
  b. dexamethasone
  c. doxapram
  d. Antisedan®

35. Nonrebreathing circuits
  a. do not have a manometer.
  b. can be set up as an open, a closed, or even a semiclosed system.
  c. do not have a reservoir bag.
  d. cannot be used with isoflurane gas anesthetic.

36. At stage II anesthesia,
  a. all reflexes except the swallow or gag reflex are present.
  b. the patient does not have a PLR.
  c. the patient may be vocalizing.
  d. more drugs must be given.

37. Ketamine
  a. provides poor visceral analgesia.
  b. is an inhalant gas anesthetic.
  c. may not be mixed with other drugs in the same syringe.
  d. may not be used in sighthounds.

38. A pressure regulator
  a. controls the amount of anesthetic gas pressure leaving the vaporizer.
  b. is attached between the patient and the anesthetic machine.
  c. controls the pressure in the scavenging system.
  d. can always be found between oxygen tanks and the oxygen flow meter.

39. Soda lime granules
  a. that have not changed color are still effective.
  b. that have changed color are still effective.
  c. absorb water from the breathing circle.
  d. generate heat as a part of the reaction with carbon dioxide.

40. A new drug is being touted as having COX-1 sparing effects, as well as blocking COX-2. Which of the following would be true?
  a. This would be a new opioid with GI tract–sparing effects and analgesic effects.
  b. This would be a new corticosteroid with GI tract–sparing effects and analgesic effects.
  c. This would be a new NSAID with GI tract–sparing effects and analgesic effects.
  d. This would be a new preanesthetic with GI tract–sparing effects and analgesic effects.

41. Suppose that a new gas anesthetic is being marketed. Its water solubility is higher than that of the gas currently being used. The patient anesthetized with this new gas should
a. induce slower and recover faster.
b. induce faster and recover slower.
c. induce faster and recover faster.
d. induce slower and recover slower.

42. A bottle of the combination lidocaine and epinephrine is used
a. for emergencies including VPCs.
b. for local analgesia and hemostasis.
c. for emergencies including cardiac arrest.
d. as a preanesthetic cocktail.

43. An anesthetic gas called X has a MAC of 2.0, while gas Y has a MAC of 2.9. If all else is the same, which of the following is true?
a. X is less potent than Y.
b. The vaporizer setting for X should be set lower, compared with Y, in order to maintain an animal's surgical plane of anesthesia.
c. The ability of X to kill microorganisms is greater than that of Y.
d. X would be less soluble in water when compared to Y.

44. In an anesthetized patient, which of the following reflexes is the last to go?
a. swallow
b. pedal
c. palpebral
d. corneal

45. Which of these drugs should be avoided in a patient that is having a seizure?
a. telazol
b. diazepam
c. propofol
d. phenobarbital

46. A closed anesthetic circuit is
a. part of a nonrebreathing system.
b. an anesthetic machine whose pop-off valve has been closed.
c. a rebreathing system where there is no waste oxygen.
d. a process in which the liver is utilized to metabolize drugs.

47. Which of the following drugs does NOT have analgesic effects?
a. acepromazine
b. domitor
c. butorphanol
d. ketamine

48. Drugs A and B both induce the hepatic enzyme system. Drug A was given to a patient daily for the past three weeks. The veterinarian is now adding drug B. Which would be expected?
a. The total dose of drug B will be increased.
b. The total dose of drug B will not be changed.
c. The total dose of drug B will be decreased.
d. The total dose will be based on the age of the patient.

49. Preanesthetic drugs are NOT given
a. to reduce pain.
b. to prevent hypersalivation.
c. to decrease the amount of maintenance drug.
d. to prevent smooth induction.

50. Barbiturates are highly protein bound. If total protein on preanesthetic blood work is higher than normal, what would you expect?
a. the dose to be increased
b. the dose to be unchanged
c. the dose to be decreased
d. the dose to be based on the patient's age

Answers and Explanations

1. b. Minimum reservoir bag size is six times the animal's tidal volume. Minimum tidal volume is 10 ml/kg. The minimum tidal volume for a 44-pound (20 kg) dog would be 10 ml/kg × 20 kg = 200 ml. 6 × 200 ml = 1200 ml or 1.2 L. Always choose a bag that is a size larger rather than smaller. A significantly larger bag would increase the circle's dead space. Of the choices given, a 2 L bag best meets the criteria.

2. a. Using a rebreathing system *increases* the risk of pressure build-up in the breathing tubes as well as CO_2 build-up. Warmer, moister, and less wasted gases are actual benefits of using a rebreathing system.

3. c. Emetics induce vomiting. They should be given to awake patients with a recent (within a couple of hours) history of ingestion of a noncaustic or corrosive substance. Activated charcoal should be administered orally after all vomiting has subsided to adsorb (adhere) toxins that remain in the GI tract and be eliminated in the feces.

4. d. The rate of oxygen consumed in this question is 10 ml/pound every minute. A dog that weighs 25 pounds uses 250 ml (10 ml/pound × 25 pounds) every minute. Since there are 700 L (700,000 ml), it would take 2,800 hours ($\frac{700,000 \text{ ml}}{250 \text{ ml}} = 2800$) to empty this oxygen tank completely.

5. d. Medetomidine is classified as an alpha-2 agonist. Ketamine is classified as a dissociative anesthetic, while morphine and butorphanol are classified as narcotics.

6. b. Diazepam is commonly mixed with ketamine in the same syringe. However, diazepam should not be mixed with other drugs because solid particles called a precipitate will form. The combination of ketamime and diazepam is neither toxic (when used correctly) nor illegal. Diazepam can lose its effectiveness if it sits in a plastic syringe too long, but that is not related to mixing it with ketamine.

7. b. The pulse oximeter monitors the percentage of hemoglobin that is carrying oxygen. It does not give the amount of oxygen in the blood. A blood sample taken and checked for blood gases will give the amount of oxygen in the blood. The probe of the pulse oximeter is attached peripherally on the animal and provides a pulse rate. This should be the same as the heart rate unless there is a pulse deficit. A pulse oximeter reading can be helpful in judging perfusion, but alone it will not determine the body's perfusion status.

8. d. The circle does not include any waste gases that are not rebreathed. The scavenging system is connected to the pop-off valve and the gases that exit the pop-off valve are waste that never returns to be rebreathed. In order to complete the circle so that air can be rebreathed, the patient must be connected and so is also a part of the circle.

9. c. The swallow reflex is also known as the cough or gag reflex. The endotracheal tube should be removed once this reflex has returned. Removal before the swallow reflex returns leaves a patient vulnerable to aspiration of contents into the lungs. Saliva, water, gastric juices, and mucus can all be present in the back of the mouth upon recovery. When a patient can swallow rather than inhale these, it is safe to remove the endotracheal tube. Brachiocephalic breeds (those with pushed-in faces) may even have their endotracheal tube removed some time after the swallow reflex has returned because they have an airway that is easily plugged. If the endotracheal tube is to be removed some time after the return of the swallow reflex, then special attention should be given to preventing the patient from biting or chewing on the tube. The other three answer choices would occur before the swallow reflex has returned.

10. c. Epinephrine is the only one of the choices that increases the strength of the heart muscle contractions, which is what a positive inotropic drug will do.

11. b. Central venous pressure (CVP) monitoring requires the placement of a catheter in a central vein (jugular or femoral) with the tip near the base of the heart. An indirect BP is usually obtained by either the Doppler method or the use of an oscillometer. Rather than psi, BP is usually measured in units of mmHg (millimeters of mercury) and when doing a CVP the units are cmH$_2$O (centimeters of water). Venous pressure monitoring is not a valid medical procedure.

12. c. Stimulation of the vagal nerve can cause bradycardia. An anticholinergic drug, such as atropine, will have an anti rest, or anti bradycardia, effect.

13. b. Under general anesthesia, barbiturates prevent the brain from perceiving pain, but they do not have analgesic effects. Barbiturates, epinephrine, or a state of hypoxia (which can result from apnea during induction) can result in an arrhythmia called ventricular premature contractions (VPC). Barbiturates depress the heart's rate and contractility. Drugs such as barbiturates induce the hepatic enzyme system to metabolize more rapidly the longer they are given, essentially building up a tolerance to all drugs metabolized by the same enzymes.

14. c. Epinephrine will stimulate all of these receptors, but the beta-1 receptors cause the heart rate and contractility to increase. This is known as a positive inotropic effect.

15. a. Solu-Delta-Cortef® contains a corticosteroid; these are kept in a crash box for their anti-inflammatory effects. Emergency anti-inflammatory drugs will be needed in some cases of anaphylactic reactions, spinal trauma, and head trauma. Corticosteroids can also provide some pain relief, euphoria, and increased urine production. However, better drugs for immediate analgesia and diuresis exist and the effects of euphoria are not of concern in an emergency.

16. d. Calcium gluconate is used for its calcium value. It can be used to treat a low blood calcium level, which is also called hypocalcemia or eclampsia. Hypercalcemia is an elevated blood calcium level. Hypoglycemia is a low blood glucose level. Hypokalemia is a low blood potassium level.

17. d. A higher MAC value means that more anesthetic gas is required in the alveoli to prevent movement when pain is present. Anesthetic gases with higher MAC values are more volatile and require use of a precision vaporizer. The precision vaporizer will have to be set on a higher percentage anesthetic gas to maintain surgical anesthetic depth. The oxygen flow when already adequate will not affect the MAC.

18. c. A review of the stages and planes anesthetic chart shows that stage III plane 3 is what best describes a patient that has a corneal reflex, no palpebral reflex, shallow respiration with some abdominal breathing, and an increased CRT.

19. a. Cardiovascular function can be assessed by checking perfusion. While all of the possible answer choices should be monitored in an anesthetized patient, only the peripheral pulse is used to help judge the patient's perfusion status.

20. b. A goal of gas anesthesia is to have a smooth procedure with no patient movement. This is accomplished by adjusting the vaporizer as needed throughout the procedure, not by keeping it at a constant level, and this cannot be predicted based on the animal's weight. The vaporizer is turned down or to zero in order to decrease anesthetic depth.

21. c. Apnea is the temporary cessation of breathing. Respiratory depression refers to the decreased quality of breaths and the decreased ability to breathe. All the answer choices are drugs known to cause apnea and respiratory depression *except* diazepam.

22. b. Greyhounds are at an increased risk of anesthetic complications when administered barbiturates (such as thiopental). Patients with a history of seizures should not be given acepromazine or ketamine. Of the choices, propofol is the only one not contraindicated for a greyhound with a history of seizures.

23. a. Induction is the period of time where an awake patient is brought to the early stages and planes of anesthesia. This has to be done *before* a patient can be intubated with an endotracheal tube. Induction can be done with a gas anesthetic, but it can also be done using injectable anesthetics.

24. b. A patient's swallow reflex is normally lost during stage III plane 3. Ketamine has the effect of retaining muscle tone and the swallow reflex longer than other induction drugs. Isoflurane, xylazine, and thiopental are similar in that they do not preserve the swallow reflex.

25. d. Capillary refill time (CRT) is delayed when perfusion is poor. Hypovolemia results in poor perfusion. Hypertension (high blood pressure), liver problems, and central nervous system (CNS) problems can lead to a sick animal that is anorectic (does not eat), loses extra fluids (vomiting, increased diuresis), and is dehydrated. Dehydration and hypovolemia are *not* the same thing.

26. b. Through a phenomenon known as the second-gas effect, nitrous oxide will increase the potency of another gas when they are used together. A more potent gas would have a lower MAC value, and means that less inhalant anesthetic agent is needed to achieve a surgical plane of anesthesia.

27. c. Diazepam is the generic name for Valium. Ketamine, carprofen, and telazol do not have antianxiety effects.

28. b. The rebreathing bag (reservoir bag) is part of the circle and can remain empty if there is a leak in the circle or the CO_2 absorbent canister (which is part of the circle too). When the oxygen flow rate is too high the bag will overinflate; conversely, if the oxygen flow rate is too low the bag will collapse.

29. c. Vagal stimulation results in stimulation of the parasympathetic (cholinergic) system. Applying pressure to the globe of the eye can stimulate a vagal response. Glycopyrrolate is an anticholinergic drug and as such will counteract the vagal stimulation. Epinephrine is a sympathomimetic, zolazepam is a benzodiazepine, and yohimbine is a reversal agent for alpha-2 agonists.

30. b. The approximate volume of oxygen in an E tank is 660 L; 660 L is the approximate volume of oxygen in an H tank.

31. c. A sympathomimetic drug will have effects that simulate a fight-or-flight response. A fight-or-flight response would include dilation of the bronchi to increase airflow to the lungs, increase skeletal muscle contraction to increase strength and speed, and increase cardiac muscle contractility to supply more blood to the lungs and the muscles. An increase in salivation occurs for rest and rejuvenation, not for fight or flight.

32. b. Halothane has the smallest MAC. It is the most water soluble and as such spends the most time in the blood, which is mostly water. It circulates through the body many more times than the other, less soluble gases. As halothane circulates through the liver and kidneys the drug is metabolized. Conversely, nitrous oxide, having the highest MAC, is the least water soluble and is blown off or exhaled the most rapidly with the least metabolization.

33. a. Since a 1:100 dilution is equivalent to 1%, a 1:1000 dilution is equivalent to 10 times less or 0.1%. It is easy to convert percentage solutions to milligrams per milliliter: just move the decimal place one to the right, so 0.1 becomes 1.0.

34. c. Doxapram stimulates the CNS's respiratory center and will counteract apnea, which means *without a breath*. Naloxone, dexamethasone, and Antisedan® are drugs that do not stimulate respiration.

35. a. Nonrebreathing systems do not have a manometer, which measures pressure within the breathing circuit, because the pressure should not increase in a properly set up nonrebreathing system. The terms *open*, *closed*, and *semiclosed* refer to the operation of a rebreathing system. Regardless of the anesthetic system, isoflurane can be used and a reservoir bag will be necessary.

36. c. Stage II anesthesia is known as the excitement stage, and the semiconscious patient may be crying, whimpering, or howling, as well as moving. All reflexes are present in stage II. While stage II is not the depth desired for anesthesia, more drugs may not be needed. The patient enters stage II on recovery, and if the patient is recovering, more drugs would only deepen the anesthesia. Also, several induction agents (barbiturates, for example) require some time to distribute from the blood into the surrounding tissues and to cross the blood–brain barrier. Time should be allowed before administering more drugs to see what depth the patient goes to after the drug has been redistributed.

37. a. Ketamine is an injectable anesthetic that is typically mixed with sedatives to counter its cataleptic (muscle rigidity) effects. While providing good somatic analgesia, visceral analgesia is poor. Ketamine may be used in sighthounds; in fact, it may be used in more animal species than any other anesthetic drug.

38. d. The pressure regulator prevents the high pressures within a tank of gas from entering the anesthetic machine at the flow meter. For oxygen, the pressure regulator limits the pressure entering the flow meter to 50 psi. There is nothing that controls the amount of anesthetic gas pressure leaving the vaporizer: the pressure that enters is what leaves the vaporizer. Breathing tubes or a breathing system would be found between the patient and the anesthetic machine. There is nothing that controls the pressure in the scavenging system, and there is no need to.

39. d. The effectiveness of soda lime granules should not be judged on color changes alone. As carbon dioxide is absorbed by soda lime, a chemical reaction occurs that produces heat and water.

40. c. NSAIDs are the class of drugs that affect enzymes COX-1 and COX-2. Newer NSAIDs attempt to block the effects of COX-2 and to leave COX-1 alone. Blocking COX-2 would block production of the prostaglandins that lead to inflammation and pain. Sparing COX-2 will allow the production of the prostaglandins that help protect the stomach lining and platelet function.

41. d. The patient would induce slower and recover slower because the gas would stay in the blood (water) longer before it would cross the blood–brain barrier (which is more lipophilic, or fat soluble) and before being exchanged from the blood to the lungs to be exhaled.

42. b. Lidocaine and epinephrine can be purchased separately or combined in a single bottle. Combined in a single bottle, they are used to provide local analgesia and hemorrhage control when injected around a surgical site. Individually, lidocaine and epinephrine are used in emergency situations for VPCs and cardiac arrest, respectively.

43. b. The lower the MAC value the more potent and more water soluble it is, so gas *X* is more potent and more water soluble than gas *Y*. A similar acronym, MIC (minimum inhibitory concentration), is used to determine an antibiotic's ability to kill microorganisms.

44. d. The reflexes in an anesthetized patient are lost in the order in which the answer choices for this question are listed, with the corneal reflex being the last one to go.

45. d. Diazepam and barbiturates are actually used to prevent seizures. Telazol contains tiletamine, a dissociative anesthetic which, like ketamine, can cause seizures in patients that are prone to this condition. Propofol is not known to cause seizures.

46. c. A closed anesthetic circuit is one of three ways to operate a rebreathing circuit. The fresh gas flow (oxygen and inhalant gas) matches the gas consumption of the patient so that there is no unused or wasted fresh gas. A closed or open anesthetic circuit (the other two ways to operate a rebreathing circuit) are not related to the pop-off valve's position as closed or open. The hepatic enzyme system is a process by which the liver is utilized to metabolize drugs.

47. a. Acepromazine, as well as all phenothiazine derivatives, do not provide pain relief. The other selections do provide pain relief for the patient.

48. a. Drug A increases the metabolism of itself and other drugs that are metabolized by the same hepatic enzyme system. Essentially, a tolerance is built up to these drugs. All else being the same, it would take more of drug B to have the same effect.

49. d. Preanesthetic drugs are used for a number of reasons, but preventing a smooth induction is *not* one of them. A smooth induction of anesthesia through stage II excitement can be accomplished by using injectable sedatives (acepromazine). Other preanesthetics can be used to prevent increased salivation (atropine) that can obscure or occlude the airway, reduce pain (xylazine), and decrease the amount of maintenance drug (morphine).

50. a. The more protein molecules in the blood that bind or hold on to a drug, the less free drug there is to cross the blood–brain barrier. More drug would need to be given to have the same effect.

12 ▶ PRACTICE TEST

CHAPTER OVERVIEW

Take this practice test after making your way through all the review chapters in this book. Like the Diagnostic Test, the following exam is based on actual veterinary technician exams commonly used today. Another practice exam is available online. Of course, none of these questions and answers are reproduced from the actual VTNE, which are kept secret, but this test has been formatted much as the national exam is.

Please use the answer sheet on page 379. Once you have completed the test in the allotted time, go to the Answers and Explanations at the end of the test and count the number of questions you answered correctly. Make note of the questions you answered incorrectly; you will want to concentrate any further review on those subjects.

1.	ⓐ	ⓑ	ⓒ	ⓓ	35.	ⓐ	ⓑ	ⓒ	ⓓ	69.	ⓐ	ⓑ	ⓒ	ⓓ
2.	ⓐ	ⓑ	ⓒ	ⓓ	36.	ⓐ	ⓑ	ⓒ	ⓓ	70.	ⓐ	ⓑ	ⓒ	ⓓ
3.	ⓐ	ⓑ	ⓒ	ⓓ	37.	ⓐ	ⓑ	ⓒ	ⓓ	71.	ⓐ	ⓑ	ⓒ	ⓓ
4.	ⓐ	ⓑ	ⓒ	ⓓ	38.	ⓐ	ⓑ	ⓒ	ⓓ	72.	ⓐ	ⓑ	ⓒ	ⓓ
5.	ⓐ	ⓑ	ⓒ	ⓓ	39.	ⓐ	ⓑ	ⓒ	ⓓ	73.	ⓐ	ⓑ	ⓒ	ⓓ
6.	ⓐ	ⓑ	ⓒ	ⓓ	40.	ⓐ	ⓑ	ⓒ	ⓓ	74.	ⓐ	ⓑ	ⓒ	ⓓ
7.	ⓐ	ⓑ	ⓒ	ⓓ	41.	ⓐ	ⓑ	ⓒ	ⓓ	75.	ⓐ	ⓑ	ⓒ	ⓓ
8.	ⓐ	ⓑ	ⓒ	ⓓ	42.	ⓐ	ⓑ	ⓒ	ⓓ	76.	ⓐ	ⓑ	ⓒ	ⓓ
9.	ⓐ	ⓑ	ⓒ	ⓓ	43.	ⓐ	ⓑ	ⓒ	ⓓ	77.	ⓐ	ⓑ	ⓒ	ⓓ
10.	ⓐ	ⓑ	ⓒ	ⓓ	44.	ⓐ	ⓑ	ⓒ	ⓓ	78.	ⓐ	ⓑ	ⓒ	ⓓ
11.	ⓐ	ⓑ	ⓒ	ⓓ	45.	ⓐ	ⓑ	ⓒ	ⓓ	79.	ⓐ	ⓑ	ⓒ	ⓓ
12.	ⓐ	ⓑ	ⓒ	ⓓ	46.	ⓐ	ⓑ	ⓒ	ⓓ	80.	ⓐ	ⓑ	ⓒ	ⓓ
13.	ⓐ	ⓑ	ⓒ	ⓓ	47.	ⓐ	ⓑ	ⓒ	ⓓ	81.	ⓐ	ⓑ	ⓒ	ⓓ
14.	ⓐ	ⓑ	ⓒ	ⓓ	48.	ⓐ	ⓑ	ⓒ	ⓓ	82.	ⓐ	ⓑ	ⓒ	ⓓ
15.	ⓐ	ⓑ	ⓒ	ⓓ	49.	ⓐ	ⓑ	ⓒ	ⓓ	83.	ⓐ	ⓑ	ⓒ	ⓓ
16.	ⓐ	ⓑ	ⓒ	ⓓ	50.	ⓐ	ⓑ	ⓒ	ⓓ	84.	ⓐ	ⓑ	ⓒ	ⓓ
17.	ⓐ	ⓑ	ⓒ	ⓓ	51.	ⓐ	ⓑ	ⓒ	ⓓ	85.	ⓐ	ⓑ	ⓒ	ⓓ
18.	ⓐ	ⓑ	ⓒ	ⓓ	52.	ⓐ	ⓑ	ⓒ	ⓓ	86.	ⓐ	ⓑ	ⓒ	ⓓ
19.	ⓐ	ⓑ	ⓒ	ⓓ	53.	ⓐ	ⓑ	ⓒ	ⓓ	87.	ⓐ	ⓑ	ⓒ	ⓓ
20.	ⓐ	ⓑ	ⓒ	ⓓ	54.	ⓐ	ⓑ	ⓒ	ⓓ	88.	ⓐ	ⓑ	ⓒ	ⓓ
21.	ⓐ	ⓑ	ⓒ	ⓓ	55.	ⓐ	ⓑ	ⓒ	ⓓ	89.	ⓐ	ⓑ	ⓒ	ⓓ
22.	ⓐ	ⓑ	ⓒ	ⓓ	56.	ⓐ	ⓑ	ⓒ	ⓓ	90.	ⓐ	ⓑ	ⓒ	ⓓ
23.	ⓐ	ⓑ	ⓒ	ⓓ	57.	ⓐ	ⓑ	ⓒ	ⓓ	91.	ⓐ	ⓑ	ⓒ	ⓓ
24.	ⓐ	ⓑ	ⓒ	ⓓ	58.	ⓐ	ⓑ	ⓒ	ⓓ	92.	ⓐ	ⓑ	ⓒ	ⓓ
25.	ⓐ	ⓑ	ⓒ	ⓓ	59.	ⓐ	ⓑ	ⓒ	ⓓ	93.	ⓐ	ⓑ	ⓒ	ⓓ
26.	ⓐ	ⓑ	ⓒ	ⓓ	60.	ⓐ	ⓑ	ⓒ	ⓓ	94.	ⓐ	ⓑ	ⓒ	ⓓ
27.	ⓐ	ⓑ	ⓒ	ⓓ	61.	ⓐ	ⓑ	ⓒ	ⓓ	95.	ⓐ	ⓑ	ⓒ	ⓓ
28.	ⓐ	ⓑ	ⓒ	ⓓ	62.	ⓐ	ⓑ	ⓒ	ⓓ	96.	ⓐ	ⓑ	ⓒ	ⓓ
29.	ⓐ	ⓑ	ⓒ	ⓓ	63.	ⓐ	ⓑ	ⓒ	ⓓ	97.	ⓐ	ⓑ	ⓒ	ⓓ
30.	ⓐ	ⓑ	ⓒ	ⓓ	64.	ⓐ	ⓑ	ⓒ	ⓓ	98.	ⓐ	ⓑ	ⓒ	ⓓ
31.	ⓐ	ⓑ	ⓒ	ⓓ	65.	ⓐ	ⓑ	ⓒ	ⓓ	99.	ⓐ	ⓑ	ⓒ	ⓓ
32.	ⓐ	ⓑ	ⓒ	ⓓ	66.	ⓐ	ⓑ	ⓒ	ⓓ	100.	ⓐ	ⓑ	ⓒ	ⓓ
33.	ⓐ	ⓑ	ⓒ	ⓓ	67.	ⓐ	ⓑ	ⓒ	ⓓ					
34.	ⓐ	ⓑ	ⓒ	ⓓ	68.	ⓐ	ⓑ	ⓒ	ⓓ					

Practice Questions

Pharmacology

1. Which of the following is NOT a side effect of ketoconazole?
   a. vomiting
   b. cartilage damage in growing dogs
   c. birth defects
   d. liver toxicity

2. Bacterial pneumonia in dogs
   a. is treated with glucocorticoids and cough suppressants.
   b. will be cured with no treatment except time.
   c. is treated with antibiotics, bronchodilators, and coupage (chest percussions).
   d. has clinical signs of nonproductive, goose honk cough, and normal appetite and attitude.

3. Which of the following drugs and routes are used to treat allergic bronchitis in cats?
   a. oral cough suppressants
   b. inhaled glucocorticoids
   c. oral antibiotics
   d. inhaled mucolytics

4. Which of the following heartworm preventatives is NOT used in cats?
   a. ivermectin (Heartgard®)
   b. milbemycin (Interceptor®)
   c. moxidectin (ProHeart®)
   d. selamectin (Revolution®)

5. Nitroglycerin
   a. is administered PO or IV.
   b. causes dilation of the veins and coronary arteries.
   c. must be handled with gloves because it is explosive.
   d. is used for maintenance therapy of heart failure in cats.

6. Safety precautions that owners of chemotherapy patients should take at home include
   a. wearing a gown and a face shield when interacting with the pet.
   b. wearing gloves when cleaning up feces, urine, or vomit.
   c. never flushing the pet's feces or vomit down the toilet.
   d. allowing soiled bedding to sit for 48 hours to decontaminate before washing.

7. Which is NOT a common side effect caused by many chemotherapy drugs?
   a. pancreatitis
   b. bone marrow suppression
   c. hypercalcemia
   d. All of the above are common side effects.

8. Which chemotherapy drug should *never* be used in cats?
   a. vincristine
   b. chlorambucil
   c. cisplatin
   d. l-asparaginase

9. Chemotherapy safety precautions in the clinic include
   a. preparing drugs in a high-traffic area of the clinic.
   b. keeping negative pressure in drug vials to decrease risk of aerosolization.
   c. administering chemotherapy drugs in the lunchroom to stay out of the way.
   d. wearing only gloves when handling chemotherapy drugs.

10. What is prostaglandin F2α used for?
    a. pregnancy termination
    b. estrus suppression
    c. open-cervix pyometra treatment
    d. both **a** and **c**

11. The mismating shot, ECP (estradiol cypi-
onate),
   a. is an injection of GnRH to prevent
      pregnancy.
   b. can cause fatal bone marrow suppression.
   c. is the preferred treatment for estrus
      suppression.
   d. is not effective until day 25 to 35.

12. What is pyometra best treated with?
   a. megesterol acetate (Ovaban®)
   b. mibolerone (cheque drops)
   c. ovariohysterectomy
   d. oxytocin

13. Which of the following is NOT a side effect of
bronchodilator use?
   a. excitability
   b. cardiac arrhythmias
   c. anorexia
   d. excessive salivation

14. Which of the following antibiotics may result
in blindness in cats?
   a. amoxicillin
   b. enrofloxacin
   c. cefazolin
   d. metronidazole

Surgical Preparation and Assisting

15. Which of the following is a synthetic,
absorbable, braided suture material?
   a. chromic gut
   b. polypropylene (Prolene®)
   c. polyglyconate (Maxon®)
   d. polyglactin (Vicryl®)

16. Which of the following is NOT a method of
onychectomy in a cat?
   a. guillotine clippers
   b. sharp dissection
   c. tenectomy
   d. laser

17. What is NOT an advantage of using a
monofilament suture material?
   a. decreased tissue drag
   b. decreased inflammatory reaction
   c. decreased chance of wicking of bacteria
   d. most can be used externally

18. Which of the following is *false* about OHE in
the dog?
   a. Animals spayed at any time in their life are
      less likely to develop mammary cancers.
   b. The shaved area should be adequate to
      ensure that no hair gets into the aseptic
      field.
   c. Incisions are usually made through an
      aponeurosis.
   d. Placing a suture or a hemostatic clamp
      around a vessel or the uterine stump is
      called ligation.

19. Which of the following is NOT an advantage of
orchidectomy?
   a. birth control
   b. prevention of testicular cancers
   c. teatment of prostate cancer
   d. treatment of perianal adenomas

20. Which of the following is NOT contained
within the vaginal tunics?
   a. the ovary
   b. the artery
   c. the pampiniform plexus
   d. the gubernaculums

21. Which of the following does NOT have retractable claws?
   a. the housecat
   b. the cheetah
   c. the lion
   d. the leopard

22. Which of the following is true of regional anesthesia?
   a. It reduces postoperative pain by preventing wind-up.
   b. Ring blocks for onychectomy should be performed at the elbow.
   c. Regional anesthesia should only be performed by the veterinarian.
   d. Surgery may be performed immediately after placement of regional anesthesia.

23. Which of the following is NOT a potential complication of general anesthesia in large animals?
   a. bloat in horses
   b. malignant hyperthermia in pigs
   c. myositis or myoglobinuria
   d. All of the above are potential complications.

24. Which of the following mechanisms of sterilization works by conduction?
   a. plasma
   b. steam
   c. direct heat
   d. cold sterilization

25. Which of the following should NOT be put in a steam autoclave?
   a. cotton muslin
   b. plastic
   c. metal
   d. glass

26. Which sterilization method requires the *least* amount of time?
   a. plasma
   b. steam
   c. direct heat
   d. cold sterilization

27. How often should an animal be monitored (TPR, mm color) during recovery?
   a. every minute
   b. every 5 minutes
   c. every 15 minutes
   d. every 30 minutes

28. Which of the following animals has complete tracheal rings?
   a. the monitor lizard
   b. the hedgehog
   c. the rat
   d. the dog

29. Which of the following is true regarding surgical clipping?
   a. You should use a #40 blade for surgical clipping.
   b. You should clip only an area large enough for the doctor to see the surgical site because appearances are important to the client.
   c. You should clip against the grain of the hair first, then with the grain second.
   d. You should use a powerful vacuum to remove the clipped hair from the skin after clipping.

30. Which of the following would NOT be a good method of scrubbing for surgery?
   a. alternating scrubs of chlorhexidine and isopropyl alcohol
   b. alternating scrubs of povidone iodine and isopropyl alcohol
   c. alternating scrubs of povidone iodine and sterile saline or water
   d. alternating scrubs of chlorhexidine and sterile saline or water

Dentistry

31. Which of the following is a periodontal instrument?
   a. a curette
   b. a Kerr file
   c. an elevator
   d. gutta percha

32. Which of the following is the correct dental formula for an adult cat?
   a. $I_3^3 \, C_1^1 \, P_2^3 \, M_1^1$
   b. $i_3^3 \, c_1^1 \, p_2^3$
   c. $I_3^3 \, C_1^1 \, P_4^4 \, M_3^2$
   d. $i_3^3 \, c_1^1 \, p_4^4$

33. Which of the following substances is the covering of the tooth below the gumline?
   a. the enamel
   b. the dentin
   c. the cementum
   d. the alveolar bone

34. When extracting the tooth, which structure must be disrupted?
   a. the gingiva
   b. the periodontal ligament
   c. the alveolar bone
   d. the cementum

35. How long does it take for tartar to form on the tooth?
   a. immediately after a meal
   b. 1 hour after a meal
   c. within 24 hours
   d. within 48 hours

36. Which of the following anaerobic bacteria has been implicated as a cause of periodontal disease in dogs?
   a. *Pseudomonas*
   b. *Porphyromonas gulae*
   c. *Aeromonas*
   d. *Clostridium*

37. Which of the following is *false* about ultrasonic scalers?
   a. They kill bacteria and remove plaque by a process called cavitation.
   b. Aerosolization of bacteria by ultrasonic scalers can lead to eye infections in veterinary technicians.
   c. Most ultrasonic scalers may be used above and below the gumline with care.
   d. Contact with the tooth surface may be maintained up to 45 seconds.

38. The extraoral approach is often necessary for the treatment of tooth root abscesses in which of the following species?
   a. canine
   b. feline
   c. murine (mouse)
   d. equine

Laboratory Procedures

39. A cat has hematuria, increased neutrophils, and large numbers of well-developed, coffin-lid shaped, clear crystals in the urine. Plain radiographs showed 3 small, radiodense stones in the bladder. Which of the following is true?
   a. The pH of the urine is acidic.
   b. The pH of the urine is basic.
   c. The stones are calcium oxalate.
   d. The stones are uric acid.

40. A dog has hyperpigmentation, obesity, alopecia, lethargy, and decreased activity level. Which of the following is the *least* likely laboratory test result for this patient?
   a. increased T_4 levels
   b. increased blood glucose
   c. decreased Na:K ratio
   d. elevated cortisol levels

41. A cat presents for monitoring of diabetes. He is under good control with insulin use. His last test was 3 months ago. Which of the following would be the best method of assessing the effectiveness of his insulin therapy?
   a. glucose tolerance test
   b. fructosamine level
   c. glycosylated hemoglobin level
   d. glucose curve

42. A vomiting dog presents at the clinic. His fecal was negative for parasites, but muscle fibers were seen in the stool. Which of the following would NOT be an important test for this dog?
   a. pancreatic lipase immunoreactivity
   b. trypsinlike immunoreactivity
   c. cobalamin and folate
   d. blood glucose

43. Which of the following electrolytes depends on the albumin concentrations?
   a. calcium
   b. phosphorus
   c. sodium
   d. bicarbonate

44. An animal comes into the clinic with elevated AST, ALT, and CPK levels. The other chemistry levels were normal. Which of the following is true?
   a. The animal most likely has kidney disease.
   b. The animal most likely has liver disease.
   c. The animal most likely has muscle disease.
   d. None of the above.

45. A cow presents with jaundice. Which of the following is NOT a possible immediate cause of jaundice in a cow?
   a. *Babesia*
   b. extravascular hemolysis
   c. intravascular hemolysis
   d. *Fasciola*

46. A miniature schnauzer puppy presents with postprandial seizures and lethargy due to portosystemic shunt. Which of the following would NOT be a common finding for this puppy?
   a. low blood glucose
   b. high serum bile acid levels
   c. normal bilirubin levels
   d. normal ammonia levels

47. A dog presents with edema. His total protein level is 3 g/dl. His urine protein is 100+ on the dipstick. His urine SG is 1.020. The sediment is negative for cells and casts. Which of the following is *false*?
   a. He has tubular disease.
   b. He has proteinuria.
   c. He has hypoalbuminemia.
   d. His BUN and Cr levels will be normal.

48. A rabbit has a bladder stone. Which of the following is the most likely?
   a. calcium oxalate
   b. struvite
   c. calcium carbonate
   d. ammonium urate

49. A rabbit has ear mites. Which of the following is the most likely?
   a. *Otodectes*
   b. *Cheylettiella*
   c. *Notoedres*
   d. *Psoroptes*

50. Which of the following parasites will NOT result in blood in the stool?
   a. *Physaloptera*
   b. *Uncinaria*
   c. *Haemonchus*
   d. *Dioctophema*

51. Which of the following parasites CANNOT be transmitted by the ingestion of earthworms?
   a. *Dioctophema*
   b. *Heterakis*
   c. *Paragonimus*
   d. *Aelurostrongylus*

52. What is the occult test for canine heartworm disease?
   a. a direct ELISA test
   b. an indirect ELISA test
   c. a filter test
   d. the modified Knott's test

53. A dog presents with cutaneous nodules. Biopsy shows small protozoal organisms in the macrophages of the skin. Which of the following is *false*?
   a. This dog has probably been in Mexico or South America.
   b. The vector for this disease is a tick.
   c. This is probably leishmaniasis.
   d. The form in the macrophages is called the amastigote stage.

Animal Care and Nursing

54. Smelly is a 6-week-old Rottweiler puppy that presented for vomiting and diarrhea of 2 days' duration. His temperature is 103.4. The diarrhea has a very fetid odor and is bloody. He has a low WBC count with a lymphopenia. What does Smelly have?
   a. parvovirus
   b. coronavirus
   c. giardia
   d. hookworms

55. Beauregard is a 5-year-old unvaccinated harrier that presented for strange seizure activity 2 days ago. He stares off into space and looks like he is chewing gum. A few months ago, according to his owner, he had a pretty severe cold that she thinks he caught from the neighbor's new puppy. The puppy had a really bad cold and then started biting the kids, so the owners had him put to sleep. What was a possible cause of Beauregard's problem?
   a. distemper
   b. rabies
   c. parvovirus
   d. lungworm

56. How are tuberculosis tests performed?
   a. IV
   b. SQ
   c. ID
   d. IP

57. Sally is a spayed female vaccinated DSH on vacation from Arizona. At home she is free roaming. The owners have a house overlooking a prairie dog colony. Sally started having a fever a few days ago and has large swellings of the submandibular lymph nodes. What is a likely cause of Sally's symptoms?

   a. lymphoma
   b. *Yersinia pestis*
   c. *Yersinia enterocolitica*
   d. *Ehrlichia*

58. Which of the following is NOT an indication of hypoxia?

   a. dyspnea
   b. cyanosis
   c. low heart rate
   d. open-mouth breathing

59. Calvin is a 7-year-old unneutered male black-and-tan coonhound. He is a show dog and is highly sought after as a stud. He has recently been having trouble walking and has been running a fairly high fever. On physical exam he is relatively normal except for pain on palpation of the testicles. What is Calvin's problem?

   a. rabies
   b. *Yersinia pestis*
   c. brucellosis
   d. Lyme disease

60. Which of the following is *false* regarding IV fluid administration?

   a. A catheter that has been in for 12 hours should be changed.
   b. Administration sets should be changed every 48 hours.
   c. Catheters should be flushed with heparinized saline.
   d. Maintenance fluid rates are calculated by % dehydration × BW(kg) × 1000

61. Rita is a 2-year-old briard that has just had her first litter. Unfortunately, she has already lost 4 of the original 8 pups. The pups looked fine initially and were suckling but died acutely with distended, black abdomens. Rita's kennelmates just got back from the National Briard Specialty show 2 weeks ago. They had mild conjunctivitis and runny noses, but Rita never showed any symptoms. What did the pups die of?

   a. canine herpesvirus
   b. mycoplasma
   c. *Bordetella bronchiseptica*
   d. brucellosis

62. Surgical fluid rates are

   a. 40 to 60 ml/kg/hr.
   b. 100 ml/kg/hr.
   c. 10 ml/kg/hr.
   d. given at twice maintenance to prevent shock.

63. Fluffy, a 12-year-old unvaccinated Persian cat, comes into your clinic. She has always been an indoor cat with no exposure to the outside (including the patio). Her owner found a kitten 10 to 14 days prior with a mild cold wandering around outside her house and brought it inside the house. She brought it to the Humane Society the next day. Fluffy liked the kitten and sniffed it a few times. Fluffy is now running a fever (104.5), is sneezing, has mild ocular discharge, and is not eating. Which of the following is NOT a possible cause of Fluffy's problem?

   a. rhinotracheitis
   b. calici
   c. panleukopenia
   d. feline leukemia

64. Which of the following is NOT a factor in calculating the energy requirements of an animal?
a. breed
b. activity status
c. reproductive status
d. whether it is herbivore or carnivore

65. On physical exam you notice that Precious has ulcerations of her tongue and palate and is drooling. She has mild epiphora (tear production) in the left eye. Fluorescein staining tests are negative, but there is blockage of the left nasolacrimal duct. She is a Persian. What would be the most likely cause of Fluffy's problem (ulcerations, fever, ocular discharge, sneezing)?
a. rhinotracheitis
b. calici
c. panleukopenia
d. feline leukemia

66. Which of the following fatty acids is essential in the dog?
a. stearic acid
b. linolenic acid
c. arachidonic acid
d. oleic acid

67. You know that most upper respiratory tract infections in cats can be easily prevented. Which of the following is NOT a good method of preventing upper respiratory tract infections in cats?
a. quarantine
b. disinfection
c. vaccination
d. antibiotics

68. Jones, an 11-year-old unneutered male DSH, arrives at the clinic. He has received his kitten series (FVRCP and RV) and yearly boosters. He has an abscess on his left rear leg and multiple healed scars all over his body. Which SNAP test will probably come up positive?
a. FeLV
b. parvovirus
c. FIV
d. giardia

69. Hogdog Ellis presents at your clinic because he just "isn't runnin' them hogs like he should be, Doc." The situation started yesterday. He had been on a 4-day hunting trip 10 days prior and he ran very well. The owner noticed the dog has been very droopy and his urine has been dark. On presentation, Ellis' temp was 104.5, P and R very elevated. His abdomen was painful on palpation as was his thoracolumbar and midlumbar spine. He has dark, reddish-brown urine. What disease should be high on his list of differentials?
a. brucellosis
b. distemper
c. leptospirosis
d. bladder stones

70. Houdini Masters is a 2-year-old intact male Jack Russell. He escaped (yet again) 7 days ago and ran down to his girlfriend's house 3 blocks over. He is fully vaccinated. His canine girlfriend just came down with parvovirus and is currently hospitalized. Which of the following is true?
a. The parvovirus vaccine is effective if given as directed, and he should be protected.
b. He should be placed in full quarantine.
c. He may go to obedience classes.
d. He should be revaccinated.

71. Which of the following is true about handling horses?
   a. They should always be approached either from directly in front or from directly behind.
   b. The horse should be haltered on the right side of the head.
   c. Horses can kick 6 to 8 feet behind themselves.
   d. Foals should be separated from the dam by placing your body between the animals.

72. How should rodents be restrained?
   a. Rats should be carried by the tail.
   b. Rats do well with a chair hold.
   c. Guinea pigs should be scruffed.
   d. Hamsters should be picked up by the tail.

73. Which amino acid is essential in a cat's diet to prevent cardiomyopathy and blindness?
   a. methionine
   b. cysteine
   c. taurine
   d. proline

74. A dyspneic cat, a collie with blunt leg trauma, a hog dog oozing blood from a shoulder wound, and a dog with impacted anal glands are in the waiting room. Which animal do you see first?
   a. the cat
   b. the collie
   c. the hog dog
   d. the anal gland dog

75. Which of the following is a cause of seizures in cattle?
   a. hypocalcemia
   b. hypomagnesemia
   c. hypokalemia
   d. both **a** and **b**

76. Which of the following is NOT a cause of shipping fever in cattle?
   a. IBR
   b. parainfluenza
   c. BRSV
   d. COPD

77. Which of the following is a cause of lymph node enlargement in horses?
   a. *Ehrlichia*
   b. *Streptococcus equi*
   c. West Nile virus
   d. tetanus

Diagnostic Imaging

78. Which of the following would NOT be included in a met check?
   a. right lateral thorax
   b. left lateral thorax
   c. VD or DV thorax
   d. right lateral abdomen

79. What is the imaging plate in digital radiography equivalent to?
   a. slow speed screen and film
   b. medium speed screen and film
   c. high speed screen and film
   d. nonscreen film

80. A dog has chronic nasal discharge. Which of the following techniques will yield the *least* diagnostic radiographs for nasal cavity and sinuses?
   a. open mouth tympanic bulla
   b. frontal or skyline
   c. open mouth VD skull
   d. lateral skull

81. Which of the following views of the cervical spine is potentially dangerous in small-breed dogs with a hypoplastic dens?
a. lateral
b. VD
c. flexed lateral
d. none of the above

82. Which of the following stifle views is the *least* desirable for assessing the stifle because it causes magnification?
a. lateral
b. craniocaudal (AP)
c. caudocranial (PA)
d. flexed lateral

83. Which of the following is *false*?
a. PennHIP should be used for evaluation of hip dysplasia in animals under 1 year of age.
b. PennHIP uses a measurement called the *distraction index* to evaluate joint laxity.
c. PennHIP can be performed without anesthesia.
d. PennHIP measures the ability of the hip joint to be luxated.

84. Which of the following may be used for myelography?
a. organic iodides
b. barium sulfate
c. air
d. none of the above

85. Which of the following allows adjustment of the speed of x-rays produced by the tube?
a. the kVp
b. the mA
c. the mAs
d. time

Anesthesia and Analgesia

86. Which of the following is true of butorphanol?
a. It is an opioid agonist.
b. It is more effective for somatic pain than for visceral pain.
c. It is long lasting.
d. Giving more of the drug will not increase its effect.

87. Which of the following is most effective for visceral analgesia?
a. ketamine
b. butorphanol
c. morphine
d. NSAIDs

88. Which of the following causes muscle rigidity and can cause seizures?
a. ketamine
b. butorphanol
c. morphine
d. propofol

89. Which of the following preanesthetics should NOT be used in seizure-prone animals?
a. glycopyrrolate
b. diazepam
c. acepromazine
d. atropine

90. Which of the following drugs is reversible with yohimbine?
a. xylazine
b. medetomadine
c. fentanyl
d. ketamine

91. Which of the following drugs is NOT metabolized in the liver?
  a. pentobarbital or pentothal
  b. ketamine
  c. diazepam
  d. medazolam

92. Which of the following is true about MAC?
  a. It refers to the volatility of the gas.
  b. It refers to the flammability of the gas.
  c. Anesthetized patients are maintained at 1.5 to 2× the MAC of the gas.
  d. The higher the MAC, the lower the percentage should be maintained on the gas gauge.

93. Malignant hyperthermia is a possible complication with which anesthetic gas?
  a. halothane
  b. isoflurane
  c. sevoflurane
  d. methoxyflurane

94. An N_2O tank pressure valve says that the tank is full. You are prepping for an orthopedic procedure that will probably require 4 hours. Which of the following is true?
  a. It is a full tank.
  b. The tank should be weighed to determine the quantity of N_2O present.
  c. The tank may be empty.
  d. You should go on with the surgery as planned using the tank.

95. The O_2 tank pressure valve says 1800 psi on an E tank. You are on a closed-circuit system and your O_2 delivery will be 1 L/minute. Your surgery should take 4 hours. Which of the following is true?
  a. You should change out your tank immediately.
  b. You should have plenty of O_2 for this procedure, plus another one of equal length.
  c. You will have just enough O_2 for the procedure.
  d. You will have enough O_2 for the procedure, but you will have to be careful not to hit the flush valve too frequently.

96. You have a faulty pressure regulator valve and no other anesthesia machine in the hospital. Which of the following is true?
  a. The anesthesia machine has to be repaired or replaced before you perform another surgical procedure.
  b. You should be very careful about your oxygen flow rate during surgery.
  c. You should keep your pop-off valve open during surgery.
  d. You should only use a nonrebreather.

97. Which of the following is true regarding vaporizers?
  a. They should be filled while the animal is connected to the vaporizer.
  b. Nonprecision vaporizers will always have the same readings regardless of environmental conditions.
  c. Precision vaporizers are generally used for the newer gases such as halothane, sevoflurane, and isoflurane.
  d. Overfilling the vaporizer will not cause damage if it is immediately drained.

98. IPPV, or assisted breathing,
   a. increases CO_2 levels in the animal during anesthesia.
   b. should be performed at a rate of 1 sigh breath per 10 seconds to maintain adequate oxygen rates.
   c. will maintain normal tidal volumes in the patient.
   d. should never be at a pressure greater than 20 cmH_2O on the manometer.

99. When using a closed circuit,
   a. the pop-off valve should remain in the open position.
   b. the oxygen flow rate should be 10 ml/kg/min.
   c. the pressures and breathing resistance are lower than in a nonrebreathing system.
   d. temperature and humidity are maintained.

100. Which of the following is Stage III plane IV of anesthesia?
   a. no reflexes, no PLR, pupils central, HR <60 bpm, pulse weak or absent, >2 sec CRT
   b. no reflexes, PLR present but sluggish, pupil beginning to appear, HR <60, breathing erratic, pulse weak
   c. no reflexes, PLR present but sluggish, pupil rotated ventromedially, HR 60 to 90 bpm, breathing shallow
   d. no reflexes (or depressed), pupil rotated ventromedially, HR >90 bpm, breathing slow and regular

Answers and Explanations

Pharmacology

1. b. Ketoconazole does not cause cartilage damage in growing dogs, but will cause other birth defects, liver toxicity, and vomiting. Enrofloxacin can damage cartilage in growing dogs.

2. c. Bacterial pneumonia is treated with antibiotics, bronchodilators, and coupage. Glucocorticoids are not generally used because they cause immunosuppression and decreased neutrophil activity. Goose honk cough is usually associated with collapsing trachea.

3. b. Inhaled glucocorticoids are used to treat allergic bronchitis in cats. Antibiotics would be ineffective and cough suppressants are generally unnecessary.

4. c. Moxidectin should not be used in cats.

5. b. Nitroglycerin is a vasodilator that is administered as a topical cream. Gloves should be worn to prevent absorption through the skin of humans applying it. It should not be used for maintenance therapy in cats because they tend to lick their skin.

6. b. Owners of chemotherapy patients should always wear gloves to prevent possible absorption of agents when cleaning up feces, urine, or vomit. These items should be flushed down the toilet and soiled bedding should be cleaned in the wash immediately. It is not necessary to wear a gown or a face shield when interacting with the pet.

7. d. Pancreatitis, bone marrow suppression, and hypercalcemia are all common side effects of chemotherapeutic agents.

8. c. Cisplatin should never be used in cats.

9. b. Keeping negative pressure in the chemotherapy drug vials (not injecting air into the vial) will decrease the risk of aerosolization of the drug. Chemotherapeutics should be prepared in a very low-traffic area to decrease the risk of potential contamination. Gloves, gowns, and eyewear should be worn when preparing chemotherapeutics.

10. d. PGF2a is used for both pregnancy termination and open-cervix pyometra treatment. It disrupts the corpus luteum, which stops the formation of progesterone. Since pyometra is a disease of prolonged diestrus, stopping the progesterone production should disrupt the pyometra.

11. b. ECP is an estrogen analog. Excessive estrogen leads to bone marrow suppression.

12. c. The best treatment of pyometra is ovariohysterectomy. Megestrol acetate and mibolerone are both oral contraceptives, and oxytocin stimulates smooth muscle contraction.

13. d. Since bronchodilators generally mimic epinephrine, excessive salivation would not occur. Excitability, cardiac arrhythmias, and anorexia are common.

14. b. Enrofloxacin can cause irreversible blindness in cats. This appears to be dose dependent. It can also cause cartilage damage in young, growing animals.

Surgical Preparation and Assisting

15. d. Prolene® and Maxon® are synthetic. Maxon® and chromic gut are all absorbable, and Vicryl® is the only braided material, so Vicryl® has the three characteristics.

16. c. Tenectomy is a procedure used to prevent the animal from using its claws, but does not remove them. Guillotine clippers, sharp dissection with a scalpel blade, or laser are all various ways to perform onychectomy.

17. b. Many monofilament suture materials cause suture reaction. The advantages of monofilament are decreased tissue drag, minimized bacterial infection, and external use.

18. a. Spaying an animal at less than 1 year of age seems to have a protective effect against the development of mammary cancers. After that time, the benefit disappears. The shaved area should be adequate to ensure no hair enters the field, incisions are made through the linea alba (an aponeurosis), and placing a suture or hemoclip around a vessel is called ligation.

19. c. Orchidectomy can help to prevent and treat prostatic hypertrophy, perianal adenomas, and testicular cancers, but is not a treatment for prostate cancer.

20. a. The vaginal tunics are found in the male scrotum and contain the spermatic cord (including the testicular artery, the pampiniform plexus, and the vas deferens), the testicles, and the gubernaculum.

21. b. The cheetah does not have retractable claws. This enables it to have increased speed in chasing prey.

22. a. Regional anesthesia prevents the wind-up effect. Ring blocks for declaw should be performed at the carpus. Regional anesthesia may be performed by the veterinary technician and should be given a minimum of 5 minutes prior to the onset of the surgical procedure.

23. a. Bloat in cattle is common with general anesthesia, but rare in horses. Malignant hyperthermia is common in swine, and myositis or myoglobinuria is common in all large animals.

24. c. Direct heat uses conduction to sterilize. Plasma causes free radical disruption of DNA, steam causes coagulation of proteins, and cold sterilization causes destruction of proteins and DNA.

25. b. Plastic will melt in a steam autoclave. Metal, glass, and muslin all hold up well in steam.

26. b. Steam requires the least amount of time of all the methods. Plasma takes several hours for venting; direct heat and cold sterilization both require several hours.

27. b. Animals should be monitored every 5 minutes during recovery.

28. a. Reptiles and birds both have complete tracheal rings. All mammals have C-shaped rings linked on the dorsal surface by the trachealis dorsalis muscle.

29. a. A #40 blade should be used for surgical clipping. The surgical area should be large enough to prevent the hair from contaminating the surgical field. Clipping should begin with the grain of the hair, then against the grain of the hair. Powerful vacuums may cause damage to the skin surface and should not be used.

30. b. Povidone iodine is inactivated by isopropyl alcohol. The other combinations should be fine.

Dentistry

31. a. The curette is a periodontal instrument. The Kerr file is used to smooth out the interior of the pulp cavity after removal of the pulp and before gutta percha placement during an endodontic procedure. An elevator is used during exodontics.

32. a. This is the correct dental formula for the cat. B is the immature cat formula, D is the immature dog formula, and C is the adult dog formula.

33. c. Cementum covers the tooth below the gumline. Enamel covers above the gumline, dentin makes up the bulk of the tooth, and alveolar bone is the maxillary or mandibular bone surrounding the tooth socket.

34. b. The periodontal ligament holds the tooth within the alveolar socket, or alveolus. The gingiva cover the alveolar bone, but should be disrupted as little as possible during extraction. The same is true for the alveolar bone.

35. d. Because it takes tartar 48 hours to form on the tooth, the AVDS recommends tooth brushing every other day in dogs and cats.

36. b. *Porphyromonas gulae* is the anaerobic bacteria implicated in canine periodontal disease. *Pseudomonas* and *Aeromonas* are aerobic bacteria, and *Clostridium* is an anaerobe rarely found in the mouth of dogs.

37. d. Contact with the tooth surface should be for less than 5 seconds. Ultrasonic scalers disrupt plaque and tartar by cavitation, which can cause aerosolization of oral bacteria that can cause infections of the eyes and nose of technicians. Scalers may be used both above and below the gumline.

38. d. The extraoral approach is often necessary for the treatment of tooth root abscesses in animals with aradicular hypsodont teeth such as the horse, chinchilla, and rabbit.

Laboratory Procedures

39. b. The stones are most likely struvite, which tend to develop in alkaline urine. The key to this laboratory diagnosis is the clear, coffin-lid shaped crystals and radiodense stones. Calcium oxalate crystals are square, with a maltese cross pattern. Uric acid crystals form in acid urine and are pigmented.

40. a. Increased T_4 levels would indicate hyperthyroidism. The symptoms of obesity, hyperpigmentation, lethargy, and decreased activity are consistent with hyperadrenocorticism and hypoadrenocorticism. Diabetes generally does not cause hyperpigmentation, but can cause all the other symptoms. Hyperthyroidism causes hyperactivity, increased metabolic rate, and thinness.

41. c. Glycosylated hemoglobin tests control over a 2 to 3 month period. Fructosamine tests control over 2 to 3 weeks. The glucose tolerance test is generally not performed in animals, and the glucose curve only monitors point values of glucose levels at the time of the blood draw. The problem with performing glucose curves in cats is that they are prone to stress hyperglycemia, which can falsely elevate the blood glucose.

42. d. Blood glucose would likely be the least helpful for this patient's diagnosis. Because he has muscle fibers in the stool (creatorrhea), it is likely that he has either a malassimilation or a malabsorption problem. PLI would be helpful to rule out pancreatitis; TLI, cobalamin, and folate would help to confirm exocrine pancreatic insufficiency or intestinal problems.

43. a. Calcium and magnesium are both affected by albumin concentrations because >98% of the ion is carried on albumin in the blood stream.

44. c. AST and ALT can be elevated with either liver, muscle, or kidney disease. If the CPK is elevated, that would probably indicate muscular involvement. If the CPK were normal, it would probably indicate hepatocellular disease.

45. c. Intravascular hemolysis would make the serum red, not icteric. Extravascular hemolysis (*Babesia*) and cholestasis (*Fasciola*) are the most likely immediate causes of elevated serum bilirubin.

46. d. Ammonia levels would be elevated in portosystemic shunt disease, while the bilirubin may be either decreased or normal, bile acids would be elevated, and the blood glucose would be low because of decreased carbohydrate processing of foodstuffs.

47. d. His BUN and Cr levels should be elevated because he has glomerular disease. The urine protein is elevated in the presence of a low to normal SG; the total protein is markedly low. Since 35 to 50% of the total protein is albumin, the albumin level must be decreased.

48. c. Calcium carbonate is the most common stone in herbivores with alkaline urine.

49. d. All rabbits should be presumed infested with *Psoroptes* and treated. *Notoedres* is a cat mite, *Otodectes* is the dog and cat ear mite, and *Cheylettiella* is walking dandruff.

50. d. *Dioctophema renale* is the giant kidney worm, which is usually asymptomatic. *Haemonchus* and *Uncinaria* are both blood-sucking nematodes that live in the small intestines and can cause bloody diarrhea. *Physaloptera* makes granulomatous ulcers in the esophagus and stomach and can cause melena (digested blood in the stool).

51. c. *Paragonimus kellicotti* results from ingestion of raw seafood such as crabs and crayfish. The other three can all be transmitted by the earthworm, which acts as an intermediate host.

52. a. The occult test for canine heartworm disease tests for the presence of heartworm antigen. This makes it a direct test. The feline antibody test is an indirect method. The filter and Knott's tests are microfilarial tests, which means they are not occult tests.

53. b. This animal has leishmaniasis. The vector is the sandfly (either *Phlebotomus* or *Lutzomyia*) and is usually contracted in Mexico or South America, although it can also be seen in the Mediterranean and in India. The amastigotes live in the cutaneous macrophages (Langerhans cells).

Animal Care and Nursing

54. a. Rottweilers and pit bulls are highly prone to parvovirus. Typical symptoms are vomiting, diarrhea, high temperature initially, and bloody diarrhea with a fetid odor. On blood work, there is a severe lymphopenia. Coronavirus can show a very similar picture, but the fever and the leukopenia would not be present. Giardia and hookworms generally have no associated temperature elevation, and giardia typically has no blood in the stool.

55. a. Beau has old-dog distemper. The initial signs are a severe respiratory illness, which may progress into neurologic signs including personality changes. The chronic sign is a chewing gum seizure.

56. c. Tuberculosis testing involves injecting a small amount of TB into the dermis. Generally, this is performed on the eyelid of cattle and primates. In cattle, this is called a Bang's test.

57. b. Sally has *Yersinia pestis*, also known as bubonic plague. It is carried by rodent fleas and is still occasionally seen in the western United States. Lymphoma is common in cats, but is not usually associated with a fever. *Yersinia enterocolitica* causes gastrointestinal disease and *Ehrlichia* does not infect cats.

58. c. Animals with hypoxia usually have an elevated heart rate because they are trying to increase tissue perfusion. Dyspnea can occur along with cyanosis (blue or grey gums) and open-mouth breathing.

59. c. Calvin probably has brucellosis. This causes orchitis (inflammation of the testicles and epididymis) which can be acutely painful. In females, it can cause abortion. This is a mildly zoonotic disease.

60. a. A patent catheter (one that flows well in a vein without inflammation) can be maintained for up to 72 hours. Administration sets should be changed more frequently and the catheter should be periodically flushed with sterile, heparinized saline to ensure patency. Maintenance fluid rates are calculated by the formula in answer choice **d**.

61. a. Canine herpesvirus causes acute death in puppies, but may be completely asymptomatic in adult dogs. Brucellosis can cause abortion, but not death within a few days of birth. Mycoplasma and *Bordetella* generally do not cause neonatal death.

62. c. Surgical fluid rates are 10 ml/kg/hour. Shock levels should only be used if the patient is having symptoms of shock.

63. c. Fluffy has an upper respiratory tract infection. Upper respiratory complex in cats consists of rhinotracheitis, calici, and chlamydia. The incubation period (2 weeks) is not long enough for feline leukemia, but the symptoms can be similar, so Fluffy should be tested. Panleukopenia presents with the same symptoms as canine parvovirus (diarrhea with blood, leukopenia, and so on).

64. d. The calculation of energy requirements of an animal is the MER × the k values (breed, activity level, reproductive status, physiologic requirements).

65. b. Although rhinotracheitis, feline leukemia, and calici should all be on the differential diagnoses list, calici is the most likely cause of her symptoms. Ulceration of the oral cavity is common with calici, but rare with rhinotracheitis and feline leukemia.

66. b. Linolenic acid is essential in the diet of the dog. Oleic acid is found in oleomargarine. Stearic acid is beef fat, or tallow. Arachidonic acid is essential in the cat.

67. d. Antibiotics will not help with viral diseases. Quarantine, disinfection, and preventative vaccination are the best methods of control.

68. c. FIV is transmitted via bite wounds *only*. It is much more common in intact adult male cats. FeLV generally affects a younger population. Parvovirus is only seen in dogs and giardia will not cause these symptoms.

69. c. Leptospirosis affects the kidneys and liver and causes hematuria, back pain, and high fevers. It is very common in animals that hunt. Bladder stones will not cause kidney pain. Brucellosis affects the reproductive tract. Distemper affects the respiratory and gastrointestinal tracts.

70. a. The vaccine is effective if given as directed, and he should be protected. He should be monitored for development of symptoms and should be kept close to home to prevent possible viral shed.

71. c. Horses can kick 6 to 8 feet behind themselves and several feet to the side. They should be approached within their field of view, haltered on the left side of the head, and foals should be separated from the dam without getting between them to avoid the dam becoming agitated and attacking.

72. b. Rats do well with a chair hold. They should not be carried by the tail because they have large bodies and their weights can cause the tail to deglove. Guinea pigs should also be placed in a chair hold and their rumps should be cupped in the opposite palm. Hamsters should be scruffed. They have no tail.

73. c. Cats require taurine in the diet. Methionine is used to increase acidity of the urine in some cat diets. Proline is essential for birds.

74. a. The cat with dyspneic disorder should be seen first, followed by the hog dog, followed by the collie, followed by the dog with impacted anal glands.

75. d. Hypocalcemia and hypomagnesemia both cause seizures in cattle. Hypocalcemia is also called milk fever, hypomagnesemia is called grass tetany.

76. d. COPD is chronic obstructive pulmonary disease. It usually occurs in horses. Infectious bovine rhinotracheitis, parainfluenza, and bovine respiratory syncytial virus are all possible causes of shipping fever in cattle, which is a huge potential income loss for owners.

77. b. *Streptococus equi* is also called *strangles* and usually infects the cervical lymph nodes in horses. West Nile virus causes meningitis; tetanus causes muscle rigidity but no lymph node enlargement; and *Ehrlichia* is mostly a hemolytic disease.

Diagnostic Imaging

78. d. In general, a met check includes a right and left lateral thorax and a VD/DV thorax. This enables visualization of potential metastases against the dark background of the air-filled lung tissue.

79. b. The imaging plate in digital radiography is equivalent to medium speed screen and film because it contains phosphor crystals that react in a similar fashion. The image can then be adjusted by changing the histogram.

80. a. The open mouth tympanic bulla technique is not a good technique for assessing the nasal cavity and sinuses because of bony and soft tissue interference and magnification.

81. c. Flexed lateral cervical spine could cause displacement of the axis and damage the cervical spine in an animal with a hypoplastic dens.

82. b. In the craniocaudal view, the plate cannot be close enough to the stifle to prevent magnification without causing hyperextension. The caudocranial view allows the patella to contact the plate directly, thereby preventing magnification of the image.

83. c. PennHIP must be performed under anesthesia in order to get the animal into the proper position. It is used to evaluate hip dysplasia in animals over 6 months of age using the distraction index as a measurement. The distraction index is the distance that the hip joint can be luxated from the acetabular fossa.

84. a. Organic iodides are the only contrast that should be used for myelography.

85. a. The kVp adjusts the speed and penetration of the x-ray beam by increasing the strength of the magnetic field between the anode and the cathode. The mA and the mAs affect the number of x-rays produced by increasing the number of electrons fired at the anode.

Anesthesia and Analgesia

86. d. Giving more butorphanol will not increase the effect of the drug. It is a very short-acting opioid and acts as an agonist/antagonist. It is more effective for visceral pain than for somatic pain.

87. c. Morphine is most effective for visceral analgesia. Ketamine and NSAIDs are more effective for somatic pain. Although butorphanol is moderately effective as a visceral analgesic, it is very short acting and is seldom used.

88. a. Ketamine can cause muscle rigidity and make it difficult to intubate an animal. It will lower the seizure threshold for many animals. Propofol, morphine, and butorphanol do not generally cause seizures and will actually cause muscle relaxation.

89. c. Acepromazine will lower the seizure threshold. Atropine and glycopyrrholate may be used in seizure-prone animals to decrease secretions and increase heart rate. Diazepam is used to treat seizures.

90. a. Xylazine can be reversed with yohimbine. Medatomadine can be reversed with atipemazole. Fentanyl is an opiate and can be reversed with naloxone. Ketamine is not reversible.

91. b. Ketamine is the only drug on the list of answer choices that is not metabolized in the liver.

92. c. Anesthetized patients are generally maintained at 1.5 to 2 times the MAC of the gas in percents. Higher MAC gases should have higher percentage on the gauge for maintenance.

93. a. Halothane is commonly associated with malignant hyperthermia in animals under anesthesia. Isoflurane and sevoflurane do not have this complication. Methoxyflurane is associated with liver toxicity.

94. b. Because N_2O is in both liquid and gas form in a tank, the tank's weight can be used to estimate the quantity of material left in the tank.

95. b. There are still 599 liters of O_2 left in the tank. 1 L/min × 60 min/hour × 4 hours = 240 L. 599 − 240 = 359 L left over, so there is enough left in the tank for a second procedure.

96. a. The pressure regulator valve changes the pressure coming from the tank to a lower pressure that can be used for the animal. If this is broken, it must be repaired. Using the machine on an animal could cause severe lung damage or death.

97. c. Precision vaporizers are generally used for halothane, isoflurane, and sevoflurane. They always have the same delivery no matter the humidity or temperature. Nonprecision vaporizers are used for methoxyflurane. They have variable delivery depending on the humidity or temperature. All vaporizers should be filled when the animal is disconnected from the vaporizer and the oxygen flow is off. Overfilling can result in saturation of dry areas within the vaporizers and should trigger a call to the repair company.

98. d. IPPV should never be at a pressure greater than 20 cmH_2O on the manometer to avoid damage to the alveoli. IPPV will decrease CO_2 levels in the animal during anesthesia. Too-frequent sighs can cause hyperventilation and respiratory alkalosis, which can cause apnea. IPPV will improve the tidal volume, but will not maintain it at normal levels.

99. d. Closed-circuit gas administration will maintain the temperature and humidity of the breathed gases better than open systems, but will have higher resistance.

100. b. Stage II plane IV is in the danger zone. This is considered extremely deep anesthesia and should only be used for very painful procedures. The animal should be monitored extremely carefully.

GLOSSARY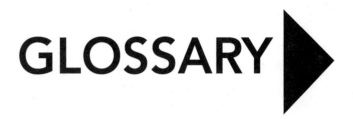

absorbable   referring to suture materials that absorb or dissolve within the body caused by enzymatic action on the suture

absorption   the uptake of drugs into or across body tissues or cells

acidosis   a decrease in blood pH characterized by an increase in hydrogen ions caused by an accumulation of acids or a depletion of alkaline substances

acoustic shadowing   an artifact seen in ultrasound imaging caused by complete reflection or attenuation of the sound beam by an object such as a calculus or gas such that deeper structures appear anechoic

agglutination   clumping of blood cells, particularly when caused by antibody binding to antigen expressed on the surface of red blood cells

agonist   a chemical or drug that has an affinity for a cell's receptor and when attached stimulates a physiologic effect

ALARA   acronym for <u>a</u>s <u>l</u>ow <u>a</u>s <u>r</u>easonably <u>a</u>chievable; a principle of radiation protection philosophy that requires that exposures to ionizing radiation be kept as low as reasonably achievable

alkalosis   an increase in blood pH characterized by a decrease in hydrogen ions caused either by depletion of acid or accumulation of alkaline substances in body fluids

alpha hemolysis   the rupture of red blood cells caused by chemicals produced by some bacteria, particularly streptococci, which results in a zone of clearing around the bacteria grown on a blood-agar plate

alpha particles   emissions released by certain radioactive nuclei that carry more energy than beta or gamma particles but are stopped quickly while passing through tissue; streams of alpha particles (alpha rays) can be used in radiation therapy to treat certain malignancies

alveoli   small air sacs at the end of bronchi in the lungs

alveolus   the tooth socket; alveolar bone is the bone surrounding the alveolus

analgesia   the absence of pain

analgesic   a drug that inhibits the sensation of pain

anechoic   lack of production of echoes from tissues in ultrasonography

anisognathic   having differing widths between the maxillary and mandibular arcades of teeth, especially in the molar teeth; such as that found with horse teeth

anode   positive electrode target of x-ray tube composed of tungsten alloy to which negative ions are attracted

antagonist   a chemical or drug that has an affinity for a cell's receptor and, when attached, blocks the action of agonists and does not cause a physiologic action

anthelmintic   a drug used to treat endoparasites (internal parasites)

anticoagulant   a substance such as EDTA or heparin that inhibits clotting in a sample of blood

anti-inflammatory   a drug used to suppress the inflammatory process

antimicrobial   a drug that works either to kill or to inhibit the growth or reproduction of microorganisms

antipyretic   a drug that reduces or prevents fever

antisepsis   removal of organisms from a living surface to a level that will not cause or transmit infection

antitussive   a drug that reduces coughing; a cough suppressant

apex   the entrance into the pulp cavity at the base of the alveolus

apnea   the temporary cessation of breathing

aponeurosis   a broad tendonlike facial plane connection; usually used to define the linea alba

arachnid   a class of invertebrate animals that includes ticks, mites, scorpions, and spiders

aradicular   pertaining to teeth that continue to erupt or grow throughout the life of the animal

arcade   a row of teeth

arrhythmia   a disturbance in the normal rhythm of the heartbeat

asepsis   without infectious organisms (a desirable state during surgery)

aspiration   the inadvertent inhalation of material into the airways and lungs

atelectasis   the collapse of alveoli and lung

auscultation   listening to sounds produced within the body, typically with a stethoscope

azotemia   a buildup of nitrogen-containing products of protein metabolism in the blood

bacillus   a rodshaped bacterium, particularly any of the genus *Bacillus*

beta hemolysis   the destroying of red blood cells by substances produced by some bacteria, particularly the beta-hemolytic streptococci

beta particles   electrons ejected from the nuclei of decaying radioactive substances and possessing more penetrating power than alpha rays but less than gamma rays

biofilm   a complex structure adhering to the surface, usually associated with bacteria; for example, as dental plaque

biotransformation   modification of a drug by the liver so that the drug can be utilized by the body

Bordetella bronchiseptica   principal bacterial cause of the canine respiratory disease complex known as kennel cough

bovine respiratory syncytial virus (BRSV)   a major viral agent in initiating bovine respiratory disease, with symptoms of clinical disease resulting from stress and concurrent bacterial infection of the respiratory tract

brachyodont   a short-crowned, well-rooted tooth that, once erupted, stops growing

BRSV   *see bovine respiratory syncitial virus*

buccal surface of the teeth facing the cheek or outside of the mouth

Bucky *see Potter-Bucky tray*

calculus oral plaque that calcifies on teeth surfaces; also called tartar

canine adenovirus type 1 (CAV-1) viral agent that causes infectious hepatitis in dogs; vaccination against CAV-2 is cross-protective

canine adenovirus type 2 (CAV-2) one of the viral agents that may cause infectious tracheobronchitis (kennel cough) in dogs, typically in comorbidity with *Bordetella bronchiseptica*

canine distemper virus (CDV) a contagious, incurable, often fatal, multisystemic viral disease that affects the canine respiratory, gastrointestinal, and central nervous systems

canine infectious tracheobronchitis *see kennel cough*

canine parainfluenza virus (CPIV) a virus that may cause infectious tracheobronchitis (kennel cough) in dogs and commonly shares comorbidity with *bordetella bronchiseptica*; causes mild to severe respiratory symptoms

canine parvovirus (CPV) a potentially fatal, extremely contagious canine virus that commonly produces vomiting and severe hemorrhagic diarrhea, depression, lack of appetite, and leucopenia

canthus the corner of the eye, either medial or lateral

caries tooth decay; often called cavities

carnassial a large, shearing cheek tooth

Caslick's procedure episioplasty or surgical repair of the vulva of a mare to reduce vaginitis (infection) or pneumovagina (air in vagina)

cast a structure observed in microscopic analysis of urinalysis formed by the precipitation of protein in the renal tubules; may contain epithelial cells, leukocytes (white blood cells), fat, red blood cells, or granular-appearing cell debris

CAT scan *see computerized axial tomography scan*

cathode a filament that provides a source of electrons; releases electrons as it is heated

caudate cell *see renal epithelial cell*

caudectomy tail amputation or tail docking

CAV-1 *see canine adenovirus type 1*

CAV-2 *see canine adenovirus type 2*

cavitation the formation of cavities

CDV *see canine distemper virus*

cementum the substance covering the root of the tooth

cestode a tapeworm

chemotaxis a process in which leukocytes are attracted by chemicals released from an area of injury or inflammation

chlorhexidine commonly used family of antiseptic chemicals possessing antibacterial, antifungal, and limited antiviral activity; used for preoperative skin preparation

cleanliness the removal of dirt and debris from a surface

closed gloving preferred method of putting on surgical gloves; hands remain inside the cuff of the gown and are not exposed to the exterior or to potential contamination

Clostridium perfringens (types C and D) the causative agent of enterotoxemia (overeating disease) in sheep and goats

collimating reducing the size of the useful beam of photons or electrons with an absorbing material; a collimator (or slit) is the mechanical device installed along the trajectory of the beam to accomplish collimating and also to help reduce scatter radiation

computed radiography a type of radiography that uses an imaging plate (IP) in place of film to create an image that is run through a laser scanner and then recovered, displayed, and can be enhanced by a digital computer

computerized axial tomography (CAT) scan three-dimensional image of a bodily structure created by computer analysis of a series of cross-sectional x-rays taken along a single axis of a bodily structure or tissue; also known as CT (computerized tomography) scan

contraindication a symptom or condition that renders a treatment inadvisable

contrast the differences in photographic density that form the image on a radiograph

coronal toward the crown of the tooth; occlusal surface

CPIV *see canine parainfluenza virus*

CPV *see* canine parvovirus

crown that portion of the normal tooth above the gumline; chewing surface of the tooth

cryptorchidectomy surgical repair or excision of retained testicle(s)

CT *see computerized tomography scan*

curette instrument with a blunt tip that is used for subgingival scaling

deciduous immature, temporary, or baby teeth that are replaced by permanent teeth as the animal ages

decongestant a drug that reduces swelling of mucous membrane surfaces

definitive host host in which the parasite or pathogen reaches maturity and undergoes reproduction

dehiscence breakdown of a repaired wound, or opening of the wound prior to healing

dentifrice a preparation used for cleaning or polishing the teeth

dentin the substance that comprises most of the tooth surrounding the pulp cavity and under the cementum and enamel

depolarization the movement of electrolytes Na^+ & Ca^+ into the cardiac cell, resulting in an electrical stimulus of heart muscle causing it to contract

diastole the period of time when heart's ventricles are relaxing and filling with blood and arterial blood pressure is at its lowest

differentiating medium a growth medium that contains nutrient substances or indicators that help to distinguish bacteria based on biochemical differences

direct digital radiography a way to produce x-rays whereby a sensitive electronic device produces images on a screen that are easier to store, copy, and send electronically than conventional x-ray films

direct radiation (primary radiation) radiation emitted from the x-ray tube that passes though the collimator opening as the primary or useful beam

disinfection removal of organisms from a nonliving surface to a level that will not cause or transmit infection

distribution the movement of drugs to the intended target tissue

diuretic a drug that reduces body water by promoting excretion via the kidneys

dose equivalent limit *see maximum permissible dose*

dosimetry badge a film badge worn by the person performing radiography for the purpose of measuring and recording the total accumulated dose of ionizing radiation that the person receives

E. coli   *see Eschericia coli*

ectoparasite   a parasite that lives on the surface of the body, such as a flea or a tick

edema   an abnormal swelling caused by the accumulation of fluid

EEE/WEE/VEE   Eastern, Western, and Venezuelan equine encephalomyelitis, respectively; mosquito-borne, potentially zoonotic (transmissible to humans) diseases characterized by disturbed consciousness, motor irritation, and commonly high mortality rates

efficacy   the intended activity or response of a drug in the body

EHV   *see* equine rhinopneumonitis

ejaculate   fluid containing semen and secretions from accessory sex glands that is expelled from the male urethra in response to sexual stimulation

elective surgery   nonurgent surgery; a surgery that is not essential to maintaining the life or function of the animal and that may be scheduled at the convenience of the owner or the veterinarian

elevator   instrument used to elevate gingival tissues for exodontics and extractions

elongation   a distortion of dental imaging in which the root appears longer than normal

embolus   a blood clot

emesis   the act of vomiting

emetic   a drug or substance that promotes vomiting

enamel   the substance that covers the crown of the tooth; it is the hardest substance in the body

endodontics   the specialty of dentistry that deals with the inner pulp of the tooth, as in root canals

endogenous   produced or caused within the body

endoparasite   a parasite that lives within the host, such as a helminth

epulis   a benign, fibrous, often-recurrent tumor of the gums of dogs

equine infectious anemia (EIA)   a contagious, incurable form of anemia, spread by biting arthropod insects, and routinely screened for in the blood test known as the Coggins test

equine influenza   a virus that usually causes mild flu-like symptoms of fever, cough, and depression, and has an increased incidence in young animals (1–3 years)

equine monocytic ehrlichiosis   *see* Potomac horse fever

equine rhinopneumonitis (EHV-1 and EHV-4)   herpesviruses that produce respiratory disease in horses and may induce abortion in pregnant mares

equine strangles   a very contagious equine respiratory disease caused by *Streptococcus equi* and characterized by abscessation of the submandibular and retropharyngeal lymph nodes causing swelling of the throat

erysipelas   a swine disease caused by the bacterium *Erysipelothrix rhusiopathiae*, which causes chronic arthritis, joint disease, heart disease, diamond-back skin disease, and death, and produces a zoonotic skin rash (erysipeloid) in humans

Escherichia coli (E. coli)   common cause of diarrhea in calves (scours) and piglets

ethylene oxide   a toxic and explosive gas agent used in specialized equipment for disinfection of materials that will melt or be damaged by other sterilization methods

eupnea   normal breathing

excretion   elimination of a drug or its metabolites from the body

exodontics   tooth extraction

expectorant   a drug that dilutes and liquefies respiratory secretions to facilitate their removal from the lungs

extubation   removal of the endotracheal tube from an animal, usually at the end of the anesthesia

facultative   having the ability to adapt to changes in the environment; a facultative anaerobe can grow in the presence or in the absence of oxygen. An obligate anaerobe can't grow in the presence of O_2.

feline calicivirus   one of the two most common viral respiratory diseases of cats; characterized by upper respiratory symptoms, pneumonia, oral ulceration (sores in the mouth), and occasionally arthritis

feline distemper   *see* **feline panleukopenia**

feline herpesvirus (feline viral rhinotracheitis)   one of the two most common viral respiratory diseases of cats; produces symptoms such as sneezing, ulcerative stomatitis, ulcerative keratitis (corneal ulcer), fever conjunctivitis, anorexia, and nasal and ocular discharge

feline immunodeficiency virus (FIV)   fatal, incurable retrovirus of cats, spread primarily via bite wounds and fighting

feline infectious peritonitis (FIP)   serious, destructive virus affecting cats; initial symptoms include upper respiratory symptoms, depression, weight loss, and lack of appetite; weeks to months later, the virus may produce a lethal form of the disease

feline leukemia virus (FeLV)   fatal retrovirus of cats that affects the immune system; transmitted primarily via saliva from fighting, sharing food and water bowls, and grooming activity

feline panleukopenia (feline distemper)   a highly contagious parvoviral disease of cats; can present with a wide variety of symptoms including depression, anorexia, fever, panleukopenia, and vomiting

feline viral rhinotracheitis   *see* **feline herpesvirus**

FeLV   *see feline leukemia virus*

fenestrated   describes a surgical drape with a hole or opening

film fog   the film darkening caused by radiation from sources other than exposure to the primary beam, such as scatter radiation or radiation in the environment

FIP   *see* **feline infecious peritonitis**

FIV   *see* **feline immunodeficiency virus**

foreshortening   a distortion of dental imaging in which the root appears shorter than normal

furcation   the gap or area where the roots of multirooted teeth meet under the crown and normally below the gumline

gamma rays   a high-energy form of electromagnetic radiation emitted by certain radioactive substances; because of their cytotoxic effects on rapidly replicating tissues, they can be utilized in radiation therapy but have potentially harmful effects on bone marrow, gonads, and the fetus

generic drug   commonly used name of a drug derived from the shortened version of its chemical name

gingiva   the soft tissue covering the interior of the mouth and covering alveolar bone; the gum tissues

gram-negative   appearing pink after the gram-staining procedure due to decolorization with alcohol and uptake of safranine counterstain by the bacterial cell wall

gram-positive   appearing dark purple after the gram-staining procedure due to retaining of the crystal violet stain by peptidoglycans in the bacterial cell wall

grid   scatter-reduction device consisting of a flat plate of thin lead foil strips and low-density spacers mounted under the x-ray table between the patient and the film cassette

grid ratio   the relationship of the height of the lead strips to the distance between them in the grid; higher grid ratios filter more scatter but also require higher primary radiation exposure

gutta percha   a rubbery latex product used as a dental filler or cement

half-life   the length of time needed for a drug to decrease by one half in its active form within the body

hardware disease (traumatic reticulo-pericarditis/-peritonitis)   intensely painful bovine condition that results from a sharp, usually metallic object penetrating the cow's reticulum (stomach) and/or diaphragm or pericardium

Hb   *see* **hemoglobin**

heel effect   unequal distribution of the x-ray beam intensity between the cathode and the anode due to absorption of the x-ray beam by the anode and the target

hematochezia   the presence of blood in the feces

hematologic indices   calculated values for the mean corpuscular volume, mean corpuscular hemoglobin, and mean corpuscular hemoglobin concentration, which are useful in determining the origin of an anemia

hematopoiesis   the process of forming and producing blood cells; takes place in the bone marrow

hemoglobin (Hb)   the oxygen-carrying protein contained within red blood cells

hemoglobinuria   the presence of hemoglobin in the urine from lysis of red blood cells in the urine or from intravascular hemolysis

hemolysis   the rupture of red blood cell membranes leading to release of hemoglobin; causes include immune reactions, bacterial pathogens, hypotonic fluids, venoms, and rough handling of blood samples

hemostasis   to stop bleeding

hydatid cyst   larval form of tapeworms of the genus *Echinococcus*, and occurring as a large fluid-filled cyst in the liver or lungs of the intermediate host

hypercapnia or **hypercarbia**   elevated carbon dioxide in the blood

hyperechoic   producing an increased amplitude of waves (echos) in comparison to another tissue in ultrasonography

hypoxemia or **hypoxia**   low levels of oxygen in the blood

hypsodont   a high-crowned and short-rooted tooth that continues to erupt either for the life of the animal or for an extended period of time of the animal's life

icterus   a yellow discoloration of the serum that is observed in jaundiced patients

indicator systems   devices used to indicate that sterilization has occurred

infectious bovine rhinotracheitis (aka bovine herpesvirus type 1)   contagious viral respiratory disease that may also produce abortions and genital infections

infectious tracheobronchitis   *see* **kennel cough**

inotropic   a drug that promotes the contractility of the heart

intermediate host   a host that harbors an immature stage of a parasite site as a larva

intraoperative   period of time during a surgery

intubation   the insertion of a tube, typically into the trachea

iodorphors   commonly used antiseptic family of iodine complexed with a surfactant (soap) that allows iodine to be released slowly and possessing antibacterial, antifungal, and limited antiviral activity

isoechoic   describes two or more tissues that are similar in echogenicity as measured by ultrasonography

isosthenuria   a condition in which the urine consistently maintains the same specific gravity as the glomerular filtrate due to the inability of the kidneys to either concentrate or dilute urine

kennel cough   the common term for canine infectious tracheobronchitis, which may be caused by a complex of bacterial and viral agents including *bordetella bronchiseptica*, CAV-2, and canine parainfluenza

kit   *see* pack

kilovolts peak (kVp)   x-ray voltage; the amount of energy (electrical potential) placed across the anode and the cathode of the x-ray tube in order to accelerate electrons toward a target

labial   the surface of the canines and incisors that face the lips

laparotomy   incision through the abdominal wall; often used to explore the abdomen, as in exploratory laparotomy

larva   immature free-living stage in the life cycle of a parasite or insect that differs from the adult stage and must undergo further metamorphosis

legend drug   a drug that is considered a prescription drug and is regulated under the Controlled Substances Act

leptospirosis   contagious bacteria that affect a variety of species including cattle, horses, pigs, sheep, goats, and dogs; potentially zoonotic; affects the liver, kidneys, and other organs

leukogram   a counting and tabulation of white blood cells

lingual   the surface of the lower teeth that face the tongue

lipemia   the presence of a lipid (fat) in the blood; occurs in postprandial samples and commonly interferes with blood chemistry tests

malabsorption   impaired nutrient absorption in the intestines; cause of diarrhea and weight loss

malassimilation   faulty uptake of nutrients by the digestive system; may be due to malabsorption or to maldigestion

maldigestion   incomplete digestion of food, such as that which occurs in pancreatic exocrine insufficiency

malocclusion   a condition in which teeth come together abnormally

mandibular   the lower jaw

Mannheimia haemolytica* (**formerly ***Pasteurella haemolytica)   a bacterium that contributes to bovine respiratory disease or shipping fever

marginating pool   a reserve of accumulated leukocytes adhered to endothelial cells that can be recruited in response to inflammation

milliamperage (mAs)   a measure of x-ray intensity that factors in milliamperes, or the amount of current passing through the cathode filaments to produce electrons, and time (in seconds)

maxillary   the upper jaw

maximum permissible dose (MPD)   the largest amount of ionizing radiation that a person may safely receive; also know as the dose equivalent limit

MCH   *see* **mean corpuscular hemoglobin**

MCHC   *see* **mean corpusculor hemoglobin concentration**

mean corpuscular hemoglobin (MCH)   the average weight of hemoglobin in a red blood cell; expressed in picograms and calculated by multiplying the hemoglobin measured in grams by a factor of 10 and dividing by the number of erythrocytes (in millions); considered the least accurate of the hematologic indices.

mean corpuscular hemoglobin concentration (MCHC)   the ratio of the weight of hemoglobin per cell to the volume in which it is contained; calculated by multiplying the hemoglobin in grams by 100 and dividing by the hematocrit; considered the most accurate of the hematologic indices

mean corpuscular volume (MCV)   a measure of the average volume of red blood cells expressed in femto-liters (fL) and calculated by multiplying the hematocrit by 10 and dividing by the number of erythrocytes (in millions)

melena   the presence of digested blood in the feces, appearing as black, tarry stool

mesial   surface toward the midline of the front of the dental arch

metabolism   the process of changing a drug to a form that can be utilized by cells or the body

microfilaria   embryonic larvae of filarid parasites such as heartworms that circulate in the blood when released from adult females

milk-and-meat withdrawal time   the period of time after administration of a pharmaceutical to a food-producing animal during which meat and/or milk from that animal should be withheld from the market for human consumption; prevents drug residues in meat and milk intended for human consumption

miosis   constriction of the pupil

MPD   *see* **maximum permissible dose**

murmur   a sound made by abnormal turbulent blood flow through the heart

mydriasis   dilation of the pupil

myelinated nerve   a nerve that is wrapped in a sheath of lipid

myiasis   invasion of the body by fly larvae; may involve the skin, nasopharynx, eyes, intestines, or urinary tract

negative feedback   a process whereby high plasma levels of a hormone or chemical messenger cause a reduction in production of that same hormone or messenger

nematode   a roundworm of the class Nematoda

nephrotoxic   destructive to the kidneys

nit   a louse egg, typically found adhered to a hair shaft on the host

nonabsorbable   referring to suture materials that are not absorbed when placed in the tissue

nonelective surgery   surgeries performed to maintain the life or function of the animal

nuclear magnetic resonance imaging (NMRI)   the image produced by the absorption or emission of electromagnetic energy by nuclei in a static magnetic field, after excitation by a suitable radio frequency magnetic field

nystagmus   a rhythmic, involuntary movement of both eyes

obligate parasite   a parasite that cannot live independently of its host

occlusal   pertaining to the chewing or masticating surfaces of the teeth

onychectomy   amputation or removal of the claw and associated third phalanx

open gloving   method of gloving in which the hands are outside of the surgical gown

orchidectomy   term for castration surgery; removal of the testicles

oronasal fistula   communicating opening between the oral and nasal cavities

Orthopedic Foundation of America   an independent organization devoted to the evaluation of x-rays of orthopedic conditions in dogs, particularly hip dysplasia

ostium   general term for the mouth

ovariohysterectomy   term for removal of the uterus, ovaries, and associated tissues; often referred to as a spay

ovum   an egg, the female reproductive cell that is fertilized

pack   a group of surgical instruments collected or assembled together for surgery; sometimes referred to as a kit

palatal   pertaining to the surface of the upper teeth that face the palate

parainfluenza type 3   one of the contributing viruses of the bovine respiratory disease complex; generally produces mild to subclinical disease

parasite   an organism that lives on or in another organism, from which it draws nutriment

paratenic host   an intermediate host that aids in transmission of the parasite without any development of the parasite taking place; the definitive host generally becomes infected via ingestion of this paratenic host

parenteral   not through the intestines; such as medication given intravenously (IV), subcutaneously (SQ), or intramuscularly (IM)

paresis   muscle weakness

Pasteurella haemolitica   *see Mannheimia haemolitica*

Pasteurella multocida   a bacterium that produces rabbit snuffles with a range of respiratory, neurologic, and dermal signs including nasal discharge, torticollis (or *wry neck*), caseous skin abscesses, conjunctivitis, ocular discharge, and dyspnea; also produces respiratory disease in bovines

pellet   in urinalysis, the compacted sediment of cells, crystals, and other solid material that settles in the bottom of a centrifuged urine sample and is subsequently resuspended after the supernatant has been poured off and observed miscroscopically

pellicle   glycoprotein in saliva that forms and covers teeth

PennHIP   an acronym for University of *Penn*sylvania *Hip Improvement Program*, a diagnostic technique for hip dysplasia which evaluates radiographs taken from three different angles

periodontium   tissues around and supporting the teeth including gingival and periodontal ligament and alveolar bone

pharmacodynamics   the resultant effect or action of a drug in a body

pharmacokinetics   the movement of a drug in a body including absorption, distribution, metabolism, and excretion

phlebotomy   the process of incising a vein, usually referring to a needle's producing a small hole in a vein through which a blood sample is collected

plaque   bacteria and salivary pellicle that begin to colonize on teeth

plasma   the liquid portion of blood in which blood cells are suspended and containing proteins, clotting factors, and other dissolved substances

polychromatophil   immature erythrocytes (reticulocytes) that stain blue-purple in Wright's stained blood smears

polydipsia   increased thirst and increased water intake

polyuria   increased production and excretion of urine

positive-pressure ventilation   giving an anesthetized patient a breath by squeezing the reservoir bag

postoperative   period of time after surgery

Potomac horse fever (equine monocytic ehrlichiosis)   rickettsial disease caused by *Ehrlichia risticii*; mosquitoes and ticks are the suspected insect vectors of this diarrheal disease

Potter-Bucky tray (Bucky)   a sliding metal tray under the radiographic table that holds the grid and the cassette

precipitate   solid particles that form in a solution

preoperative   period of time just prior to surgery procedures

primary beam   beam of particles that passes through the window of the x-ray tube and strikes a target

primary radiation   *see direct radiation*

proglottids   the segments composing the body of a tapeworm

prophylaxis   preventive treatment to preserve teeth and surrounding tissues

proprietary drug   a drug that has a brand or trade name protected by patent

protons   subatomic particles possessing a positive charge and found within the nucleus of an atom

protozoa   a group of free-living, single-celled organisms that includes parasites such as coccidia, cryptosporidia, toxoplasma, and others

pulp   internal canal of the tooth containing vessels and nerves

pupa   the second stage in development of an insect, falling between the larval stage and the adult stages usually taking place in an inactive structure such as a cocoon

rabies   acute viral fatal encephalomyelitis caused by a lyssavirus of the Rhabdoviridae family and capable of affecting all species of mammals; zoonotic and spread via bite wounds

radicular   pertaining to teeth that erupt for a long period of the animal's life but eventually the apex closes, hindering further tooth growth; typically seen in herbivores such as horses or cows

radiodense (or **radiopaque**)   a substance such as metal or bone that will appear white on a plain radiograph

radiolucent   anything that permits the penetration and passage of x-rays or other forms of radiation; appears black on x-ray film

regimen   proper drug usage, including the right patient, drug, dose, frequency, route, and withdrawal time

renal epithelial cell (or **caudate cell**)   a type of cell, occasionally seen in the urine sediment, that is slightly larger than a leukocyte but much smaller than squamous or transitional epithelial cells; these cells line the renal tubules and may indicate kidney tubule disease

repolarization   the movement of potassium out of cardiac cells, resulting in heart muscle relaxation; it follows cardiac depolarization

respiratory minute volume   the number of breaths per minute multiplied by the patient's tidal volume

reticulocyte   immature, anucleate erythrocytes that contain RNA and are distinguishable when new methylene blue stain is utilized; may appear macrocytic or polychromatophilic with Wright's stain.

retropulse   the driving back of a tooth or other tissues

reverberation   artifactual images containing multiple bright bands that appear due to repeated reflection between the transducer surface and the tissue under study

Salmonella   zoonotic bacterium that can cause severe enteritis in humans, and typically harbored by poultry species and reptiles; also a cause of diarrhea in calves and foals.

scaler   instrument with a pointed tip and one cutting edge that is used for supragingival scaling

scatter radiation   x-ray beam that changes in direction while passing through the patient; it has a negative effect on image quality

scours   diarrhea in calves

selective media   a bacterial growth plate that has substances added to it either to promote or to inhibit growth of certain bacteria

serology   the identification and measurement of antibodies, antigens, and other immunological substances in the blood

serum   the clear, straw-colored portion of blood fluid that remains after blood has clotted; does not contain blood cells or fibrinogen, but retains other substances dissolved in the blood such as electrolytes, glucose, enzymes, and other proteins.

specific gravity   a measure of the weight and thus the concentration of a substance; usually measured as compared to water, which has a specific gravity of 1.000

spirochete   a type of coiled bacterium such as *Leptospira interrogans*, *Borrelia* species, and *Treponema* species

squamous epithelium   a layer of platelike superficial cells, such as the outermost layers of mucous membranes and the skin

sterility   removal or destruction of all living organisms including bacterial spores; the state of being sterile

stomatitis   inflammation of the membrane surfaces of the mouth

sulcus   the groove between the tooth surface and the gingival (gums); around all teeth

supernatant   in urinalysis, the liquid overlying the pellet of solid material after centrifugation of the urine sample

symbiote (or **symbiont**)   an organism that lives in close association with another organism either to the advantage or to the disadvantage of the second organism

systole   the period of time when the heart's ventricles are contracting and arterial blood pressure is at its peak

tartar   oral plaque that calcifies on teeth surfaces; also called calculus

tetanus antitoxin   a source of passive natural immunity to naïve animals; it neutralizes unbound toxin of the *Clostridium tetani* organism

tetanus toxoid   a vaccine that induces active immunity to the toxin produced by the causative bacterium of tetanus, *Clostridium tetani*

therapeutic index   the difference between a safe therapeutic dosage and a toxic dosage

therapeutic range   the dosage of a drug needed to create the desired drug action safely

thromboembolism   a blood clot

thrombus   a combination of blood factors, including platelets and fibrin, that forms a blood clot

transducer   an instrument housed within an ultrasound probe that converts electrical energy into sonic energy, and vice versa, acting as a transmitter and receiver of ultrasound information

transitional epithelial cell   the type of epithelial cell that lines the urinary bladder and may be seen in the urine sediment

trematode   an unsegmented, leaflike worm; a fluke

traumatic reticulo-pericarditis/-peritonitis   *see hardware disease*

turbidity   cloudiness of a solution such as urine

uremia   an excess of nitrogen-containing products of protein metabolism in the blood; distinguished from azotemia by its producing symptoms of chronic renal failure

urine sediment   the centrifuged solid portion of urine that is examined microscopically for the presence of bacteria, cells, casts, crystals, parasites, and the like

Vacutainer®   the brand name of a vacuum-evacuated blood-collection tube produced by Becton, Dickinson and Company; the term has come to mean any vacuum blood collection tube

vagal tone   the effect produced on the heart when the vagus nerve is stimulated and starts parsympathetic actions in the body

vector   a carrier, usually an insect, that transmits a pathogen from one animal to another

venipuncture   the process of puncturing a vein with a needle for the purpose of intravenous injection or blood sample collection

ventricular premature contractions (VPC)   a heart arrhythmia in which the ventricles contract before the sinoatrial (SA) node and atrium

viscosity   a measure of the thickness or resistance to flow of a liquid

West Nile virus (WNV)   a mosquito-borne equine encephalomyelitis that occasionally also produces disease in humans; symptoms include weakness and muscle tremors

withdrawal time   the period of time in which a drug must not be administered to animals intended for food or milk production

WNV   *see* **West Nile virus**

zone of inhibition   the clear area on a blood-agar plate surrounding a paper disc that is impregnated with an antibiotic in which susceptible bacteria do not grow

ADDITIONAL ONLINE PRACTICE

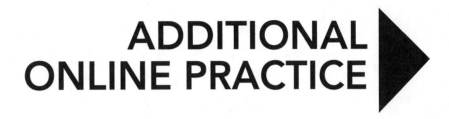

Whether you need help building basic skills or preparing for an exam, visit the **LearningExpress Practice Center**! On this site, you can access FREE additional practice materials. This online practice will also provide you with:

- **Immediate Scoring**
- **Detailed answer explanations**
- **Personalized recommendations for further practice and study**

Follow the directions below to access your free additional practice:
- Email **LXHub@learningexpresshub.com** for your access code. Please include your name, contact information, and complete book title in your email.
- Write "Free online practice code" in your email subject line.
- You will receive your access code by email.
- Go to **www.learningexpresshub.com/affiliate** and follow the easy registration steps. Be sure to have your access code handy!
  - ❑ If this is your first time registering, be sure to register as a new user.
  - ❑ If you've registered before with another product, be sure to follow the steps for **returning users**.

The email address you register with will become your username. You will also be prompted to create a password. For easy reference, record them here:

Username: _____

Password: _____

With your username and password, you can log in and access your additional practice. If you have any questions or problems, please contact LearningExpress customer service at 1-800-295-9556 ext. 2, or e-mail us at **customerservice@learningexpressllc.com.**

NOTES

NOTES

NOTES

NOTES